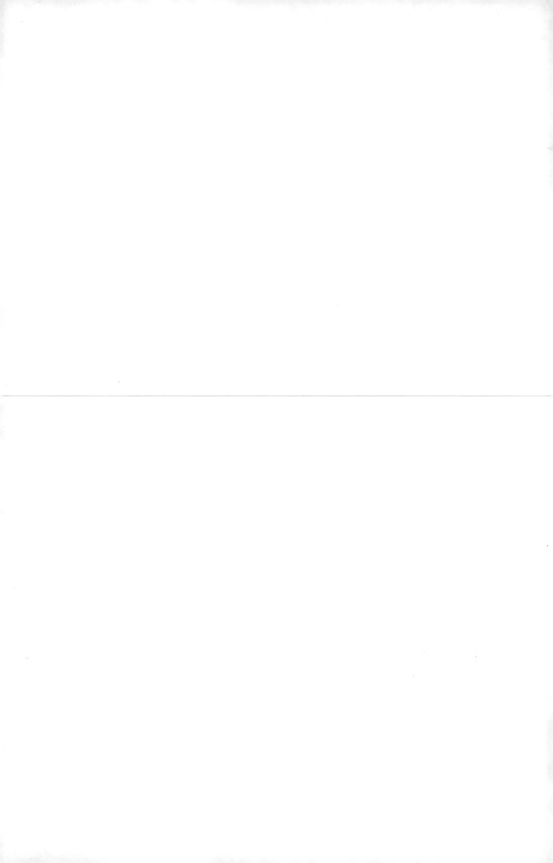

Drawing Blood

Drawing Blood

*Technology and Disease Identity in
Twentieth-Century America*

Keith Wailoo

The Johns Hopkins University Press
Baltimore & London

This book has been brought to publication with the generous assistance of the American Association for the History of Medicine.

The Johns Hopkins University Press
2715 North Charles Street
Baltimore, Maryland 21218-4319
The Johns Hopkins Press Ltd., London

Library of Congress Cataloging-in-Publication Data will be found at the end of this book.
A catalog record for this book is available from the British Library.

ISBN 0-8018-5474-1

Contents

Preface

Problems of disease, medicine, and medical technology touch all of us on intensely personal levels. A few years ago a crisis involving my father crystallized, for me, the problem of technology in medicine—something I had been studying, up to that point, from a historical distance. The drama involved my entire family, as well as a cardiologist, and an "abnormal" electrocardiogram (EKG) reading. This particular case centered on the meaning of the diagnostic test, but in its broader aspects the dilemma evokes the core issues of this book—the ways in which technologies have become props for working out larger problems of disease identity, patient identity, and professional identity in twentieth-century medicine.

In an unexpected phone call from my mother, I learned that my father was in the hospital with a "kidney problem" and possibly a heart ailment. His doctor suspected kidney stones, but the diagnosis was far from definite. A routine test showed that my father had an abnormal EKG, and this could mean that he also had a heart problem. He was in pain and anxious. During one family conversation, I found out that my father had been hospitalized with a kidney disorder as a child and that he was concerned that this ghost had somehow reappeared. As a very athletic man in his early fifties, he was also disturbed to hear of the possibility that he had a heart condition. His doctor was being cautious, holding him in the hospital for tests and observation.

When I arrived at the hospital—a teaching hospital—I found my father nauseated by the painkillers. I stayed with him for a while and then headed for the hospital's library. I sought out some cardiology textbooks, photocopied a few pages of EKG charts, and brought them back to his room, intending to suggest that an abnormal EKG test did not necessarily mean that he had a "bad heart" or a disease and that there was a big gap between the representation and the actuality of a "diseased" body. I was both concerned and genuinely curious about how his doctors would draw the connection between technical finding and "disease."

A cardiologist consultant appeared in the semiprivate room. He did a quick physical examination and asked my father questions about symptoms and complaints. I don't remember the consultant volunteering information, but just before he turned to leave he noticed the stack of EKG photocopies. "Oh," he said, "I see somebody's been looking at EKGs."

Tentatively, I asked, "What exactly is wrong with my father's EKG?" The cardiologist replied, "Your father has what's called an 'inverted T-wave.'" It happened, by chance, that I had just read about inverted T-waves, and I recalled these few points: "It says that there are several interpretations for inverted T-waves. One is something called 'biker's heart.' It says that, in very athletic people, this sometimes happens quite normally. My father has run quite a number, about six, of marathons. And he still runs a lot. Do you think this could explain the EKG?" The specialist confirmed that this was possible. Then, turning to my father, he asked: "How much do you run now?" My father explained that he had stopped running marathons a few years ago. "Now, I run about eight miles a day." After taking this in, the specialist decided, "You'd have to run a lot more than that to explain this." I recalled another point: "It also says here on a separate page that this kind of thing is often found as a normal variation in black men." "That's true," came the response, "but it's usually younger black men."

My next question seemed obvious enough. "How do you tell whether this is a heart problem—which is something my father should worry about—or something that he shouldn't worry about?" The specialist's conclusion was not particularly definitive: "I suppose the only way is to check an older EKG and to compare the two. If this showed up recently, I'd be worried about it. But if it was there earlier, then I'd be less worried." We determined that there had been another EKG a few years back and that one kind of "diagnosis" would involve a simple comparison of charts. One thing was clear: there were so many questions about my father's past, his athletic routine, and his very identity that we had collectively obviated any additional invasive cardiac diagnostic tests. As the cardiologist left, I was relieved and I knew my father was, too—but not because anything had been definitely settled. Was my father at risk for congestive heart failure, or was he just another person with an inverted T-wave? The difference between a "bad heart" and a "normal heart" had become more complex, but reassuringly so. A few days afterward, it had become clear that my father did have a kidney stone, but his so-called heart problem continued to be, ambiguously, both "real" and "unreal."

Consider this clinical scenario as an example of how technologies are used (somewhat ritualistically) to create meaning, to shape identity, and to construct diseases. The EKG itself did not determine the clinical outcome; rather, the EKG presented a sign. The sign could work on many different levels—psychological, professional, economic, clinical, and social. A pessimistic reading of the inverted T-wave could produce new anxieties about hidden disease, but another reading could reassure us about the patient's ethnic identity or athletic achievement. On a clinical level, one interpretation of the T-wave could chart a course toward yet another, more costly, diagnostic intervention, but a nonpathological interpretation pointed to early discharge from the hospital. The art of reading such technological indicators, performed in many private rooms throughout the hospital, could enhance the status and income of the specialty (particularly if the test was perceived as finding "hidden" disease). But if the ambiguities of the EKG were made evident, this could erode confidence in the specialist, highlighting the instability of disease concepts and perhaps undermining professional and institutional growth.

The use and interpretation of technologies in such closed clinical settings raise a larger question about the construction of knowledge in modern medicine. This question is at the core of this book. How have technologies been used to distinguish and classify authentically sick people? How dependable have those classifications been, and how have they evolved? How have technologies of blood reading and blood manipulation, in particular, been used to create disease identity and professional identity? What implications have these technologies had for particular specialists, particular groups of patients, and medical institutions—pharmaceutical companies and research hospitals? In what follows, I focus not on cardiology but on hematology; this book explores a handful of blood diseases that exemplify not only the history of technology in twentieth-century medicine but also the ways in which questions of gender, race, lifestyle, and professional politics were inevitably linked to the construction of medical knowledge. By telling the story of these blood diseases, I hope to illuminate the complex cultural role of technologies in our lives.

Acknowledgments

Countless friends, colleagues, and family members helped make this book possible. First, I must thank my dissertation advisor, Charles E. Rosenberg, who introduced me and many others to the historical problem of disease, medicine, and society and who has taken continued interest in my evolving project. Thanks also to Robert Kohler, Rosemary Stevens, Mark Adams, Judith McGaw, Nathan Sivin, and Henrika Kuklick for their comments on early versions of this work. Over the years, many others have given time, attention, and intellectual support to me and my work. They include Jeff Brosco, Marta Hanson, Gabrielle Hecht, Susan Speaker, Shari Rudavsky, Elizabeth Toon, Jennifer Gunn, Lynne Snyder, Maneesha Lal, and Julie Johnson. Particularly warm appreciation for their gracious readings and sharp insight must go to Chris Feudtner and Nina Lerman. An early stage of this work was supported by a graduate fellowship from the National Science Foundation.

At the University of North Carolina, valuable readings on portions of this book came from Nancy King, Sue Estroff, Larry Churchill, Gail Henderson, and others in the truly interdisciplinary Department of Social Medicine. Carolyn McIntyre, Kay Hill, and Becky Eatmon provided important administrative and secretarial support along the way. Others at UNC also gave feedback on ideas and chapters; they include Megan Matchinske, John Kasson, Bill Kerwin, Jerry Calleson, Paul Godley, Tera Hunter, Lloyd Kramer, Don Reid, Leon Fink, and Judith Farquhar. For their seemingly bottomless reservoir of advice, opinion, and commentary, Michael McVaugh, Don Madison, Kendrick Prewitt, and Barry Saunders are owed much more than a "thank you." The book took shape (through suggestions on particular chapters, selected arguments, or points of information) with help from Gert Brieger, Sy Mauskopf, Harry Marks, Ed Morman, Mary Fissell, Joel Howell, Jane Maienschein, Jon Beatty, William Schneider, John Harley Warner, Rob Aronowitz, Todd Savitt, Gerard Fergerson, David Rosner, Kenneth Ludmerer, Naomi Rogers, Margaret Humphreys, and Peter English.

This book benefited from commentary in numerous scholarly forums. These include the Yale University Institute for History of Medicine; Stanford University Department of History; University of Arizona Department of Zoology; University of Minnesota Program in History and Philosophy of Science and Technology; University of Michigan Bentley Historical Library; East Carolina University Department of Medical Humanities; Johns Hopkins University Institute for the History of Medicine; University of North Carolina Department of History (and the Triangle Workshop in the History of Science, Medicine, and Technology); National Library of Medicine; Marine Biological Laboratory at Woods Hole; and University of Pennsylvania Department of History and Sociology of Science.

Barbara Rosenkrantz's comments as a reader helped to bring clarity and purpose to an early version of this work, as did the comments of another anonymous reader. Jacqueline Wehmueller, my editor, provided advice at just the right times, improving the manuscript in both subtle and dramatic ways.

Numerous archivists provided assistance in my research. Among them were the professional staffs at the Marriott Library at the University of Utah; the Countway Library at Harvard University; the Mississippi Valley Collection at the McWerter Library at University of Memphis; the Bentley Historical Library at the University of Michigan at Ann Arbor; the William Osler Library at McGill University; the Philadelphia College of Physicians; the Regenstein Library at the University of Chicago; the Hagley Library Center for Business, Technology, and Society; and the Schlesinger Library at Radcliffe College.

The subtle influence of my parents (Bert and Lynette Wailoo) and my brother (Christopher) is scattered throughout these pages, and so (I would like to believe) is the influence of the spirited storytelling of my grandfather, Stanley Adolphus Lewis.

Finally, a few words of appreciation to my wife, Alison Isenberg, who deserves more thanks than a paragraph can hold—for her patient readings, her editorial suggestions, and her own historical scholarship (a model that has inspired me in many ways). Alison's love, support, and fine example have certainly helped bring this book to life.

Drawing Blood

Introduction
Putting the Question to Technology

In the twentieth century, doctors have learned to think and act through their technologies. That is, two key features of twentieth-century medicine have been the deployment of technologies by specialists and the ways in which technologies such as EKGs and fetal heart monitors have assigned coherent meaning to particular symptoms and bodily features, guiding the physician's mind and hand. Such technologies have played a large role in assigning an "identity" to diseases. For example, as new diagnostic and therapeutic technologies emerged in the last ten years, the identity of acquired immune deficiency syndrome (AIDS) evolved rapidly. AIDS began not as AIDS, per se, but as a fragmented assortment of rare diseases in the early 1980s (patients died from Kaposi's sarcoma, pneumonia, tuberculosis, and other opportunistic infections). Only with the creation of an antibody test for human immunodeficiency virus (HIV) and after contentious debate about its meaning did AIDS become a discrete, immunologically defined entity.[1]

Did the HIV test clarify our understanding of the disease? Yes and, surprisingly, no. While the HIV test has assured many of us that these disparate ailments have an underlying unity, contemporary medical science also acknowledges that the test identifies only a *latent* disease state. The HIV test locates a spectrum of diseases waiting to happen, but not a disease itself. Partly because of this diagnostic ambiguity, the use of the test to assign meaning has engendered contentious social, political, moral, and medical debate. When should it be used? On whom? What does the test really tells us? It has become clear that the social and political turmoil surrounding AIDS (the context) shapes the meaning of any HIV test. For some observers, the HIV test appropriately identifies a "sick" and dangerous individual. For others the test itself has become dangerous, a vehicle for labeling, perpetuating social discrimination, marking the spread of a "gay disease," or designating an insurance liability.[2] The test has also become a key tool of public health administration—preventing thousands of transfusions that would have resulted in new HIV infections. Depending upon its user, its interpreters, and the context, such a technology can have both oppressive and liberating effects.

A complex relationship exists between the HIV blood test and the disease called AIDS. Diagnostic technologies (such as the HIV test) do not *define* diseases so much as they stand in some relation to disease phenomena, framing and giving a particular coherence to lived experience, labeling sets of symptoms, and directing social policy. Further complicating matters in the case of AIDS is the problem of newer technologies. Enter the AIDS vaccine. Researchers are aware that any persons who agree to receive an experimental AIDS vaccine (even those uninfected) undoubtedly would later test HIV positive, with many unintended consequences.[3] Thus, the advent of new technologies inevitably alters the meaning of old ones—sometimes making these old technologies more difficult to interpret, easier to decode, or obsolete. What is true for AIDS has been true for diseases throughout the twentieth century: in addition to simplifying and resolving our knowledge of disease, technologies have been one of many factors *constituting, creating,* and *complicating* diseases in our time.[4]

The story of technologies and AIDS is one contemporary example of a twentieth-century drama, an ongoing dialectic between technology and disease. In this century more than any other, physicians have pursued a technological understanding of disease—allowing their technologies to structure their thoughts, while often pondering the imprecise correlations among their technologies, clinical symptoms, and disease as an experiential, emotional, epistemological, personal, or social concern. Physicians and students of twentieth-century medicine have seldom appreciated the full range of problems that arise when technology confronts disease. Today, for example, the question of technology is often reduced to an economic problem, frequently characterized as *technology assessment.* (Some studies in this genre examine the financial costs of technology; others evaluate the ethics of technology—the imperative to treat or withhold treatment. Some explore technology's systematic "depersonalization" of medicine, while others highlight, whether through statistics or anecdotes, particular technological triumphs and failures.[5])

This book confronts many of these familiar problems from a historical perspective, taking (however) a broader cultural view of technology and technology assessment.[6] It explores how technologies have influenced the identity of particular blood diseases over many decades, using as its case material chlorosis, splenic anemia, aplastic anemia, pernicious anemia, and sickle cell anemia. Some of these disorders existed as legitimate diseases for only a few decades, but were widely discussed in their day. The meaning and identity of each changed over time, shaped by technological fashions, by the evolving politics of technological medicine, and by evolving social and political assumptions about patients and disease.[7]

One might assume that changes in thinking about blood diseases in the twentieth century were influenced primarily by the tools and insights of specialists in hematology, just as our thinking about AIDS has been steered by the tools and insights of immunologists and virologists. But the production of knowledge about the blood involved more than the expert manipulation of instruments. The evolving identity of hematology itself—the practice and the specialty—is a key part of the story. Indeed, the knowledge hematologists produced was always closely related to transformations in their own lives, their social and economic relations, and their professional culture. Professional identity and disease identity were mutually constitutive.

The late nineteenth century was an era dominated by the family doctor and by a culture of medical individualism. Even as hospitals grew in size and number and doctors migrated there to work, family-centered practitioners produced much of the existing knowledge of disease. Yet it was clear to family doctors that the organization and production of knowledge was changing dramatically, becoming increasingly located in hospitals, medical schools, state bureaucracies, and research-oriented corporate enterprises.[8] Academic hospitals and research institutions like the Rockefeller Institute for Medical Research appeared in the first decade of the century. These centers for knowledge production challenged independent producers of knowledge, offering them the benefits of incorporation into a new order. The bulk of this book examines this transformation and its implications for the use of technology and for thinking about disease. Refracted through the histories of chlorosis, splenic anemia, aplastic anemia, and pernicious anemia, we see the story not only of family doctors, but also of pathologists, surgeons, and others coping with economic and organizational change, and we discern how their professional ideals and technological practices shaped what they said about these diseases.

Each chapter examines one dimension of the cultural transformation in hematological thought. Chlorosis—an anemia of young girls—had been a central medical concept of family doctors for centuries, but by 1920 it was regarded as a defunct disease concept, an old-fashioned way of thinking about women and about disease. In chapter 1, I suggest two reasons for its disappearance: the decline of the family doctor as a producer of legitimate knowledge and the changing politics of American womanhood. The chapter also explores the afterlife of chlorosis and the ways in which changing attitudes toward technology and womanhood have reconstructed medical memories of chlorosis.

Splenic anemia emerged as a new disease in the late nineteenth century, only to suffer a fate similar to that of chlorosis. Chapter 2 portrays its rise as a poignant reflection of the rising status of abdominal surgeons and their tools and of the strength of their diagnostic autonomy. Its fall signaled the surgeons' reluctant incorporation into the newly emerging order, where diagnosis became a more corporate exercise. In chapter 3, I examine how aplastic anemia was transformed by several factors—by the departmentalization of the pathologist, by his new role as scientific manager in the hospital economy, and by developments in industrial life and labor relations well beyond the pathologist's awareness and control. Chapter 4 analyzes the production of a "cure" for pernicious anemia and its commercialization in the 1920s, which resulted in the 1934 Nobel Prize for three American university-based researchers. This, too, was an outgrowth of the new order, indicating the ways in which close relations between universities and pharmaceutical industries had reshaped the production of hematological knowledge since the era of chlorosis.

These four diseases tell the story of how, by the 1920s, a vast technology-based system had emerged for the production of knowledge about the blood and its diseases, with diverse implications for physicians, different groups of patients, and the culture of American medicine. Chapter 5 turns to the production of knowledge about sickle cell anemia, a disease associated with "Negro blood," a disease through which hematologists sought to work out troubling questions of race, race relations, miscegenation, and Negro identity using the new tools of scientific medicine. As our discussion of these diseases makes clear, the trajectory of hematological thought was not determined by specialization and technology in any narrow sense. Rather, hematological thought was a specialized response to clinical, as well as social and economic, challenges.[9]

Taken as a group, the anemias—like AIDS—earned a collective identity with the advent of new tools of blood analysis in the nineteenth century—the hemocytometer and the hemoglobinometer.[10] During this period of increasing public regard for experts, physicians began looking at the blood through these instruments, counting corpuscles, estimating hemoglobin, and recognizing new phenomena that might be correlated neatly with patterns of debility and death. But, unlike the greatly feared scourges of the nineteenth century, the anemias were not dramatic diseases with which patients rapidly identified. Neither did they evoke widespread fear. To most patients, the anemias were unknown and unappreciated until specialists identified and explained them. Indeed, it was the privileging of hematological symptoms by a handful of physicians that established the legitimacy of "the anemias" as diseases in their own right. According to the blood specialists, anemia was an insidious presence, crippling workers, women, black people, and other people in the prime of life. These anemias were by-products of a new age in medicine, created *ab initio* from the insights of a generation of self-conscious, technologically invested practitioners.

All of these curious blood depletions highlighted crucial problems of moral decay, social integrity, and identity. Were such blood diseases caused by the individuals themselves, originating somehow in their failing constitutions? Were women and Negroes somehow more predisposed to anemia, and if so what should be done? Was overexertion or particular moral excesses like drunkenness to blame for anemia? Were these diseases somehow the by-products of economic and social problems—such as the exploitation of female labor in modern factories, malnutrition, poverty, economic downturns, and exposure of factory workers to dangerous chemicals? What was the most judicious and justifiable way of alleviating the symptoms of such sufferers—medical treatment or social reform? Physicians of the time acknowledged that the anemias inculpated the moral character of particular patients as well as the state of society, and these diseases suggested the need for a specialist to examine the relationship of medical knowledge and social policy. Throughout the heyday of the anemias, clinical thought and social thought flowed naturally from blood—the "river of life."[11]

Blood analysis has always had a powerful symbolic place in medical practice and social thought. As Michel Foucault and many others have observed, familial relations were traditionally conceived as "blood relations," and physicians continued to see blood as a motive force in heredity, racial identity, and disease.[12] Thus, when the nineteenth-century hematologist took the blood as his focus, he chose a rich symbol of individual identity, social health, and group relations. Writing in 1905, physician Richard Cabot associated the hematologist with the title character in Rudyard Kipling's novel, *Kim*. Just as the spy Kim could understand what was happening in society by "reading" and "interpreting" the social makeup of traffic along Burma's Grand Trunk Road, so too could the hematologist understand the whole body by counting "monocytes" and analyzing "leukocytes."[13] Even with the increasing specialization of medicine, blood study continued to have metaphorical appeal, offering the practitioner a role as a "secret agent"—producer of both specific and generalized knowledge.[14] A half-century after Cabot wrote, a 1957 television health program promoted blood as "an elixir, still mysterious, yielding some of its secrets but retaining many others."[15] In 1978, one eminent hematologist admitted that "even hematologists in their daily talk confuse and assign genetic, racial and other features to the blood. We are creatures of habit, and habits have a way of lasting."[16] Whether because of habit or because "power speaks *through* blood," this fluid has continued to be mysterious and potent, containing for doctor and patient alike a wealth of vital yet hidden information about disease, the body, and society.[17]

The modern hematologist possesses the ability to read this "passive vehicle" as a microcosm reflecting problems in the body as a whole, illuminating the "true" reasons for lethargy, debility, pallor, and death.[18] To some of Cabot's generation (the first to make a specialty of hematology), blood analysis defined pragmatic roles in patient management by bringing a somatic rationality to hospital work. For others, it had a transcendent meaning. More than just another body fluid, blood was (as one author put it) "the law upon which . . . physical integrity depends."[19] Whatever the particular meaning of hematology they seized upon, hematology-oriented practitioners used these conceptions to define a place for themselves among the growing numbers of early twentieth-century medical specialists. Blood work evolved with the changing social structure of medicine—with hospital practice, public health work, and academic research—integrated into the thought and practice of many practitioners, reaching far beyond hematology proper.[20]

Technology plays a large part in the story of specialty formation. From the late nineteenth century to the World War II era, hematologists produced a wide range of tools with which to read and manipulate the blood—each tool bringing its own clarity and complexity into the cultures of medicine. In the late nineteenth century, microscopic instruments for measuring the size and number of blood cells (hemocytometers and hemoglobinometers) found their places in office and hospital practice. Along with these, general physicians used numerous methods for manipulating the blood of sick patients *in vivo* (arsenic compounds, iron pills, tonics, and dietary supplements). After the turn of the century, techniques of blood manipulation multiplied along with the self-defined "hematologists." Such specialization brought conflict, especially among those who used competing techniques and tools of blood manipulation. At the same time that hematologists proliferated, industrial toxicologists and public health workers implicated a wide range of chemicals like lead and benzol in the "poisoning" of the blood. The following chapters consider tensions among these various "blood specialists" over the proper use and interpretation of chemical agents, transfusions, the surgical removal of organs, x-rays, and other methods of blood testing and manipulation.

From 1900 through the 1950s, blood testing and manipulation became increasingly varied and sophisticated. Emmel's test for sickle cell anemia was, for example, thought of as a dependable genetic test; blood transfusions became more widely used; splenectomy (a useful method of blood manipulation) enjoyed a high status for a time; liver treatment seemed to be a tool of unmatched specificity and consumer appeal in blood manipulation; and bone marrow biopsy emerged as a promising but painful type of hematological diagnosis, controlled by hospital-based pathologists (much to the chagrin of a later generation of hematologists). In our assessment of each of these technologies, it becomes clear that professional status, economic competition, and consumer appeal featured centrally in their use and in the production of hematological knowledge. Technology assessment, therefore, cannot be done apart from a careful consideration of specialty identity.

What were the identity politics of those who defined, managed, and in a sense "owned" these blood diseases? For a time, for example, hematological tools were a friend to the family physician and to his reform ideals in the late nineteenth century. In his 1887 treatise, *Anaemia*, Philadelphia physician Frederick Henry wrote that blood analysis justified a rethinking of the very nature of American women. Women who were stereotyped to be "constitutionally delicate" were in fact "suffering—if such a term may be applied to a condition which brings with it so great a freedom from responsibility—from a light grade of chronic anaemia."[21] The technology of blood analysis allowed Henry to identify this biological anomaly and to redefine women as victims of cultural and social stresses. For family doctors like Henry, the techniques of diagnosis and disease management were all part of the reformers' role.

In this era of dramatic shifts in American gender roles and expectations, technology appealed to doctors like Frederick Henry in no small part as a tool for responding to social change and guiding women's social relations.[22] Henry insisted upon removing young, anemic girls from their friends and unhealthy surroundings and placing them in special clinics—where physicians could monitor their blood, direct their treatment, and guide the rejuvenation of their blood. Such "moral management" enjoyed fashion in the 1890s. By the 1910s, however, physicians agreed that moral management was outdated. At the same time, they agreed that chlorosis did not exist. If we wish to understand what made this mysterious disease "real" in its time, we must examine Henry's technology, how it was used, and what it meant to reform-minded physicians as they tried to fix their own identities even as they sought to redefine the identity of women in a period of extensive cultural change.

Splenic anemia became a new disease linked to the identity of another professional group—the abdominal surgeons. Its emergence reveals how blood analysis and innovative surgical technique provided a compelling basis for the creation of a disease. The existence of splenic anemia in turn endorsed a daring professional persona that enjoyed wide cultural appeal in the 1910s. Yet persistent debates about the disease's "reality" reflected the struggles of abdominal surgeons to maintain their surgical individualism in an era of incorporation and bureaucratic reform. By 1930, surgeons—succumbing to institutional trends of the era—agreed that splenic anemia (like chlorosis) probably did not exist.[23] To explain the history of this disease, one must examine not just the craft of abdominal surgery and the techniques of blood analysis, but also the surgeon's changing role in the culture of scientific medicine.

Aplastic anemia rose to public prominence at the same time that chlorosis and splenic anemia faded. Determining the identity of aplastic anemia became a crucial question within modern hospitals, in industrial factories, and in numerous workmen's compensation hearings. Was this an organic entity, originating somewhere in the body of its victims? Was the disease a by-product of the reckless exposure of workers to new chemicals like benzol? Was it best managed by more rational hematological work in the hospital, by industrial regulation, or by removing "susceptible workers" from the factory workforce? In these new institutional contexts, hematological specialists became valued experts, and they cautiously embraced the role of scientific managers and technological arbiters—using blood analysis not only to diagnose in hospitals, but also to assign legal blame and moral responsibility in courtrooms and on factory floors.

The rise of pharmaceutical enterprise and academic research meant yet another expansion of hematological knowledge and a further shift in disease identity. In 1926 two Harvard researchers (George Minot and William Murphy) discovered a new liver treatment for the deadly, if little-known, pernicious anemia. Their collaboration with the Eli Lilly pharmaceutical company yielded a supposed cure, brought them popular acclaim, and eventually earned them the 1934 Nobel Prize. Careful blood analysis in the aftermath of liver treatment seemed to validate their discovery. Yet some physicians questioned this definition of pernicious anemia, for it seemed to highlight how modern pharmaceutical companies had gained control of the academic researcher's mind. One Harvard-affiliated physician later saw this as one example of "how the articles of medical men . . . often take on the flavor of advertisements for commercial nostrums."[24] Was this corporate conquest of pernicious anemia a feat of modern advertising? The construction of pernicious anemia in this period illuminates the role of hematology in raising the status of scientific medicine and in cementing relations among pharmaceutical industry, university research, and the consumer.

By the 1920s, blood analysis technology had gained considerable currency in medical thought and practice. It had also become a key tool in what sociologist Erving Goffman called "the management of spoiled identity"—the sick, the deviant, the marginal.[25] For some specialists during this period, for example, blood analysis offered direct insight into vital questions of racial identity and hereditary character (much as genetic testing does today). Consider the early history of sickle cell anemia. For white physicians concerned with the biological integrity of their own race, it seemed obvious that this new disease was caused by "Negro blood," a characteristic that could be detected using a technique created in 1917. Their use and interpretation of Emmel's blood test highlights the ways in which blood analysis could speak not only to problems of industrial work and pharmaceutical advertising, but also to problems of racial intermarriage, segregation, and race relations in America.

Such cultural preoccupations played a determining role in the trajectory of hematological thought.[26] Chapters 1 through 4 are meant to explore the interdependence of disease identity and medical identity and the role of technology in that relationship. *Disease* is often presumed to be the physician's nemesis, and *technology* is seen as the physician's tool in combatting this enemy. In this classic sense, both disease and technology stand essentially apart from the doctor. The histories of the anemias suggest otherwise. Anemia, as it turns out, was an amorphous disease category *given coherence* by the rising status of blood analysis technology in medicine, and *giving coherence* and legitimacy to medical roles. Medical pronouncements on disease identity helped to legitimate physicians' tools and legitimated their own identities, whether as reformers, healers, scientists, advertising men, or racial theorists. As a disease category, anemia could incorporate a wide range of patients—anyone with a low blood count, lethargy, or a variety of other complaints. Such a category proved to be sufficiently labile to remain intact for generations and to serve the needs of different practitioners. Anemias could be shaped by the specific rules of conduct, intellectual preferences, and social relations of different specialists at different times in the twentieth century.

World War II marked a major transition in the history of technology in medicine and in this system of knowledge production. In the aftermath of the war, federal patronage of science skyrocketed, promoting the proliferation of powerful new technologies and new relationships among doctors, patients, technologies, and diseases. The federal government, as a major new patron of medical research, brokered the rise of new disciplines like molecular biology and reshaped older patterns of technology use. As a result of federal patronage, a variety of new "basic sciences" and their tools (radiation, chemotherapy, electrophoresis, antibiotics) became incorporated into medical education, practice, and research. These developments brought new disciplines and their tools into tension with established medical thought. As hematologists embraced new tools of blood analysis, they saw that new technologies meant new concepts about blood and disease. "Anemia" seemed to be deprived of its former coherence. Hematologists sought to bring the identity of "their" diseases and their goals into line with the new tools of scientific medicine. "Anemia is no longer a disease," wrote one specialist, "only a symptom of other diseases."[27] Chapter 6 examines the implications of this new system of knowledge production, which was sustained by the rise of the federal government as a major patron and broker of technology in medicine.

In the 1940s, 1950s, and 1960s, the new tools of radiation, chemotherapy, electrophoresis, and antibiotics signified for hematologists that they had achieved new levels of insight into the blood. The initial enthusiasm for such technologies led blood analysis in fundamentally novel directions. As Bernard Seeman wrote about pre–World War II hematology, "one of the most persistent myths involving blood—and one that has taken an incredible human toll—is the belief that blood not only contains life but also the qualities of a being."[28] In the hands of molecular biologists in post–World War II America, the new technology of electrophoresis provided liberation from previous patterns of hematological thought by focusing not on blood, per se, but on the hemoglobin molecule as the site of disease. The conception of sickle cell anemia as a "molecular disease" (rather than a disease of "Negro blood") was revolutionary, providing a compelling new model and suggesting that these new tools brought new insight into human identity and a reconstruction of cultural sensibility. Yet the medical embrace of these new technologies also raised new problems. One problem raised by electrophoresis, for example, was that, by focusing on hemoglobin analysis, it identified and constructed pathological conditions that often did not, and *might never*, exist in a clinical sense.[29]

The advent of federal patronage and the proliferation of new technologies also posed challenges for hematology as an organized subspecialty and raised the question of who would control these powerful new tools. No sooner had hematologists organized and identified themselves as a field than they encountered competition with aggressive new disciplines for federal funding and popular appeal. One leading hematologist called on his colleagues to understand "the forces that are molding us" and to shape their discipline accordingly. Fields such as oncology and human genetics, as well as molecular biology and pathology, had also turned their sights to the blood. By the middle and late 1960s, hematologists believed they were suffering because of this increased competition—unable to speak effectively on blood-related matters. The story of their struggle for control of leukemia (was it a blood disease or a cancer?) and hematologists' responses to other controversies provide us with a window on competing constructions of the blood and on the hematologist's evolving identity amidst a new politics of blood, disease, and technology. The rise of vocal patient advocacy, the tug of federal policy, and ever-increasing specialization were among the new forces that redefined hematological knowledge, blood diseases, and hematology as a field. A final chapter examines these forces in our own time and their influence on the thought of hematologists and other specialists who speak on matters relating to the blood and disease.

Hematology has always been a fragile specialty, without distinct boundaries. In contrast to other specialties that can claim to have distinctive tools (radiology), special clients (pediatrics), particular diseases (diabetology), or an organ-based integrity (cardiology), hematology's claims were never firmly established. Hematologists have always even debated among themselves whether blood could be considered an organ. In his 1929 book, *Diseases of the Blood*, Paul Clough suggested that "the blood is not a living tissue, but is merely a passive vehicle for the transportation of materials . . . Abnormalities in the blood corpuscle must, therefore, be regarded as symptoms of disease elsewhere in the body."[30] Hematologists never created an impenetrable tool-based specialty, partly because of the wide dissemination of blood analysis tools across the porous boundaries of the field. Hematology's supposed turf was always vulnerable to the claims of competing specialists. Decades after Clough wrote, another observer proclaimed that "hematology is not a unified subject or discipline in the same sense as neurology and cardiology . . . There is no agreement on who should be its exponents, whether clinicians, pathologists, or transfusion officers."[31] By the late 1960s and early 1970s, the political context of medical thought and practice had been radically transformed and hematologists saw their inability to compete for ownership of such lucrative blood diseases as leukemia as failure.[32] The subsequent merger with cancer specialists (to form hematology-oncology) only confirmed their tenuous control over the meaning of blood.

This book offers, then, a cultural history of hematology and hematological thought in late nineteenth-century America. It explores the ways in which some blood diseases were owned, controlled, managed, and lost by specialists amidst a changing social context. It traces subtle transformations in the way that human experiences—lethargy, pallor, blood poverty, debility, and death—were being rationalized by the new tools, patterns of thought, and expanding authority of scientific medicine. It touches, therefore, on the politics of twentieth-century specialization and on the use of technologies in the process of building specialties, institutions, research programs, and social policy.

The history of hematology also highlights problems of professional identity, patient identity, and disease identity. These are not, of course, necessarily commensurate uses of the term *identity*. Certainly, the history of identifying diseases is very different from the history of creating specialty identities. The creation of a *patient identity*—whether through social processes that stand outside of medical practice or through the acts of diagnosis and labeling—can be considered a third, distinct problem of identity. Yet, as I will suggest throughout this book, these various questions of identity must be considered together. How physicians style themselves, how they identify diseases, and how they characterize patients are closely related. Many of the physicians appearing in the pages of this book saw this interrelation, and, for them, technology played a significant role in working out these problems of identity.[33] To study this relationship—the construction and management of disease identities and medical identities—is not simply to reject, *a priori*, these constructions. It is, rather, to see these constructions as dynamic entities, shaping medical practice and social behavior, evolving with the cultural relations of biomedicine, and existing alongside (and often in conflict with) experiential, social, political, or spiritual constructions of self and disease.

Technologies were only one among a variety of factors aggregating to shape the identity of these specialists and to constitute and create concepts of disease. But technologies also have their own characters, which should not be lost in the seamless web of interactive factors. Moreover, I define *technology* broadly as "knowledge-producing tools," and I therefore consider not only instruments but the vastly expanding number of new drugs, surgical techniques, clinical facilities, and formalized research protocols, such as randomized clinical trials, as technologies. Perhaps the term *technological system* might be more appropriate to describe such an assemblage.[34] All such knowledge-producing tools have provided hematologists—and physicians in general—with varied ways of identifying biological anomaly and subjecting it to disciplined analysis and management. From this perspective, technology assessment becomes the study of a cultural interplay of practitioners, tools, and diseases in diverse and changing contexts.

What, then, is a disease? How are diseases related to the physicians who study them, the technologies doctors deploy, and the larger social relations of knowledge production? These are key concerns of this book. And these are not new concerns. Writing in 1928, one British physician noted that "the problem frequently arises whether changes in the clinical characters of the disease are real . . . whether apparent alterations are due to modifications in description rather than in fact—in other words, whether the change has been in opinion only."[35] It would be too simple to insist that these anemias were merely opinions, social constructions, cultural artifacts, or products of technological fashion within particular specialties. The challenge for historians of disease is to explore not only *how* disease identities were constructed, but also the *consequences* of these constructions for patients, physicians, and society as a whole. Precisely how did disease constructions evolve through time, what economic and social interests did they serve, and how did they affect the lives of patients, physicians, and researchers?[36]

Diseases are undeniably powerful human concerns, personal and physical crises in a crucial sense. Indeed, the disease experiences of particular patients—industrial workers, African Americans, women's groups, and middle-class men—are important themes in this book. Yet, diseases must also be thought of as cultural products, changing over time with technology and social relations, with the institutional and organizational politics of specialties, and with changing cultural assumptions and evolving medical identities. Among these forces, technology has undoubtedly become central to disease thought in the twentieth century, and technology has also become central to the management of patients, to the making of professional careers, and to the assignment of a reality to disease. The drama of technology in medicine is not a simple narrative—it involves many conflicting stories. Whether those stories are successes, failures, farces, or misadventures, it is clear that technologies have become central props in the play of modern medicine.

Let me return to the problem of AIDS to make a final point about technology, context, and the identity of disease. Would the HIV virus in a different context, without our modern technologies—blood transfusion, HIV tests, and syringes—have produced the disease AIDS? In a previous era would the people with HIV have been hemophiliacs and intravenous (IV) drug users? No. Without our elaborate system of blood transfusion and without the availability of syringes (modern technologies of routine fluid exchange), a nineteenth-century virus would not have affected either hemophiliacs—who often depend on blood transfusions—or IV drug users. HIV could not have manifested itself in nineteenth-century society as it does today. It would not have been the same as AIDS. Should we see these technologies as part of the AIDS problem? Yes. Is AIDS, at least partly, a consequence of the dramatic growth of blood transfusion networks in post–World War II industrial societies? Certainly. The popular dissemination of the syringe is also certainly part of the disease profile.

Today we understand that, to control the disease, we must deploy new technologies to monitor and regulate this now-expansive technological system. Otherwise, hemophiliacs and patients needing routine transfusions are put at risk. Contaminated syringes are clearly conduits for the disease, and some argue that circulating sterile syringes among IV drug users should be part of an enlightened approach to AIDS. The regulation of transfusion and syringe practices—two twentieth-century technologies—has provoked intense moralizing, and the perceived identities of these populations (as "innocent victims" or "self-indulgent criminals") have influenced how we choose to monitor and regulate these technologies. In the last ten years, however, we have accepted that such technological systems are undeniably part of the character of the pathology.

We must, of necessity, develop a broad view of the relationship of disease identity and technological development. These technologies (syringes, blood transfusions, HIV tests, and other laboratory instruments) alone do not fully identify the phenomenon we call AIDS. They provide only limited windows on the disease (a theme I will expand upon in the following chapters). Most students of HIV and AIDS quickly see that, without the gay liberation movement and the congregation of gay men in urban centers in the 1960s and 1970s and without the patterns of so-called unsafe sex, the virus would not have manifested itself in public consciousness as a "gay disease." This label (like the labels placed on hemophiliacs and drug users) has also structured social debates and social policies. In short, the politics and culture of late twentieth-century American life—a constellation of technologies, attitudes, and social relations—have made HIV "AIDS" and inform how we define disease.

At the same time, we encounter a potential paradox: we depend upon technologies to interpret and give meaning to this complexity. We depend upon laboratory technologies, for example, to provide clinical portraits of AIDS, to show us a complex biopathological entity (at once signified by a decimate population of white blood cells, a crippled immune system, the presence of HIV antibodies indicating the presence of the HIV virus, and a variety of opportunistic infections). This multiplicity of technologies brought to bear on a sick person makes up another representation of AIDS, giving clinical identity to the disease, shaping patient management, and defining broader social policies.

Indeed, throughout the twentieth century, such technologies have depended upon a broader set of symbolic, political, and social relationships to endow them with the power to identify disease. In another cultural context such technologies might have no value. In the nineteenth century, for example, an identical human immunodeficiency virus would have manifested itself differently, as tuberculosis, pneumonia, or some other infectious disease. HIV would have taken its identity from the disease context of the time, fading into the background of the diseases we associate with nineteenth-century urbanization, industrialization, and poverty (i.e., it would be so contextualized as to be virtually meaningless). Indeed, were we able to place the HIV test into the hands of the nineteenth-century practitioner with instructions for its use, it would probably remain on his shelf, bearing little relevance to the disease problems at hand and playing no role in the process of giving identity to the disease, to the patient, or to the medical practitioner. HIV would probably have been identified as tuberculosis. It would have been given an identity based upon the tools, assumptions, and broader social context of the time—and the same is true today. The deployment of technologies like the HIV test is part of larger cultural processes, which this book examines.

The question of what makes a disease "real" in any period is no idle philosophical concern; it is, rather, a problem that lies at the center of ongoing medical, public health, and social debates—ranging from questions of moral responsibility to financial reimbursement and technology assessment. Do fetal heart monitors detect crises that are vital, insignificant, or epiphenomenal? Do EKGs detect latent disease? Is the discovery of the prostate-specific antigen blood test and its use in screening a step forward in early prostate cancer detection? Is it a premature diagnostic device, promoted by urologists and leading us toward therapeutic disaster? To even begin to answer such questions, we must understand the patterns by which particular interests and practices shape the use of technologies and construct the identity of disease in place and time. Such an assessment of technology and disease identity acknowledges the existence of suffering and at the same time seeks to illuminate the factors that inevitably shape the perception, treatment, and alleviation of that suffering in twentieth-century America.

1

"Chlorosis" Remembered

Disease and the Moral Management
of American Women

What are we to make of a disease that occupied a central place in medical thinking for many decades and then disappeared in the early twentieth century? Chlorosis was such a disease. The chlorotic girl was all too familiar to the family doctor of the 1890s. Her poor appetite, gastric disturbance, and faint green pallor could be noted by close friends, family, and eventually by the family physician. An intense lethargy often left her unable to do household chores or perform any physical labor. As the renowned William Osler wrote in 1894, "headache is common in the early stages, and dyspnoea and palpitation are not often absent . . . More often still an anxious mother brings a daughter whose menses have ceased, and the physician is begged to direct his treatment toward the restoration of this function."[1] For novelists like Henry James and W. Somerset Maugham writing in the early 1900s, the chlorotic girl was a pathetic and enigmatic figure, a generations-old character presenting a vague complex of symptoms.[2] By 1920, however, the chlorotic girl had disappeared.

Some physicians and historians have suggested that the chlorotic girl vanished because of advances in early twentieth-century medical technology. The ailment evaporated when confronted by the more precise diagnostic tools of a "modern" medical era. Improvements in diagnostic hematology (the close analysis of blood cells) supposedly made vague symptom-based diseases like chlorosis obsolete and brought into being more precise hematological descriptions of disease. Others have argued that advances in iron therapy (that is, *drug* technologies rather than *diagnostic* technologies) vanquished chlorosis. Yet other writers have suggested that technologies had nothing to do with its disappearance, that chlorosis was nothing more than ideology—it represented an artifact of Victorian opinions about women, their bodies, and their place in society. As Victorian assumptions waned, so too did chlorosis. Finally, a few historians have asserted that some of the very technological innovations that focused medical attention so intensely on the blood in the nineteenth century may have contributed to the diagnosis of this false and imaginary disease.

What was the relationship between medical technologies and this mysterious disease? This chapter begins by exploring what chlorosis meant to American physicians from 1880 to 1910, and it explores the ways in which hematological technologies played a central role in both the construction and the demise of the chlorotic girl. How physicians used and interpreted technology shaped the history of this disease, as did other historically specific social and cultural forces. The desire of late nineteenth-century family doctors to be "moral managers" and social reformers informed their use of technology and informed their construction and reconstruction of the chlorotic girl. After recounting the heyday of chlorosis, I turn to the construction of memories about chlorosis through the rest of the twentieth century. These memories reflect changing debates about the social status of women, the role of technology in medicine, and the continuous reshaping of modern medical identity.

For centuries, chlorosis had a secure place in standard medical thinking. In the sixteenth and seventeenth centuries, it was widely believed to result from delays in marriage. Chlorosis could be remedied, wrote Johannes Lange in 1554, by expedient marriage and coition.[3] In this view, chlorosis was a disease of virgins and women who failed to adopt familial roles appropriate to their stage of life. Women became chlorotic *because* they were out of step with social mores.

Subsequent generations of physicians would develop their own explanations of chlorosis, its origins, and appropriate therapy. By the late nineteenth century, the definition of chlorosis had shifted markedly from that of Lange's time, reflecting contemporary attitudes about women and disease. In this new era, physicians attributed chlorosis to the increasing pace and character of modern society. Many believed that the

disease—characterized by lethargy, pallor, nervousness, gastric disturbance, and menstrual abnormalities—was brought on by hard physical
labor in industrial jobs, stresses of higher education, and other changing
social demands. As the turn of the century neared, chlorosis was seldom
labeled a "virgin's disease," for now it appeared in well-to-do married
women and in adolescent working girls. The malady now encompassed
a more expansive array of symptoms than in Lange's time. All agreed that
this was an illness originating in modern feminine maladjustments to
economic, social, and cultural dilemmas.[4]

For many physicians of the time, chlorosis was an elusive problem
illuminated particularly well by new technologies. Frederick Henry, in
his 1887 study of *Anaemia,* offered one view. He suggested that insensi-
tive doctors too often mistook chlorotic and anemic women for
hypochondriacs or regarded them as constitutionally delicate. But many
of these women were "suffering . . . from a light grade of chronic
anaemia."[5] Henry and his colleagues insisted that chlorosis (too often
dismissed as constitutional weakness or imaginary disease) could be recognized using the tools of blood analysis as a hematological disorder.[6]
These women, said Henry, customarily "played the role of amiable
drones in the hive of busy workers."[7] With proper hematological diagnosis and "moral management," they would return to more productive
roles within the family. He prescribed regular diets containing meats,
routine doses of Blaud's iron pills, and a bit of arsenic for particularly re-
calcitrant cases. But for Henry and a small coterie of northeastern medical authors, the first step in the recognition of this disease was the use of
cutting-edge diagnostic technologies—the hemoglobinometer and
hemacytometer.

The hemacytometer was both microscope and a blood-counting instrument. To use it, one placed a drop of blood onto a sterile glass slide
and observed the magnified blood cells. The individualized cells could
be counted against a grid background on the slide. Early hemacytome-
try therefore involved meticulous counting of blood cells per grid and
thus an estimate of the patient's blood count. Hemoglobinometry also
involved microscopic analysis, but here the observer focused on the pig-
menting, oxygen-carrying material—the hemoglobin—within the red
blood cells. The blood color would be matched against a standard chart.
Variations from a norm would be recorded, as would changes over time.
The color could be translated into an estimate of the hemoglobin per-

centage, thus indicating the oxygen-carrying capacity of the patient's blood.

Despite their focus on the blood, no thoughtful physician of this era would deny that chlorosis had its origins in problems of productivity and womanhood in America.[8] Chlorosis afflicted working-class women and their middle-class counterparts. While medical advertisements for "blood-building" pills and tonics depicted sallow, respectable-looking chlorotics, physicians spoke of the high prevalence of chlorosis among immigrant women who frequented dispensaries and outpatient departments of large urban hospitals.[9] In 1890, one Boston doctor speculated that "twenty percent of the immigrants become chlorotic within a year of their arrival here . . . This is a familiar fact, and is commonly explained by a change of manner of living from the out-of-doors to the confined work of domestic servants."[10] Looking around at American society, physicians saw increasing numbers of immigrant women working in factories, young middle-class women attending institutions of higher education, and women of every class involved in social and political causes. To these physicians, chlorosis grew out of these trends. "Why were our women semi-invalids, and their male companions healthy and strong?" wondered Chicago surgeon Franklin Martin.[11] He concluded that "every thoughtful gynecologist was pondering these problems in the [eighteen] eighties." Chlorosis merely highlighted the sad consequences of social change in women's lives, and most of this sad tale could be chronicled by examining the transformation of the blood.

Even in the 1890s, chlorosis was not a stable, well-defined entity. In late Victorian America chlorosis was at once a collection of changing symptoms and part of a medical rationale for the moral supervision of girls. Whatever chlorosis had meant before the 1890s, during this decade the diagnosis became intertwined with the broader goals of uplifting and morally reforming American women, and technologies of hemoglobin analysis were crucial to this agenda. Although it is tempting to argue that the decline of chlorosis signaled the emergence of laboratory skills in medicine, I will argue that technologies had been central to its diagnosis in the 1890s. To comprehend chlorosis, we must consider the subtle shift in technological interpretation, in doctors' roles and patients' identities during this era, and in the place of technology within the cultural relationship of doctor, patient, family, and disease.[12] Chlorosis was a problematic and evolving construct—a disease shaped by a changing encounter between doctors, their technologies, and their patients.

Technology and the Moral Management
of Girls in the 1890s

In his 1887 book *Anaemia*, Frederick Henry implied that too many so-called delicate women were "treated with excessive consideration by friends and relatives of their own sex" and pampered in their afflictions.[13] Moreover, they were "often regarded by the average practitioner as lucrative humbugs." This system of medical and social relations needed reform because this pampering concealed the actual prevalence of a disease. Henry called on his colleagues to acknowledge the existence of disease and to enforce a strict seclusion from these negative influences. "A complete control of the patient is essential," he said, "and to this end, the seclusion insisted upon by Dr. Weir Mitchell is of great importance, for by it an important obstacle to recovery is at once removed, to wit, the demoralizing sympathy of injudicious friends."[14] In Henry's estimation, the disease called for isolation from sympathetic relations in the form of Mitchell's famous rest cure. With such treatment, these "amiable drones" of the household might take on more productive roles within the family. Henry was one of many physicians who believed that the problem of degenerating and nonproductive womanhood demanded such thoroughgoing isolation and careful therapeutic reform.[15]

For these physicians, chlorosis and anemia resulted from a variety of biological maladjustments to modern society.[16] In 1882, the Boston physician Robert Edes speculated that "cases seem to originate in two almost diametrically opposed conditions, which may be briefly named, *underwork* and *overwork*." High-pressure education and high-stress labor were also key causes: "If, as I believe, our system of education is responsible . . . for an important proportion of the chronic female invalids, the remedies are easily seen . . . They are: moderate and carefully regulated bodily exercise; less study for prizes and more for knowledge; . . . and perhaps most important of all, lucrative employments beside teaching which shall be considered respectable for women."[17] Edes did not oppose women's education per se but endorsed a moderate "moral and hygienic" schedule to ease the stresses created by education. New York gynecologist T. Gaillard Thomas believed that chlorosis was a maladjustment to the onset of puberty, but a manageable one. "Those who suffer from it usually menstruate regularly for a time after they first arrive at the age of puberty, and then this trouble begins to develop. As a general rule, it seems to be originally due to some strong mental or emotional disturbance, and nostalgia [for childhood] is regarded as one of its most frequent causes."[18] Chlorosis almost always involved poor eating habits, faulty menstruation, and gastric disturbances, all traceable to the demands being heaped upon America's young girls and women. Chlorosis was the female body's rebellion.

Medical writers insisted that they were well positioned to diagnose chlorosis and to guide these girls and their families through this treacherous path to womanhood. According to Lionel Beale, in his 1887 book *Our Morality and the Moral Question,* modern physicians had supplanted even religious authorities in such matters. Religious advisors were too much like indulgent friends. "The practice of habitual confession," Beale argued, "is calculated to do irreparable mischief . . . Medical practitioners are more likely to be of real assistance to the patient than the clergy, or secular, classic, or science instructors. Our position as family advisers as regards bodily and mental health, and on the general hygienic management of the young would seem to point us out as the fit persons who should be consulted."[19] Moral management by physicians provided an alternative to injudicious sympathy, nostalgia, or indulgence. Who better than the family doctor to oversee the bodily, mental, and hygienic management of the young? Disorders like chlorosis proved the point, neatly legitimizing this medical ideal.

Chlorosis reflected the essential biological and social continuity of disease, as well as the essential biological and social focus of the family doctor. Accordingly, curing chlorosis demanded an attack not on a germ or on a particular biopathological entity, per se, but on this corrupting system of social relations. The chlorotic girl had learned to be "capricious" in habits and behavior and had been indulged by reassuring female friends, by family members, and by physicians. Many such "slight ailments," wrote Beale, were "likely to be made worse by the concentration of the sufferer's attention upon them, as well as by the expressed concern of female friends and relations . . . Practitioners, and notably those who make the diseases of females their special concern, have . . . actually contributed to increase the evil."[20] A strict daily regimen and isolation from the pressures and indulgences of society would cure the disease.

In calling for extended moral supervision in special clinics outside the patient's accustomed environment, such physicians styled themselves as a particular type of social reformer. In removing girls from the home, the treatment for chlorosis differed dramatically from the treatment for simple anemia. T. Gaillard Thomas suggested that, in cases of anemia, "iron is of the very highest service . . . [but] this is not the case where chlorosis is present." Chlorosis required a more systematic control. "The patient requires something more, and I feel sure that if she could only have a complete change of scene, with something new constantly to engage her attention, for a number of months, she would recover more quickly than if any other course were pursued."[21] Thomas advocated a systematic deployment of technologies and medical inducements—constant dietary regulation, therapeutic use of iron and nerve tonics, regular exercise, and frequent bowel movements. He offered such a regimen in his own clinic for women—opened in mid-Manhattan in 1881. This pattern of institutional care was a variation on S. Weir Mitchell's rest cure and represented not indulgence but careful clinical management—an appealing conjunction between Thomas' entrepreneurial interests and the therapeutic desires of middle-class families.[22]

By the last decade of the nineteenth century, such clinics and hospital wards offered a small clientele the uplifting influence of this wide-ranging moral management.[23] In an 1894 issue of *New England Kitchen Magazine,* Ellen Richards could speak positively of the "hospital diet," suggesting that "no better school of diet can be found than an intelligently managed hospital."[24] Away from supportive friends and parasitic doctors, chlorotic patients benefited from controlled circumstances, close monitoring of all their physical and nervous signs, and a regimen that regulated their bowel movements, oxygen intake, and blood count.[25] New York's Francis Delafield used a regimen of Blaud's iron pills (six to twenty-four times a day), oxygen gas inhaled for ten to fifteen minutes a day, bowels moved at least once a day, and blood measured every few days.

> Now, all this can probably be done for this girl if she enters the hospital, and that will probably be the best place for her . . . It will not be enough to give this girl some iron and let her go to work. She needs rest in bed; she needs diet, besides iron, oxygen, and enemata to relieve constipation . . . The moral condition comes into play largely; . . . they are cases for management rather than anything else—the moral management, the regulation of diet and the mode of life.[26]

These physicians defined the disease essentially as a moral matter and saw themselves as moral supervisors and surrogate parents to the girls placed temporarily in their clinical care.

In cases of chlorosis and anemia, the centerpieces of moral management were the technologies of blood monitoring. Using the newly developed hemocytometer or hemoglobinometer, physicians could monitor the number of red blood corpuscles in their patients or measure the amount of hemoglobin within these blood cells.[27] Subtle changes in blood color revealed the apparently beneficial effects of the diet, exercise, proper eating, and hygiene. According to Delafield, proper treatment could transform the hemoglobin (the coloring agent in the blood) dramatically. "It will take, probably, two or three weeks before she will be well enough to go to work. By the end of two or three months, one can say beforehand with considerable certainty, that the blood will have changed in about this way: Instead of having 20 per cent haemoglobin, it will have about 80 per cent."[28] Restoration of the hemoglobin was but one of the measurable results of moral management.

Despite their reliance on the technology of blood monitoring, such physicians recoiled at the suggestion that technologies fully *defined* the disease—that chlorosis was nothing more than a hemoglobin deficiency. As Frederick Forcheimer of Cincinnati wrote, "unfortunately [in] this definition, the term chlorosis is to be looked upon as an essentially clinical one."[29] The implication was clear. Physicians should use hemoglobin as a scientific *indicator* of the progress of disease and of the patient's recovery, but this indicator was only a symptom of the real problem and should not be mistaken for the disease itself. Was medicine to be a narrow clinical undertaking focusing on blood measurement or an integrative technological, moral, and social practice? Clearly, how doctors used and interpreted their technology had sweeping implications for their own practice and their own moral position in society.

Even when physicians embraced a more clinical definition of chlorosis, they continued to believe that chlorosis had moral and social origins. For Charles Simon, a young physician at the newly created Johns Hopkins Hospital, chlorosis could be called a hemoglobin deficiency without fear of losing the big picture.[30] In the 1890s, Hopkins had become a national exemplar of the new scientific medicine, with its emphasis on laboratory-based diagnostics and research. Yet Simon employed laboratory methods of blood analysis precisely to bring into sharper focus the moral question. He spoke of the failure of families to control their adolescent girls, and he emphasized the valuable role physicians played in guiding moral development. Simon reviewed the extensive literature on chlorosis, arguing that chlorosis originated in "capricious appetites," in "perversions" of diet, in "malnutrition" of girls *and* boys, and in the all-too-common practice of masturbation.[31] The lower classes became chlorotic because, too often, they imitated the "aristocratic" eating habits of the wealthy. Simon asserted that control of these habits through moral management and blood monitoring was essential to the disease's eradication.

Institutionalized moral management meant that "the patient is obliged to eat what is placed before him," said Simon. In his view, the modern democratic hospital made the benefits of this moral management available to all, independent of class. The hospital was probably the best place for the "the poor, hard-worked, and ill-fed shop girl," as well as for her middle- and upper-class counterparts.

> Experiments are not necessary to show that the same girl's diet at home is widely different from that which she receives in a hospital . . . At the Johns Hopkins Hospital the writer had occasion to study three chlorotic girls—intimate friends—who invariably carried with them a box containing pepper and salt. Of this they partook with apparent relish. It is not the writer's intention to dwell upon this form of capricious appetite, but to point out the fact that a similar perversion exists regarding staple articles of food.[32]

In the hospital, these poor shop-girls as well as their middle-class counterparts found a uniform and strict regimen and isolation from noxious social influences. Simon prescribed five meals a day, moderate exercise, "ten hours of sleep, warm salt-water baths twice weekly, dry friction in the morning, avoidance of society, etc."

Illnesses with a moral or social etiology (as Lionel Beale observed) offered physicians a chance to play out their roles, to reaffirm their identity by exerting moral pressure on the sick. "During illness, it need scarcely be said, we have abundant opportunity of learning and judging of the facts and of investigating the circumstances which have led to the commission of offenses against morality."[33] For family doctors as well as hospital-based physicians, a diagnosis of chlorosis suggested these technologies of moral management. Facing apparent upheaval in the lives, expectations, and behaviors of young girls, physicians seized upon chlorosis as a reliable disease category and as a clinical rationale for transforming capricious and ill-fed girls into models of regulated, controlled, and well-behaved young women. The monitoring of blood, appetite, and habits conferred scientific legitimacy on moral management.

Contemporary handbooks for young women echoed the need for

moral management in chlorosis, yet these books often distributed the burden of moral management between parents and physicians. In her 1898 book, *What Women Should Know,* Eliza Bisbee Duffey advised that in chlorosis "the attendance of a physician is absolutely necessary, but, aside from this, there is much that parents can do." As the disease reflected failures of parental oversight, parents had an obvious role in its treatment. "This disease is almost always the result of too close confinement, prolonged sedentary employment, innutritious diet, improper dress, late hours, unnatural excitements and general bad habits, so that a course of life the reverse of all this is the proper one to pursue in order to avoid the disease."[34] In her self-described "woman's book about women," Duffey echoed medical proscriptions: chlorosis was a disease of capricious girls. But for her, the responsibilities for its prevention and treatment rested equally with parents, physicians, and society.

The lifestyles of working girls and college women engendered vigorous debate during the last decades of the nineteenth century. Between 1880 and 1910, the percentage of women in the labor force rose from 14.7 to 24.8 percent of all workers.[35] In 1890, women accounted for less than 25 percent of college graduates; by 1900, the figure was 40 percent.[36] As historian Kathy Peiss has argued, the unregulated working girl and woman posed a special problem for middle-class moralists and social reformers.[37] Physicians' ideas about chlorosis echoed and legitimized this strain of middle-class anxiety. In this context, physicians portrayed chlorosis as an embodiment of much that was wrong with American womanhood, a disease that revealed the precise hematological dangers of freedom, capricious behavior, mutual female indulgence, and collective women's activities.[38] Chlorosis highlighted the dangers of sympathy and indulgence, stressed the value of moderation in work, and highlighted the role of family doctors in technology-based moral supervision, guidance, and uplift. The disease, the treatment, and the social reform mission reinforced one another. The identities of doctor, patient, and disease were affirmed in the lens of the microscope, reified by blood analysis technology. The evolving identity of chlorosis would depend upon this nexus of social concerns.

The Death of Chlorosis in the Modern Hospital

Already in the 1890s, the chlorosis construct showed signs of weakness and fragility in the face of changing medical agendas and social concerns. Not all parents shared the late Victorian moralist's concern about moral degeneration, masturbation, illicit sexual practices, and capricious behavior. Charles Simon of Johns Hopkins noted that parents often recoiled at the doctor's suggestion that their daughter's disease was caused by masturbation, by failures of parental oversight, or by some other moral failing. "In the case of girls . . . he will frequently hesitate to communicate his suspicions to the parents. They would be shocked were they told that their daughter is a masturbator. The mere insinuation of such an idea would undoubtedly frequently drive the family to a more 'gentlemanly' physician."[39] While some saw the biological and social scope of the chlorosis diagnosis as a strength, others—envisioning a more limited medical moralism—saw it as a problem. As David Rosner has noted of New York's hospitals in the early years of the twentieth century, "efficiency" replaced moral guidance as a new hospital ideal. As a result, "no longer were patients present . . . long enough for trustees to assume responsibility for the social and moral improvement."[40] In such contexts, blood counting and blood monitoring took a new role, becoming not a tool for moral management but a tool for creating presumably amoral, biologically specific classifications of disease and thereby increasing the economic efficiency and rationality of patient care. As hospitals multiplied, the growth of this new style of hematological thinking and the ideal of efficiency in patient management threatened to make chlorosis obsolete.

In the new concept of *hypochromic anemia*, many physicians found a disease term that was crafted not for the moral economy of family-oriented practice and social reform, but for the moral economy of hospital work. If chlorosis disappeared because parents recoiled from the label, it also disappeared because hospital-based physicians were turning away from moral management toward "scientific management," creating new roles for technology in medicine. This new view of disease, too, would have its own heyday and its own fall from grace.

The use of hemoglobinometers and hemacytometers to measure variations in the appearance of blood (in conjunction with staining methods to create sharper gradations in color) suggested that the term *chlorosis* could be replaced with more precise categories of blood disease—based on minute observations of the different kinds of blood cells that were present in illness.[41] As a proponent of this diagnostic style wrote, "the invention and employment of the hemacytometer and the hemoglobinometer has enabled us to . . . know that pallor may be due to too few corpuscles or too little hemoglobin."[42] A decrease in corpuscles might be thought of as one disease, whereas the decrease of hemoglobin—a phenomenon that resulted in pale-centered red blood cells—might be thought of as another disease. But physicians did not all embrace this clinical vision of disease. One skeptic wrote that "it has . . . been established that this view of the blood-change in chlorosis is *altogether too narrow* . . . The essential point is that the percentage of hemoglobin is reduced in this affection, [but] . . . *this is common in many forms of anemia.*"[43] Even advocates of this "narrow" view—the view that chlorosis was essentially a hemoglobin/blood disease—admitted that there was no necessary relationship between the blood picture and chlorosis and that similar blood changes were found in a wide range of disorders.

Essentially, the two visions of disease represented two distinct visions of the doctor's place in society. One was a social vision of disease, and the other was narrowly hematological. Even in the 1890s, however, a reductionist trend was clear. Charles Simon suggested that physicians use their tools to create a new disease identity devoid of explicit moralism. "The question arises: What is the smallest amount of hemoglobin that may be met with in health?" Simon wrote. "Percentages lower than 70, when associated with a fairly normal number of red corpuscles . . . should be regarded as indicating a condition of chlorosis, or a simple anemia, a term which the writer prefers."[44] The data produced in hospital work suggested that chlorosis could be reduced to hemoglobin values. But if chlorosis *could* be diagnosed by a simple blood test, why not abandon the term altogether and simply speak of *hemoglobin deficiency* or *hypochromic anemia?* Simon asserted that "it would be better to discard the term 'chlorosis' altogether, as it has reference to a symptom only, viz., the greenish yellow hue of the skin."[45] Renaming disease became a vehicle toward avoiding the moral questions surrounding chlorosis, redefining disease as a specific hematological problem, and embracing a purely clinical problem of patient management.

Physicians of the 1890s asked themselves what their purpose and role in society should be. Linked to this social dilemma were questions of disease identity: Was the blood picture "the symptom" or "the disease itself"? On one side stood the doctor as moral guide to family and society; on the other, the doctor as clinical manager. In the early years of the twentieth century, the clinician was ascending in status and prominence. Diagnostic styles and interpretations of technology changed accordingly. Features such as the hue of the skin, the capricious habits and behavior of a young girl, and her family's failure of oversight figured less and less in the diagnosis of "disease." As one upstate New York general practitioner determined in 1902, chlorosis was simply a less than optimal hematological state detectable by the staining of cells and their analysis under the microscope: "the centers [of the red blood corpuscles] may not take eosin stain, indicating a deficiency of hemoglobin, which is chlorosis or grave secondary anemia."[46] No mention was made of the moral question or of moral management.

Critics of this view thought that it was the hemoglobin that was "merely symptomatic" and that the "real disease" originated in the moral and social realm. Distinguished older physicians like England's T. Clifford Allbutt urged all physicians concerned with chlorosis not to retreat into technical narrowness, noting that "the physician will not forget, so far as in him lies, to rectify such disadvantages of life as he may be able to ascertain. Over pressure at school, unwholesome conditions of work or amusement, late hours, worry, tight lacing [of the corsets]."[47] In moving diagnosis away from this realm, clinical scientists adjusted their diagnostic standards to changing institutional and consumer expectations. They styled themselves as disinterested experts treating all patients equally according to their blood values and thereby raising their own social and epistemological status. Such a shift had egalitarian, and even democratic, overtones for, in the modern hospital, shop-girls and wealthy women would both be evaluated by the same scientific standard. Chlorosis thereby became a symptom rather than a disease, a vestige of an old-fashioned medical subjectivity.

Yet chlorosis did not disappear everywhere and for everyone. It continued to be a vital concern for experts in childhood and development, appearing in a wide range of advice literature for parents. Scholars who were interested in the family and adolescent life continued to see it as a crucial warning sign. In his 1904 book, *Youth: Its Education, Regimen, and Hygiene,* the leader of the new adolescent psychology movement, G. Stanley Hall, noted that, "in this time of sensitiveness and perturbation, when anemia and chlorosis are so peculiarly immanent to her sex, remission of toil should not only be permitted, but required."[48] Hall saw chlorosis as linked to puberty and as a caution to parents to avoid overworking their children. Chlorosis continued to intrigue psychologists and some general practitioners. In her 1926 text, *The Adolescent Girl: A Book for Parents and Teachers,* psychologist Winifred Richmond defined chlorosis as a typical disease of puberty. Years after clinicians ceased to recognize the existence of this disease, Richmond wrote that "though rest, good food, and air are important adjuncts they will not alone correct the deficiency in the blood, and the girl in whom chlorosis is suspected should always be under the care of a competent physician."[49] Despite these psychologists' observations, knowledge production about disease had shifted away from family doctoring and sites of moral management into modern hospitals and laboratories. "Chlorosis" had become anathema to the modern clinical scientist and, insofar as they were now dominant in the production of medical knowledge, its demise seemed assured.

New technologies of blood analysis do not explain how and why chlorosis disappeared. Rather, a changing medical culture prompted new interpretations of existing tools and hastened the disappearance of chlorosis. The symptoms that made up chlorosis—lethargy, blood diminution, gastric and menstrual disturbance—continued to exist but would be recategorized into new disease constructs. As medical practice became increasingly institution based in the early twentieth century, a new style of scientific disease management emerged, focusing on efficiency and rationality. To clinicians, moral management seemed inefficient, old-fashioned, and punitive. The concerns of late nineteenth-century medical moralists about appropriate womanhood had given way to a new faith in efficiency and bureaucracy as proper modes of disease management and social reform. Experts, reformers, politicians, and physicians of the era celebrated the efficiencies of large-scale management, in the hospital as in other realms of life. Chlorosis, it appears, simply did not fit within this new system.

The rise of modern hematological management and the advent of newer diagnostic categories like hypochromic anemia celebrated a new form of expertise. But subsequent advances in medicine and society would undermine even this construction, producing yet more reformulations of this disease. Such reformulations (or memories of chlorosis) were informed by ever-changing attitudes toward women, technology, and the nature of disease. Aware of the disease's symptomatological vagueness, twentieth-century authors have continued trying to resolve the mystery of the disease. An analysis of their writings allows us to understand something more about the presumptive power of technology in twentieth-century medicine and its limits in constructing memories of the past. Chlorosis had not been gone for a decade when some writers began to perform imaginative postmortems on the disease.

Explaining the Death of Chlorosis

Gender

Shortly after chlorosis's demise, some physicians argued that women's emancipation, not technology, accounted for its disappearance. Chlorosis became a symbol of the progress of women in the twentieth century. In his 1920 *Layman's Handbook of Medicine*, Richard Cabot speculated, "Why it occurs only in women in this particular age, why it is now apparently disappearing from America are questions that have never been answered."[50] After the Great War, these "pasty-faced girls" were nowhere evident.[51] In 1938, Cabot wrote, "forty years ago it was common; now it is seen rarely; some say never."[52] Seeking reasons for its decline, many in this generation pointed to the virtual revolution in the status of women in Western societies.

Ironically, where earlier physicians had blamed the young girl's freedom, lax and capricious behavior, and loose morality for chlorosis, many who had witnessed women's suffrage in the United States (bringing with it political freedom and changing sexual mores) associated these developments with chlorosis' demise. They constructed a new postsuffrage identity for the disease, an identity that underwrote women's emancipation in their time.

Even in 1915, in the pages of the widely read textbook, *Modern Medicine*, Cabot described how chlorosis had been most prevalent among Boston's Irish domestic workers. Reviewing some two hundred cases from his own practice, he asserted that "among our cases a majority occurred in the Irish race, which ten years ago (when chlorosis was common) supplied the larger number of recently immigrated domestics."[53] The immigrant woman's confrontation with American work and lifestyle had caused chlorosis.[54] "It is hardly credible," Cabot wrote, "that the occupation of the domestic [alone] predisposes to chlorosis, and it seems more likely that the occurrence of the disease is favored by the sharp change of habits and surroundings which many girls undergo at the time they enter domestic service."[55] Chlorosis was partly a product of the constitutional inadequacies of immigrants and partly due to the working conditions they encountered. The identity of chlorosis had reflected these convergent forces. But according to the new story, as immigrant women and girls adjusted over time to the new demands of work, chlorosis had declined.

Some physicians retrospectively linked chlorosis directly to labor conditions themselves and portrayed its sufferers as the victims of labor confinement and exploitation. Women's unions, social reformers, industrial health advocates, and many physicians (singing from the same page) made the improvement of women's labor conditions a prominent part of a Progressive Era political agenda. Some physicians therefore chose to remember chlorosis not as a disease of underwork, school, puberty, or bad habits, but as a disease "common among ill-fed girls of large towns, who are confined all day in close, badly lighted rooms."[56] In an early work on industrial disease, Sir Thomas Oliver suggested that "anemia and chlorosis are maladies most notable in the early years of womanhood from 15–20, [caused by] long continued sitting when at work, or its opposite much standing, deprivation of fresh air and too short intervals for taking food."[57] To these reformers, chlorosis was a disease generated by female exploitation. This was a potent image of disease and exploitation, resonating with contemporary events—such as the 1911 Triangle Shirtwaist Company fire, in which 146 women locked in the factory had perished; the resurgent women's suffrage movement; and the Supreme Court's 1910 ruling upholding the right of state governments to restrict women's working hours. Most medical authors in the 1910s and 1920s recalled with certainty that "overworked girls confined in close, badly lighted rooms" were in fact the disease's chief victims.[58] The cultural importance of working women's confinement had pushed this dimension of chlorosis to the forefront of medical memory.

There were also those who remembered that chlorosis had affected *all* classes of women, and these physicians pointed to *general* improvements in the lives of women to explain its decline.[59] In a 1931 essay, physician-historian David Reisman stated that it was only natural that diseases like chlorosis should rise and fall with intellectual, social, and political change. To Reisman, diseases were not static entities, but evolving ones. "Many of them," he wrote, "are like human beings . . . They are born, they flourish, and they die." Chlorosis was "one of the most interesting examples of how such factors influenced the life of a pathology."[60] It disappeared because of the emancipation of women: in diet, work, dress, lifestyle, and politics. "The disappearance of the green-sickness," said Reisman, "is due to a variety of causes; to a change in our habits of living—a healthier, freer mode of life, in which women have their full share, shorter working hours, athletics, the disuse of the tightly laced corset, modes of dress and outdoor life giving sunlight a better chance, and a better balanced diet."[61]

Reisman did not associate the decline of chlorosis with the movement toward hospital practice and new uses of technology, but with the disappearance of a Victorian past. Physical constraints (corsets, limited exercise, and an indoor life) and social hardship (long working hours, industrial exploitation) for women had caused this disease. To Reisman, modern society had become enlightened and chlorosis had disappeared. Other writings in the 1920s and early 1930s concurred with this self-congratulatory view of chlorosis as a disease of late Victorian society, a disease intricately connected to the identity and daily rituals of Victorian women.[62] These writers rarely specified whether *emancipation* meant female suffrage, economic self-determination, sexual liberation, or the abandonment of corsets. More often, they congratulated themselves and their society, praising the freer mode of life that a previous generation had sought to condemn.[63] For British physicians, the corset—that archetype of Victorian constraint—had retrospectively become the key culprit.[64]

Physicians fell in line with the beliefs of their time, revising former attitudes about the control of women and constructing a new picture of chlorosis that endorsed freedom. Few would have agreed with their late nineteenth-century counterparts, who believed that chlorosis was a disease caused by too much freedom, demanding as its cure stricter technology-based oversight of women. As one British physician observed, "there has probably been a greater change in the life and habits of civilized girls during the last twenty years than . . . during the previous twenty centuries . . . The cult of fresh air, along with free movements and exercise in the open air have been welcome changes in the habits of girls. The tight corset, important as it was as a causative agent, was, I believe, only one amongst several causes."[65] Despite the enormous changes that had taken place in diagnostic technologies in their time, few of these physicians disputed the centrality of this *social* transformation in the history of the disease. Even after its demise, the disease's identity and the story of modern women continued to be closely intertwined.

Even today (perhaps especially so, given the heightened social interest in women, technology, and medicine), this view of chlorosis as a disease of Victorian society—as a product of social *assumptions* and *behaviors*—continues to inform historical writing about the disease.[66] The emancipation motif has continued to be influential in how we explain the movement of this, and many other, diseases through time. In the 1980s, for example, historian Joan Brumberg offered a story of chlorosis as an episode of women's emancipation from nineteenth-century norms, a story similar to that of early twentieth-century physicians.[67] To Brumberg, however, chlorosis disappeared because women themselves—mothers and daughters alike—had "moved beyond invalidism" as a cultural ideal.[68] Her story created a chlorosis that pointed to the role of cultural norms in disease construction, a story that supported the freer movement of women in society. Unlike her predecessors, however, Brumberg emphasized that girls chose for themselves these disease labels and cultural norms. Such narratives of disease as cultural liberation have had an enduring appeal, particularly in the 1920s and the 1980s, when such stories spoke to contemporary concerns. Yet this motif has been only one among the preferred themes in reconstructions of chlorosis.

Technology

In contrast to these gender-centered stories of chlorosis, other reflections on chlorosis have focused on the identity politics *within* laboratory medicine. For some writers, gender was of limited importance in the disease's demise. Advances in therapy played no role in its demise. Chlorosis' demise depended essentially upon the availability of new diagnostic techniques, improved physiological knowledge, and other factors internal to medical practice. Others, including myself, have refuted these claims. It is important, however, to explore why this story has endured. The analysis highlights a continuing debate in twentieth-century medicine about the proper place of technology in medical thought, medical progress, and the profession's sense of itself.

With the proliferation of hospital diagnostic laboratories in the early 1900s (the increasing use of x-rays, chemical tests, microscopic exams, and other tools), it seemed only natural to some physicians that ideas about diseases in the past had faded in the light of new knowledge and practice.[69] The new twentieth-century physician—working in the laboratories of hospitals and research institutes and performing increasing numbers of blood tests in the pursuit of scientific precision—spoke of disease in biological, somatic, or organic terms. To such specialists, the peculiar paleness at the center of red blood cells was evidence of a specific type of blood disease—a "hypochromic anemia."[70] Chlorosis had simply been a vague approximation of what laboratory tests now identified as hypochromic anemia, as tuberculosis, or as numerous other diseases.

Even during its demise, chlorosis continued to reflect debates between the traditional doctor and the technology-oriented specialist. Their disagreements revolved around whether physicians should give in to the allure of new technologies and to new modes of knowledge production.[71] New terms like *hypochromic anemia* stirred intergenerational conflicts over diagnostic rules of conduct, skill, acumen, and professional identity. In 1925, British physician F. Parkes Weber rejected the "modern physician's" chauvinistic dismissal of his elder brethren.

> It is true that formerly in general practice countless troubles in women of all ages were attributed to "anaemia" without any blood count being made . . . It is therefore quite natural that some modern physicians of a younger generation, experts in blood examination . . . should question the alleged former frequency of chlorosis, suggesting that it was due to want of knowledge and insufficient or careless examination of the blood. But no one who was a house physician in London about 1890 can admit the justness of such an accusation.[72]

Technology lured younger physicians unjustly to denigrate doctors in the previous generation. But, in fact, said Weber, "the ordinary features of chlorosis were well known. Indeed, one could make the diagnosis with practical certainty when one passed girls and young women in the London streets."[73] If anyone was deluded it was the modern laboratory expert, who believed that he alone enjoyed privileged insight into disease.

Technological change has often engendered such conflicts over the nature of disease and diagnosis. This has been a recurring tension in twentieth-century technology-dependent medicine. As one group of physicians have embraced a new tool, using it to foster new and privileged insights into disease, they implicitly (and often explicitly) have questioned the judgment of other diagnosticians. The upholders of the diagnostic status quo, challenged by technological novelties, have responded defensively. The outcomes of such confrontations have never been obvious. The outcomes of such debates—essentially about professional status, hierarchies of knowledge, and professional identity—have been determined by the historically specific factors.

In the 1920s and 1930s, physicians like Weber regarded the problem of chlorosis as a historical referendum on the increasingly technological character of medicine in this era. How one remembered chlorosis became a vital matter of professional practice. In a 1937 article, A. L. Bloomfield of Stanford University tried to be diplomatic amidst these tensions about "chlorosis" and "hypochromic anemia," and he analyzed their competing "claims of definite identity."[74] He regarded the two diseases as phenomenologically identical, stressing "the impossibility of differentiating chlorosis in the late nineteenth century sense from the hypochromic anemia of modern writers."[75] He emphasized that anyone who argued that one diagnosis was more correct than the other was being "dogmatic."[76] To Bloomfield, the debate between old and new diagnostic practice was put to rest by a humbling realization. *Both* diagnostic categories stood on equal, but equally shaky, footing.

Medicine's alleged technological progress and its scientific rationality had merely replaced one vague taxonomic category with another, moving from one style of knowledge production to another. According to Bloomfield, both chlorosis and hypochromic anemia were hopelessly imprecise, and their champions made exaggerated claims. The symptoms that defined them—breathlessness on exertion, weakness, digestive disorder—were found in many disorders, and therefore both categories were arbitrary, outdated, and even sentimental.[77] Of hypochromic anemia, he noted: "No sooner had [modern physicians] laid down criteria [for the definition of this new disease] . . . than exceptions and variations begin to appear in great numbers . . . it will serve no useful purpose to set up a definite disease on the basis of criteria to which so many and such obvious exceptions exist."[78] The categories of chlorosis and hypochromic anemia were both misguided attempts to create a concrete terminology for symptoms that varied widely from one case to the next. New technology did little to clarify this complex problem.[79] The modern laboratory-based doctor was no better or worse, it seemed, than his nineteenth-century counterpart.

In a 1936 article entitled "Chlorosis—An Obituary," W. M. Fowler suggested that modern practitioners, depending on new diagnostic tools, were somewhat like blind men touching different parts of the elephant. They had gradually reordered and reclassified what had been chlorosis into separate disease entities. "Some cases, which would previously have passed for chlorosis, are now undoubtedly being recognized by improved diagnostic procedures as early tuberculosis, Bright's disease, or chronic hemorrhagic anemia . . . it is possible that this shift in terminology and the withdrawal of certain cases to other categories may account to some extent, but not entirely, for the lessened incidence."[80] Fowler admitted that this version of chlorosis' demise was mere speculation and that theories of its demise were "as inadequate and . . . as fanciful as were the theories of its etiology."[81] Fowler understood what few fellow physicians comprehended—that retrospective diagnosis, using the medical tools of one era to explain diseases in another, was full of conjecture and speculation, especially given the vagueness of "chlorosis" in earlier times. Chlorosis was, in many respects, a disease from a different era, and modern physicians were poorly equipped (precisely *because* of their wealth of diagnostic technology) to understand it.

This was an irony of modern medical technology. The diagnostic developments of the 1920s and 1930s gave rise to an increasingly fragmented, unstable, and speculative set of historical identities for chlorosis. For many physicians of this generation, the relationship between technology and disease was by no means clear. *Disease* evoked the image of an ideal-type classification, a set of normally associated symptoms with small variations from the norm. Many diseases were not clearly defined entities, but contingent classifications of symptoms that might blur into each other. Moreover, the identity of "the disease" depended upon fashions in diagnostic technique. (This relationship is particularly evident in the history of pernicious anemia; see ch. 4.) Greater accuracy of tools was no guarantee of more dependable disease diagnoses. Thus, many physicians believed that some of the diseases constructed by modern physicians (like hypochromic anemia) were no more real than chlorosis.[82] There was little consensus about the status of terms like *hypochromic anemia* or their superiority to older views of disease. With technological progress came diagnostic diversity, and also considerable confusion.

This too has been a recurring theme throughout this century: the story of chlorosis has been seen as a kind of referendum on technology-based laboratory medicine, and particularly on the benefits and drawbacks of hematological diagnosis. For some, like L. J. Witts, the story had a progressive moral: "the recession of chlorosis, like a retreating tide, revealed the presence of other cases of unexplained hypochromic anemia which had previously been subsumed in it."[83] Others have praised the fact that "laboratory medicine sprouted and flourished in the very years that chlorosis languished and disappeared."[84] But the profession's own ambivalence toward the laboratory and deep cultural ambivalence about laboratory medicine have lingered. Writing in the 1980s, Irvine Loudon suggested that laboratory medicine was not the solution to chlorosis but was part of the confusion. He argued that "the era of laboratory medicine, which on the whole was so triumphantly successful in clarifying our understanding of disease, actually confused the picture so far as chlorosis was concerned."[85] Loudon sided with a traditional view of disease over what he portrayed as diagnostic myopia.

With the rise of a laboratory-based style of diagnosis, Loudon argued, nineteenth-century medical practitioners began to rely too heavily on blood counts.[86] The characterization of chlorosis as an "anaemia of adolescent girls" replaced what had been a more complex psychosocial disorder involving nervousness, gastric disturbances, and eating problems.[87] Technological innovation and precision in hemoglobin analysis diverted physicians away from these complexities. Thus, modern technology did not necessarily clarify our understanding of disease, nor did it necessarily lead to better treatments. By relying on the microscope, physicians merely reordered their perceptions—constructing temporary and unreliable taxonomies, narrow conceptions like "hypochromic anemia," which ignored the epistemological, social, and psychological complexities of disease.

Was technology central to the rise and fall of chlorosis? If so, how? Or were changing gender beliefs and behaviors its undoing? Those who debated the role of technological change in chlorosis have not for the most part engaged with those who have insisted on the centrality of the gender question. The two styles of analysis represent dominant cultural concerns since early in this century, concerns that have reemerged in the latter part of the century along with anxieties about the nature of technology and medicine. Before these cultural anxieties reemerged, a third story of chlorosis appeared in the middle part of this century, reflecting the beliefs of yet another cohort of specialists about technology, gender, and disease in America.

Iron and the Gender Question in Hematology

In 1987, William Crosby suggested that the rise of laboratory medicine was merely part of a much grander story of women, doctors, and disease. Better diagnosis by itself had not conquered chlorosis. Rather, the twin forces of diagnosis and therapy in the twentieth century had brought about the disease's rapid decline. "The ability to diagnose anemia before it became severe permitted early therapeutic intervention."[88] The view that diagnosis and treatment worked hand in hand to overcome the suffering of women became a dominant motif only after World War II, given legitimacy by the therapeutic achievements of that era. With the production of antibiotics during the war and the "conquest of polio" in the fifties, physicians grew confident about their therapeutic power. Memories of chlorosis constructed during this era featured doctors and iron (the drug) as their heroes. Simply put, the prescription of iron had caused the disease's decline.

These stories emphasized that chlorosis was nothing more than an "iron deficiency anemia" and that the prescription of iron supplements had caused its gradual decline.[89] In an introductory essay to the 1963 *Clinical Disorders of Iron Metabolism,* the textbook's three authors wrote that "perhaps the most significant factor [in the disappearance of chlorosis] was the growth of rational medicine and the corresponding change in the taxonomy of disease . . . 'chlorosis' gave way to 'simple anaemia.' This in turn was soon replaced by 'iron deficiency anemia.' The old clinician's diagnosis could no longer withstand the assault by the new terminology of the new science of blood morphology."[90] This generation of physicians (unlike their predecessors in the 1890s or the 1930s) claimed to see clearly that chlorosis had been a simple problem of iron intake and iron metabolism. This was, moreover, a problem especially prevalent in women because of their unique physiology.

This new identity for chlorosis revealed less about chlorosis as described in the 1890s and much more about a particular culture of hematological thought that had grown and expanded by the middle of the twentieth century. By knitting together observations about iron metabolism, modern therapeutics, and female physiology, hematologists constructed a chlorosis that reflected the growing chauvinism of their times. By the 1950s, they celebrated the power of "wonder drugs," the virtues of the new science of iron metabolism, and the central place of these technologies in giving an identity to midcentury women, their diseases, and medical practice.

This drug-centered reconstruction of chlorosis expanded upon and revised what physicians had long known—iron was, in fact, a tool of limited power in the treatment of chlorosis.[91] Physicians had always steered away from therapeutic reductionism. In the 1890s, iron was merely one component of the overall "moral management" of patients. As one New York physician had written in 1889, "The particular medicine which you give them is not of so much consequence. The changes in the blood, the anemia which these patients have, does not, as a rule respond very readily to the use of iron; it responds much more readily to the mode of life, to diet, and exercise."[92] Therapeutic successes came because of doctors' particular skills at moral and therapeutic management.[93] Of course, some physicians did celebrate iron.[94] But it was the method of using iron in treatment, rather than iron pills per se, that physicians celebrated when speaking of chlorosis.[95] Any physician understood that *iron alone* was not curative, that iron treatment frequently caused constipation, and that this side effect also required its own delicate treatment.[96] For the traditional doctor, iron was no magic bullet; it was merely one part (and not even a necessary part) of an extended therapeutic oversight.[97]

Gradually, even broad-minded physicians found it appealing to think of iron as a specific cure for chlorosis.[98] This tendency stemmed from the growing influence of pharmaceutical enterprises in medicine and the practitioner's inclination to use such drugs as if they were diagnostic technologies (treating patients first and then using their responses to determine the diagnoses). For one Chicago physician in 1917, the increasing market availability of iron pills explained why "we do not see more cases of the disease than we do . . . it is common among the poorer classes to buy, without prescription, one of the many advertised remedies for 'anemia' when it is apparent from the pallor that such is the diagnosis . . . and, as most of such preparations contain iron, a recovery is usually effected."[99] This culture of drug consumption prompted physicians to underwrite the notion of "specific remedies" and to reconfigure their ideas about diseases around their patients' responses to drugs.[100] (Ch. 4 explores this trend and its relation to consumerism in greater detail.)

By the 1930s, Russell Haden captured the new attitude when he wrote that "now every clinician recognizes the value of iron and the need for giving large doses."[101] Another practitioner bemoaned the fact that doctors were prescribing drugs first and then waiting for a response before diagnosing diseases. "The time to establish the diagnosis," he warned, "is before, not after, the blood picture has been obscured by indiscriminate therapy." While decrying these tendencies to use drugs as diagnostic tools, the same author advocated a classification of anemias based on the very practice he had criticized. "Anemias," he wrote, "may be divided for therapeutic purposes into two main groups . . . the anemias of the first group respond brilliantly to the administration of the proper therapeutic agents, whereas for those of the second group there is no specific drug therapy."[102]

Iron pills, in other words, had become not only widely marketed consumer items, but also useful "diagnostic" tools. Instead of using a hemacytometer to diagnose blood deficiency, physicians in the 1930s and

1940s were simply prescribing iron pills diagnostically.[103] Iron pills had replaced hemoglobinometers and hemacytometers as the diagnostic tool of choice for many general practitioners. As one author wrote in the mid-1950s, "currently iron holds a prominent place in the medical armamentarium and is now incorporated in an astounding variety of proprietary preparations."[104]

As iron gained that "prominent place" among diagnostic technologies, hematologists called upon their experiences with iron therapy and iron metabolism in women to construct a compelling new identity for chlorosis. Old themes concerning appropriate womanhood, work, and lifestyle resurfaced, given renewed legitimacy by a new science of iron metabolism. The measurement of iron and iron metabolism seemed to be a powerful means of studying the woman in sickness and health—her diet, her lifestyle, and her unique physiology from puberty, through menstruation, fertility, pregnancy, and menopause. In this context, it seemed quite obvious to many authors that chlorosis was essentially a maladjusted iron metabolism.[105]

A wide range of iron studies from the 1930s through the 1960s suggested that women were essentially products of a physiological drama featuring iron as its lead actor. Some focused on the role that iron played during pregnancy in the health of the fetus.[106] For others, the measurement of a "hemoglobin value" could be used to establish parameters for determining normal activity during girlhood.[107] While men absorbed enough iron to maintain a normal amount of hemoglobin, women became anemic very easily—because they "lose blood at each menstrual period, . . . require large amounts of iron during pregnancy . . . and again during lactation." Iron deficiency became characterized as an elemental fact of womanhood—a timeless disorder, requiring constant medical vigilance. "For women, then," wrote one author, "the amount of iron in the diet is not enough . . . Anemia . . . has been in the past and is still today a common source of ill-health in women."[108] A knowledge of iron metabolism was essential for guiding the woman in her tortuous journey through life.

French feminist philosopher Simone de Beauvoir unmasked this style of biological thought in her 1953 book, *The Second Sex*. Diseases like anemia and chlorosis were constructed by biologists as acts of a play, in which the woman as individual and the woman as organism were two characters brought into dramatic conflict. According to "the data of biology," she wrote, the desires of the prepubescent girl did not conflict with

her needs as an organism. "[But] at puberty the species reasserts its claim
. . . Not without resistance does the body of woman permit the species to
take over; and this struggle is weakening and dangerous . . . At this period frequently appear such diseases as chlorosis, tuberculosis, scoliosis
. . . and osteomyelitis . . . From puberty to menopause woman is the the-
ater of a play that unfolds within her and in which she is not personally
concerned."[109] De Beauvoir insisted that such portraits of women were
overly deterministic. She conceded that "the biological facts . . . are one
of the keys to the understanding of woman," but denied "that they establish for her a fixed and inevitable destiny."[110] Medical writing on diseases like chlorosis promoted an image of the woman as naturally limited by her body. Hematology (through the science of iron metabolism)
provided one compelling part of that modern portrait.[111]

Hematological accounts of women and iron gained a wide cultural currency, both within medicine and in wider circles—as some theorists
sought to justify a domestic model of American womanhood in the
post–World War II decades. One portrait of anemia and the American
woman appeared in a 1962 *Time* magazine and focused on first lady
Eleanor Roosevelt—a controversial public figure and a high-profile example of activity both inside the first family and in political life. Her bout
with anemia, her failure to heed her doctor's warning, and her death
from miliary tuberculosis became an occasion for reminding women (according to the magazine) that her life, death, and very identity had been
determined by the quality of her blood. Entitled "Too Busy to Be Sick,"
the article began, "For at least two years, Mrs. Roosevelt had been anemic. [But] she was as contemptuous of fuss and feathers in regard to her
health as in other matters . . . [she] was unfit by temperament to be an invalid. She liked to say: 'I'm too busy to be sick.'" As her blood count fell
below the "danger level," however, she was forced to submit to medical
treatment that "carried the risk of lowering her resistance to infection."
Still "doggedly trying to carry on her work from the hospital bed," Mrs.
Roosevelt fell victim to tuberculosis and died. Although a drug-induced
"lowered resistance" had been partly to blame for her death, the article
concluded that "in anybody as determined to keep going as she was, it is
not surprising that the TB germs . . . were able to multiply and damage
the lungs."[112] The conflict between the individual female (however determined she was to remain active) and the organism resulted in tragedy.
Pushed beyond its limits by Mrs. Roosevelt's choice of lifestyle, her body
supposedly rebelled.

During this era few would have questioned the logic of this portrait of anemia or of the hematologist's decision to link "anemia" and "chlorosis" with such dilemmas of womanhood. As if a historical pendulum had swung, the midcentury reconstruction of chlorosis endorsed limitations on women's freedom. Medicine's support for emancipation had changed with the times to an endorsement of a more confined life for American women. All of this was reflected in the choice of a disease name and in the historical equation of iron deficiency anemia with chlorosis. According to one 1978 thesis, late nineteenth-century physician Ralph Stockman invented the idea of iron insufficiency "[but] he did not extend the idea to a new concept of disease—that of nutritional anemia."[113] It would be left for twentieth-century hematologists to solidify the connection.[114] For those who accepted the equation of chlorosis with iron deficiency, all other explanations of this disease seemed to be fundamentally mistaken. The capricious appetite, corset wearing, masturbation, moral laxity, emancipation, shifts in disease nomenclature, positive responses to Fowler's solution, or negative responses to iron therapy—all of these could be characterized as misguided attempts to identify the disease. The construction of chlorosis generated within the culture of mid–twentieth-century hematology was unabashedly drug centered. The historical identity of chlorosis had also become closely bound to the attitudes of the modern hematologist and his use of iron to paint a deterministic, but culturally compelling, portrait of physiological womanhood.

Technology's Narratives: Stories about Chlorosis

What insights might we gain from these stories of chlorosis in the nineteenth and twentieth centuries, and in particular about gender, iron pills, and hemacytometers? Physicians and historians leaned heavily on state-of-the-art technologies and on the social values of their era to construct "chlorosis," both in its heyday and well after its demise. Chlorosis has meant many different things during the last century. Three dominant motifs, each with its own ambivalent message, have shaped the life, death, and afterlife of this disease construct: changing gender ideologies, changing assessments of diagnostic tools, and the problem of evaluating iron.[115] Focusing on these three areas, historians and physicians have refined, revised, and extended late nineteenth-century ideas of chlorosis, producing radically different and constantly evolving portraits of womanhood, medicine, and disease.

Medical practitioners themselves and their technologies have been part of the historical drama of disease construction and reconstruction. Historians have created yet other narrative reconstructions of chlorosis and anemia. (I have already mentioned Joan Brumberg and Irvine Loudon.) In 1977, historian-physician Robert Hudson revisited the problem of chlorosis and Victorian clothing style, suggesting tentatively that the tight, binding corset must have had something to do with anemia and the green symptoms of the disease.[116] Another physician, A. Clair Siddall, suggested that enthusiasm for bloodletting (common in the nineteenth century, he argued) *must* have produced a great deal of iron deficiency.[117] Moreover, Siddall suggested that the increase in bloodletting reflected the expansion of obstetricians and gynecologists and their increasing competition with midwives.[118] Thus, the disease continues to be a powerful repository of ready historical lessons—about the nature of disease, the practice of medicine, and the consequences of technological innovation.

My concern in this chapter has not been to explore the truth of these claims, but to examine the ways in which these stories have been constructed and the purposes they serve. In a recent essay, Donna Haraway asked, "Are biological bodies 'produced' or 'generated' in the same strong sense as poems?"[119] The history of chlorosis suggests not only that bodies are produced, but also that their modes of production can be studied historically. I have made no universal claims about what chlorosis "really was." Rather, my analysis has emphasized that it was the *interaction* of technologies, gender ideals, and a changing culture of medicine— that is, the culture of moral management, the culture of laboratory medicine, the promoters of iron metabolism research, or the advocates of women's emancipation—that shaped the changing identity of chlorosis. One can see this disease as the product of a particular interaction between medical technologies and culture: in the 1890s, the disease's changing identity reflected shifts in the identity of the family doctor and in the role of the hemacytometer in medical practice; the reconstructed chlorosis of the 1950s represented a convergence of repressive attitudes about the woman's body and the place of iron in legitimizing her role in society.

Clearly, there is no single disease called *chlorosis*. Technologies have played a key role in giving many different identities to this complex phenomenon.[120] Assigning one universal identity to chlorosis would be both meaningless and arrogant. In retrospect, we can see that some cases of chlorosis may have been identical to iron deficiency anemia and others may have mirrored anorexia nervosa, but we can only speculate about how widely these statements apply. Retrospective diagnosis, using the technologies of a given moment to explain the past, has many pitfalls. One must conclude that diagnostic tests and drugs have been among many significant factors aggregating to constitute and reconstitute the disease. These technologies themselves have been products of particular cultural moments. The privileging of one technology over another (iron pills over hemacytometers) in the construction of disease cannot be understood apart from broader cultural assumptions about professional identity, patients' identity, and the nature and location of disease.

Ultimately, to understand "disease," we must be prepared to critically assess twentieth-century technological medicine and the cultures that have deployed and interpreted technology. Although some physicians may claim that technologies uncover a timeless reality of disease, the history of chlorosis makes clear that technology by itself is not a reliable guide to understanding what diseases are and how diseases move through time. Rather, the users of diagnostic and therapeutic technologies have described diseases that suit contemporary concerns. Theirs have been contingent, and historically bound, portraits of disease, linked to a politics of medical practice and to particular problems of womanhood in their time.

Assessing technology in medicine necessarily involves understanding that technology's scripting of disease has carried diverse implications for culture and identity. This analysis of chlorosis (as described, experienced, and remembered) leads to several (by now obvious) conclusions about technology: (1) technology has the capacity for either the confinement or the emancipation of its subjects; (2) technology can both clarify and confuse disease identity; and (3) technology has, in the twentieth century, an enduring role in legitimizing diverse medical attitudes and identities. The life, death, and afterlife of chlorosis make clear that the interpretation and use of technology can reflect, legitimate, or undermine any number of cultural beliefs. The story of chlorosis also highlights medicine's enduring desire to define, through technology, a legitimate female identity. The meaning of technology in medicine is inevitably structured by other cultural concerns—professional ideals and anxieties, patients' stories, and other disease narratives. The following chapters turn to four other blood diseases, whose claims to existence in the twentieth century were much stronger than that of chlorosis and whose various trajectories illuminate other aspects of twentieth-century medical technology and its relation to problems of identity.

2

The Rise and Fall of Splenic Anemia
Surgical Identity and Ownership of a Blood Disease

In 1901, two Chicago surgeons described a disease called "splenic anemia" in a Swedish woman, aged twenty-two. Her constant fatigue and pallor had long attracted the attention of doctors, and at an earlier date "she [had been] given arsenic (a blood-building treatment), and improved much in general health." But medicinal treatment worked only temporarily. Gradually "she became pale, reduced in flesh, and so weak that at times she was unable to continue her work." Most doctors might have diagnosed this as "chlorosis" and treated the young woman with tonics and arsenic or with the moral management characteristic of the period. But these Chicago surgeons—Malcolm Harris and Maximilian Herzog—saw things differently. In May 1899, the young woman had visited Dr. Harris, who had noted her severe anemia and the conspicuous enlargement on the left side of her abdomen. He "recognized the case as one of so-called splenic anemia . . . and splenectomy [removal of the spleen] was advised as a curative measure."[1]

The futility of cautious medicinal treatment was only too obvious to Harris. "The treatment of splenic anemia from a medical standpoint has not proved successful . . . Attention is therefore particularly directed to the value of splenectomy in this class of cases." Despite the novelty of this diagnosis, both surgeons were convinced "that the changes in the spleen must in some way be responsible for the blood deterioration . . . otherwise removal of the changed [enlarged] spleen would not be such an excellent therapeutic measure as it appears to be."[2] On the basis of such assumptions, the woman's spleen was removed. Although her recovery was somewhat tortuous, Harris and Herzog stated that she had returned to full health by early 1900. Such bold interventions, they believed, distinguished abdominal surgeons clearly from the cautious and pampering doctors of their time.

By the 1930s, however, splenic anemia had become obsolete. This chapter examines the rise and fall of splenic anemia, situating this story in the context of the emerging culture of abdominal surgery, its use of hematological tools and other technologies, and the ethos of scientific exploration, disease discovery, and colonization of the body. Surgeons had believed that their view of disease was more "real" than the views of other physicians because of their "direct observation" and manipulation of the body in illness. The patient with splenic anemia was defined by leading-edge techniques of blood analysis, antiseptic surgical practice, and postoperative statistical studies. This powerful set of tools engendered new strategies for giving identity to practitioner, patient, and disease. But surgical ownership of the blood and the spleen did not endure. Other blood and body specialists used these tools differently. We must look to the disciplining of individualistic surgeons and their incorporation into the hospital in the 1910s and 1920s—that is, to social and institutional forces—to explain the disappearance of splenic anemia as a legitimate disease.

Through history the spleen had been an organ enshrouded in popular and medical folklore. Physicians trained in the humoral tradition knew that the spleen produced black bile and that it was a linchpin in preserving a healthy balance of humors. Its precise function, however, remained unsettled. Into the nineteenth century, learned doctors recalled that even Galen accepted that the spleen was "full of mystery."[3] At best this organ was incompletely understood, and some physicians believed that perhaps God and tradition had intended it to be so.[4] As anatomical knowledge advanced, the spleen seemed to be the last mysterious organ. To some, its unwillingness to be subdued by modern medicine demonstrated the divine mystery of the body.[5] But in the late nineteenth century, this common belief yielded in the face of medicine's technical innovations. Developments in the craft of abdominal surgery and hematological measurement made the patient's abdomen a novel site for surgical adventure and scrutiny. Pioneering surgeons of the era claimed to have unlocked some of the spleen's mystery. For a few decades spanning the turn of the century, the mystery of the spleen succumbed to modern technologies of blood analysis and organ manipulation.

In retrospect, this period of increasing certainty in "splenic thought" is an aberration. Today's physicians readily admit to being puzzled about many features and functions of the organ. The encounter between turn-of-the-century surgeons and the spleen provides us, then, with a glimpse of how these specialists used techniques and technology to construct a new identity for an unknown organ and a new disease and to fashion a new identity for themselves.

Traditionally, surgeons had taken little interest in the spleen or the abdomen. The advent of antiseptic surgery in the late nineteenth century stimulated a long-dormant curiosity.[6] The new practices of sterilizing instruments and cleaning wounds had so lowered the risk of mortality following abdominal operations that a handful of surgeons began to make the investigation and repair of internal organs a profitable specialty. In an America with dangerous factories and mechanized industries, industrial surgeons gained valuable experience patching internal organs that had been ruptured in industrial accidents, creating something of a cottage industry in abdominal surgery. The abdomen, according to Philadelphia surgeon and popular writer William W. Keen, had become "the surgeon's playground." By other accounts, this was "the golden age of abdominal surgery." Critics, on the other hand, would speak of the "highway robbery of the abdomen" to describe what they saw as increasingly unwarranted violations of the body.[7] The suturing and removal of internal organs attracted wide acclaim and notoriety—these were tour-de-force operations with life-saving popular appeal. For the first time in history, new developments in the techniques of antiseptic surgery allowed a generation of surgeons to make a workplace of the human abdomen.

While the spleen itself continued to be shrouded in medical and popular mystery, the modern surgeon's technical skills opened such mysteries to exploration and reevaluation and fostered an exploratory ethos among these craftsmen. Removal of the spleen—splenectomy—became a symbolically important, if rare, operation in the 1880s and 1890s. In the aftermath of these operations (often performed after accidents had ruptured the spleen beyond repair), surgeons noted a curious response in their patients. Using the hemacytometer, they witnessed an immediate increase in the numbers of red blood cells. Where the red blood count had been low, it shot upward after splenectomy. Surgeons reasoned that, in patients with damaged and enlarged spleens and a low blood count, the spleen must have had a role in blood destruction. Thus was born the theory of splenic anemia, a disease in which the spleen (enlarged and sensitive to the doctor's touch) had caused anemia.

In a characteristic description, one author stated that "the [splenic] enlargement is uniform, smooth, painless, usually reaches to the navel . . . and may occupy the whole of the left half of the abdomen. It may exist for years without any symptoms other than the inconvenience . . . [but] sooner or later the patient becomes anemic." Disease onset was rarely sudden. "More commonly pallor is gradual and the patient may come under observation for the first time with swelling of the feet, shortness of breath, and all the signs of advanced anemia." This blood depletion could be chronicled in several ways. "The red blood cells may fall as low as two million and in an average of a series of uncomplicated cases the leucocyte count was under 3,500 per c.mm. . . .Some patients have permanent slight anaemia . . . others remain very well except for recurring attacks of anaemia of great severity."[8] The spleen's removal, many of these experts asserted, provided a daring technique for alleviating this severe blood depletion.

Rochester, Minnesota's William Mayo, a pioneer in abdominal surgery and a leader among American surgeons of his time, was one of those who vigorously endorsed the existence of this disease. The spleen, in Mayo's estimation, could no longer be thought of as a mysterious organ. It could now be assigned a particular identity, and the suffering of these patients could be named. In patients whose anemia was accompanied by enlargement of the spleen, Mayo reasoned, the spleen was clearly the "agent of blood destruction . . . set into motion by influences over which it has no control."[9] Removal of this fragile, bloody, ductless organ—which often adhered fiercely to adjoining abdominal tissue—promised to be curative. In an age when the mysteries of disease seemed to be receding in the face of advances in surgery and laboratory science, the concept of splenic anemia represented the propitious wedding of hematological observation and surgical craft in the fight against disease.

Where the family doctor embraced hematology and seized upon the disease "chlorosis" in the name of moral management, surgeons pursued another strategy of disease construction and management. As they moved into this uncharted terrain, surgeons used hematology to legitimate surgical practice, styling themselves as the first generation of scientific surgeons, a generation on the verge of the discovery and conquest of new diseases. They portrayed themselves as akin to explorers, traversing vast, mysterious, and forbidden frontiers. As one surgeon recalled in 1925, the new surgery called for a masculine and adventurous sensibility: "Sea captains of old sailed in waters that were uncharted. Their guides were nebulous and doubtful; their dangers great . . . The surgeon of today is like the sailor of a past age. He, too, is embarked upon oceans that are unmapped and wide. For ever, and with much labor, feeling his way with the lead, as it were, he is beset with incessant troubles. Innumerable are the surgical disasters with which he is menaced."[10] Here was a portrait of modern surgeons for the new century—intrepid explorers of a dark continent, venturing forth with scalpel in hand, "feeling [their] way with the lead," thinking as they navigated but fortified in their quest by hematological science. Indeed, it was in this era that surgeons coined the term *exploratory surgery*. In their novel explorations of the human abdomen, surgeons began to see diseases that no explorers had ever before encountered.[11]

"Splenic anemia" became a new disease, reflecting the ascendance of abdominal surgeons in the culture of early twentieth-century scientific medicine. For some thirty years, splenic anemia would remain alive in surgical thinking and then it would fade. By the 1930s, it was seldom mentioned. Today splenic anemia does not exist. From today's vantage point, its architects are viewed with a mixture of awe and ridicule. In 1980, hematologist William Crosby suggested that splenic anemia was a "phantom disease," a figment of surgical imagination and a by-product of limited knowledge applied overenthusiastically. At best, it was a "waste-basket term" (just as chlorosis had been), a vague catchall diagnostic category for a constellation of other syndromes and diseases. In this view, splenic anemia represented a temporary surgical enthusiasm. According to current thinking on the spleen, the splenectomy removed a vital part of the patient's immune system, resulting (under the worst circumstances) in what physicians now label "overwhelming post-splenectomy infection."[12] Thus, for Crosby, the story of splenic anemia recapitulated medicine's slow transition from mystery and ignorance through a temporary and misguided enthusiasm to the understanding we hold today.

In 1981, Alastair H. T. Robb-Smith cautioned against dismissing outright the reality of splenic anemia. Perhaps Mayo and his peers were heroes after all, and their enthusiasm should not be ridiculed. Robb-Smith suggested that this disease and the related splenic disorder called Banti's disease (where splenic enlargement and anemia were associated with cirrhosis of the liver) are quite legitimate. Where Crosby looked with skepticism upon these surgeons, Robb-Smith praised them for bringing an entire family of splenic abnormalities into clear focus. "From this tangled skein of splenic pathology," he wrote, "we have for years been trying to unravel one definite thread and it looks as if, at last, the attempt has been successful."[13] In this view, William Osler's first clinical description of splenic anemia was a tentative but visionary step along a daring path of progress, a bold move in the adventure of modern medicine. Surgeons also deserved credit for initiating research on the spleen.

By focusing on redeeming individual reputations, however, such historically minded physicians as Crosby and Robb-Smith have missed an excellent opportunity to study the social processes whereby a disease achieved and lost its status as a "real" entity and how the identity of a disease became linked to the identity of practitioners. The construction of splenic anemia depended in part on the use of hematological tools by surgeons, and its movement through time depended upon evolving debates about the proper use and interpretation of such tools. To explain what made splenic anemia "real" in its heyday and why it disappeared, we must examine the deployment of such tools within the cultural matrix of surgeons, hematologists, and their patients.

To understand splenic anemia, we must consider the masculine, rugged, and individualistic surgeon of the late nineteenth century. He was an independent craftsman who readily embraced blood analysis to improve his work. He also came to regard his skill at surgical excision as a superior tool of knowledge production—a technology in its own right. Yet, even with the surgeon's rising stature in hospital work and knowledge production, the prospect of cooperation with other specialists posed significant challenges. Abdominal surgeons had developed autonomy in matters of diagnosis and treatment, and after the turn of the century they struggled to retain this autonomy in the face of institutionalization and bureaucracy. The identity and fate of one disease was linked to these developments. Ultimately, the modernizing hospital—the same institution that figured prominently in the disappearance of chlorosis—also hastened the demise of splenic anemia.

This chapter portrays splenic anemia as a product of a particular moment in surgery's cultural history and suggests some of the general ways in which institutionalization and technical specialization direct the movement of diseases through time. The issues of professional identity and technical autonomy are central here. Writing in 1922, Keen acknowledged that "the spleen is anchored, sutured, or even removed at will . . . We wonder why there should be an appendix, gall-bladder, or spleen for the patients seem to get along quite well without them as with them." In the first decades of the new century, surgeons answered this question as individual craftsmen. Keen suggested, with only a hint of humor, that "possibly they persist . . . incidentally, for the benefit of us surgeons."[14] This was an era when surgeons explored many of the internal organs for the first time and claimed an expanding jurisdiction over the appendix, the gallbladder, the gastrointestinal tract, the kidney, and the spleen. Splenic anemia became a symbol for some surgeons of their own autonomy in an increasingly corporate medical world.

Surgery's Encounters with the Mysterious Spleen

In a 1901 paper read before surgical colleagues and later published in the *Annals of Surgery*, Boston surgeon J. Collins Warren placed splenic anemia high on his list of fifteen "diseases of the spleen." "This was a disease," he noted, "which has lately been brought into prominence . . . and it seems to me one which holds out promise of good results from surgical treatment."[15] He cited the eminent Johns Hopkins surgeon A. C. J. Kelly, a vigorous advocate of splenectomy in splenic anemia. Kelly was also known for his disdain for ineffectual "medical" treatments. Moral management and watchful waiting were scorned by such bold practitioners. Both Warren and Kelly believed that surgical technique held the key to understanding and treating disease. In splenic anemia, Warren wrote confidently, "the enlarged spleen is the essential feature of the disease." Quoting Kelly, he wrote, "'Medicinal treatment is hopelessly inefficient. In but a few cases has temporary improvement followed regulation of the diet, iron, arsenic, and the like . . . ' [Kelly] advises operation as soon as the physician can become assured of the correctness of the diagnosis."[16] To these experts, *splenic anemia* was a plausible, if debated, diagnostic term that embodied the best that the healing professions had to offer.

The new surgery, in Warren's thinking, was clearly superior to medicine in matters of diagnosis and treatment. Such a claim contrasted sharply with surgery's traditional cautiousness, especially where the abdomen was concerned. Before the 1880s, theories about the spleen were rarely tested by experiment or practice. Rather, the mystery of the spleen was deepened by the surgeon's characteristic reluctance to open the abdomen. But in the last third of the nineteenth century, the surgeons' ability to perform abdominal operations with lowered risk of mortality opened new theoretical and technical possibilities. Antiseptic surgery turned "mere theories" about internal organs into "testable hypotheses," making abdominal surgery into an experimental science.[17] Splenic surgery was but one small innovation among an explosion of abdominal operations. To British surgeon William Evans, surgery had inevitably pushed aside the undependable snake oil potions and tonics of the old-fashioned doctor: "While some consider that drugs are of the greatest importance in the treatment of disease, others look upon them as almost valueless . . . For it has been found possible by surgical operation to cure many conditions which at one time could be treated by the means of medicine, and even then the results were unsatisfying."[18] Even in the vaguely defined area of splenic abnormalities, modern surgeons believed that their boldness would eventually win the day.

As early as the October 1889 issue of *Harper's Magazine,* William W. Keen had begun to popularize this view of the new surgery. "In no department of medicine has there been more rapid and . . . astonishing progress in recent years than in surgery," Keen wrote. "This progress is due chiefly to two things—the introduction of antiseptic methods, and to what we have learned from laboratory work and experiments on animals." The modern surgeon went forward where his predecessors would have hesitated or retreated. "During the war of the rebellion," Keen recalled, "a gun-shot in the abdomen was looked upon as almost necessarily fatal. Surgeons did not dare to open the abdomen either to search for the ball, to close a fatal perforation of the bowels, or to check hemorrhage."[19]

But with the tools of antiseptic surgery and an aggressive spirit, "surgeons have dared to open the abdominal cavity to verify a probable diagnosis, or to perform an operation." *Daring* became a key term in the new surgeon's vocabulary. Daring surgery produced new knowledge of the body's workings in health and disease. Because of his daring, the modern surgeon prepared to "go still further and . . . open the abdomen to *make* a diagnosis." Surgeons expanded their practice into traditionally medical realms. As a consequence of surgery's new adventurous spirit, Keen argued, diseased and damaged organs could be more easily identified, treated, and removed. Human lives could be saved. The benefits to knowledge and mortality could be demonstrated statistically. "In 375 cases of entire removal of one kidney," wrote Keen, "197 lives were saved."[20] In some 90 cases where the enlarged spleen was removed, 51 patients recovered. By taking over the care of medical cases and venturing into the body, modern surgery was "gradually throttling disease at its very birth, and preventing its onslaught upon the health of the world."[21] Modern surgery was on the verge of a total victory over disease.

Even as the practices of abdominal surgery expanded, some lay and medical observers protested against these trends.[22] It seemed to many of them that technical acumen threatened to overwhelm established theories and modes of therapy, to violate the integrity of the human body, and to undermine traditional morality. For some of these observers, bodily integrity was a spiritual rather than a surgical matter. At least one author pointed out the key paradox of this new surgical mind-set: while surgeons could now remove the spleen at will, they did not (nor did they claim to) actually *understand* the organ. In a short 1878 tract entitled "The Spleen," Lucretia Hubbell suggested that the spleen was a mystical and unknowable machine, one of the last organs to resist the onslaught of medical science. "As all the medical schools have failed to discover for what purpose this organ was made and what its office is—being the only organ that has not been fully explained—and as God must have had some object in creating this organ," Hubbell wrote, "I have been led to study and investigate it."[23] Hubbell gave the spleen a heroic, divine identity, pointing to the body's place in a divine plan. Splenectomy raised the specter of surgery overrunning God's fine work.

Practitioner, spiritualist, and patent medicine entrepreneur, Hubbell portrayed the spleen itself as the limiting obstacle to the hegemony of scientific medicine. Addressing the prospective patient, Hubbell asked, "Would you put your clock in the hands of a man to repair who did not understand the pendulum? did not know its use? Indeed you would not; yet you put yourself in the hands of a doctor to repair the beautiful machinery of your body, when he tells you that he is unacquainted with the operations of the spleen, does not know what the Creator meant it for." Surgeons were "experimenting" with a system that baffled them. Even when their experiments failed miserably, killing their patients, they remained blind to their misadventures, never finding fault with their own contrivances. She warned patients that "by some experiment he [the surgeon] may shut off the currents of the battery and kill you at once, as millions of others have been . . . for do not patients die suddenly under the treatment of doctors every day . . . They say the patients have a relapse, but the true cause is they had shut down the battery unawares."[24] Hubbell's message gave a mechanistic yet divine identity to this organ. The spleen represented a mystery that should be respected and regarded with spiritual reverence. Throughout the decades of surgical innovation, similar objections remained implicit in popular literature, and even in medical writing.

A few surgeons admitted their physiological ignorance of the spleen, but surgical experimentation continued. Large numbers of abdominal injuries in industrial and everyday accidents and steady improvements in surgical mortality provided opportunities for perfecting the technique of splenectomy. New York surgeon Francis Markoe acknowledged in 1894 that, even though surgeons were mastering splenectomy in cases of injury, their knowledge about the spleen in disease remained speculative at best. Splenectomy in cases of disease showing splenic enlargement could be justified only as a last resort. Clearly, an enlarged spleen by itself was not a justification for splenectomy, and splenectomy had already proved unwise in leukemia and malaria. In one case, Markoe stated, only after "medical measures failed to check the progressive enlargement of the spleen which now threatened by mechanical pressure the life of the patient" could he advocate splenectomy. Even then, he proceeded only after consulting with his colleagues and the patient's family.[25] Other surgeons echoed Markoe's caution. New surgical skill was not, by itself, a reason for expanding the surgeon's practice. James P. Warbasse of Brooklyn, New York, acknowledged that surgical acumen had moved far ahead of surgical theory: "Unfortunately, [while] our knowledge of the physiology of the spleen is still in a state of confusion . . . the surgery of that organ is on a more established basis."[26]

Zealous surgeons addressed this gap between advancing technical ability and "confused" physiological understanding by turning to the scientific tools of their day. By embracing hematological observation and statistical analysis, surgeons self-consciously fashioned themselves as surgeon-scientists. They used these tools to show that they could regulate themselves, legitimate their practice, and put splenectomy on a more rational basis. Careful blood analysis separated the overzealous craftsman from the scientific surgeon, according to Warbasse. "This is not for those gentlemen to treat who, in the fullness of their operative zeal, would extirpate whatever abdominal tumor is removable. The examination of the blood and a study of statistics are matters of prime importance."[27] Warbasse suggested that, with hematological studies, surgeons could bring rationality to the use of splenectomy in disease. Detailed blood counts of patients before and after operations proved that splenectomy produced a surge in the body's red blood cell production. By analyzing the postsplenectomy hematological profiles of various patients, surgeons believed that they could distinguish between beneficial and detrimental operations after the fact. Such knowledge would then be useful in refining the diagnosis of true splenic diseases and guiding the rational selection of patients for operation.

Through such investigations, the scientific surgeon would escape the moral outrage that society often leveled against overzealous craftsmen and undisciplined experimenters. As Warbasse noted: "Forty years ago Kuchler, of Darmstadt, ventured to remove an hypertrophic malarial spleen. His patient died, and he was sharply criticized by the medical societies of his day . . . Vulpius, of Heidelberg [in 1894], who has compiled an immense number of statistics on this subject . . . has shown that at the present time . . . the number of cures has been about 50 per cent; and that the diseased spleen is no longer a *noli me tangere* [a thing that must not be touched] for the knife of the surgeon."[28] Hematological observation and statistical analysis permitted surgeons to touch the spleen, and to remove it, without fear of criticism.[29] At the turn of the century, the use of splenectomy in conjunction with hematological observation and statistical studies allowed the surgeon to style himself as a scientist, rather than as the crude zealot others thought he was. Bringing these new technical practices together in his work (splenectomy, hematological observation, statistical analysis), a new surgeon emerged, producing new concepts of disease.

As early as 1894, several of America's eminent practitioners supported the existence of the disease called splenic anemia. Its appearance marked the application of these state-of-the-art techniques to the clinical problem of disease identification. In his 1894 textbook, the prominent Johns Hopkins clinician William Osler endorsed the "provisional" existence of such a blood disease. He stated that the term *splenic anemia* did not connote causation, but merely the *association* of anemia with splenic enlargement. Six years later, however, Osler was prepared to grant splenic anemia a more provisional existence, writing that "doubt has been expressed as to the existence of a separate and distinct disease to which the term splenic anaemia should be given. We do not know whether the anaemia is the result of the enlarged spleen, or whether, as seems more probable, both are secondary to some cause as yet unknown."[30] Leaving the question of causation aside, however, Osler acknowledged the postoperative successes of surgeons. Splenectomy had been shown to alleviate cases of intractable anemia, and based on these findings a disease called splenic anemia must be said to exist. "Provisionally," Osler decided, "until we have fuller knowledge, it is useful . . . to label the condition splenic anemia." Such a provisional allowance, coming from the premiere diagnosticians of the era, carried weight with medical and surgical practitioners alike. As the new century unfolded, a handful of equally prominent abdominal surgeons would parlay Osler's provisional allowance into a more far-reaching professional program.[31]

What were the origins of splenic anemia? The surgeon of 1900 would have argued that the origin of splenic anemia lay in the diseased spleen itself. But splenic anemia had indisputable origins in changing diagnostic conduct and in the rise of a culture willing to support surgical experiment and adventure. A new disease born in the waning years of the nineteenth century, splenic anemia was a by-product of scientific surgery, the disease's identity crafted by a novel constellation of tools. For this generation of practitioners, technologies of blood counting using hemacytometers and techniques of abdominal surgery legitimized this leading sector of scientific medicine.[32] The public and the medical professional alike marveled at the ways in which abdominal surgeons ventured aggressively into terrain long considered off limits. Rising in status, abdominal surgeons were well positioned to argue for the existence of splenic anemia—as they did for other new diseases like "appendicitis." Such diseases represented, they knew, not unambiguous biological realities, but a defensible surgical claim staked on a particular body part. Splenic anemia's existence depended upon the tools, the diagnostic practices, and the evolving place of abdominal surgery among the cultures of scientific medicine.

Explorer and Hematologist:
The Persona of Abdominal Surgeons

At the heart of much writing on splenic anemia was the surgeon's use of hematological tools to shore up his belief in the moral superiority of splenectomy. The combination of these tools sustained a bold persona. Presenting the case of the young Swedish woman at the Chicago Surgical Society, Malcolm Harris and Maximilian Herzog heard a chorus of praise from their fellow surgeons. These surgeons also ridiculed medical objections to splenectomy. The formidable A. J. Ochsner "thought the danger of splenectomy in such cases had been overstated . . . patients did not die on account of the operation per se, but owing to the fact that the operation was done under conditions in which almost any serious operation would be fatal." Christian Fenger, doyen of surgery and pathology in Chicago, also gave his blessing to this practice. It was a necessary experiment and a commendable aspect of surgery's scientific quest: "If surgeons should not operate on any case of secondary enlarged spleen, then how were they to know on what spleens to operate and those on which not to operate?"[33] From this standpoint, splenectomy and hematological investigation were noble experimental measures. The existence of splenic anemia became closely associated with the surgeon's desire to venture into this uncharted terrain.

Surgeons portrayed the operation itself as an unpredictable journey into the diseased body. Every operation posed a test of the surgeon's skill and acumen at navigation and exploration. The spleen, sitting on the left side of the abdomen, was a blood-engorged, ductless mass that might easily erupt into hemorrhage if mishandled. In a 1906 issue of *Surgery, Obstetrics, and Gynecology*, Dr. B. Brinkley Eads told a characteristically dramatic story of an injured machinist with a ruptured spleen who was rescued from certain death by a splenectomy. The man had been working in an elevator pit when the elevator descended upon him, causing severe internal injuries. "He was carried home, a few blocks distant, and about six hours later was taken to the Cook County Hospital."[34] Having captured the horror of the injury, Eads turned to the operation. A colleague described Eads's exploration of the abdomen, his discovery of splenic hemorrhage, and the intricacies of the splenectomy.

> The spleen was the next organ sought, and upon examination a rupture was disclosed, with complete pulpification of the lower third, and almost complete separation of the organ from its pedicle . . . [Eads] immediately grasped the splenic artery and vein in his finger, arresting the hemorrhage, and followed by the application of a large artery clamp. He ligated the lower portion of the pedicle and removed the pulpified lower third . . . [and eventually] removed the remainder of the organ.[35]

Eads closed the patient's abdomen shortly afterward, completing the successful operation. Fourteen days after his accident, the machinist was discharged from Cook County Hospital, having made an "uninterrupted recovery."

In cases of splenic disease, the surgeons focused on their technical battle with the organ itself; in such cases, the adventure was not always heroic. The spleen's boundaries with adjoining tissue were often so imprecise that surgeons had great difficulty telling where the spleen ended and the rest of the body began. Eads's contemporaries acknowledged that "adhesions may be so extensive and firm that the spleen may be practically continuous with its own bed . . . Extensive and firm adhesions may be a contraindication to continuing the operation."[36] The organ's very existence as a separate entity often depended on surgical skill at cutting. This intimate connection between "the organ itself" and adjacent tissue set the stage for numerous disasters. In a 1901 discussion of a case, Dr. M. L. McArthur recalled a tragic mishap.

> [I] had attempted to remove an enormous spleen reaching down into the pelvis, and because of the slipping of the organ from the hands of an assistant after raising it up to ligate the pedicle, a clamp being on, the vessels were torn, and the case terminated fatally . . . this made [me] think that the technique would not be considered simple . . . when enlargement of the organ exists, it was one of the difficult procedures in surgery to safely grasp the pedicle.[37]

Focused as surgeons were on the proper deployment of technique, to McArthur this was not a human tragedy but an indication of the extreme difficulties of the procedure. There was no question of the surgeon's moral culpability here. According to Berkeley Moynihan, the most prominent British abdominal surgeon of this era, "the operation is one which may call forth all the resources of the surgeon."[38] Before he opened the abdomen, no surgeon could foresee how diseased the spleen might be or whether this particular spleen would be lifted easily from its bed or adhere fiercely to the body.

The modern surgeon confronted the elements of the body in bold and individualistic fashion, guided by a steady scalpel and reassured in his righteousness by the hematological evidence. As with any occupational group, surgeons constructed a collective identity—as daring but gentle men of science who "courted disaster" and held life in their hands.[39] As sociologist Charles Bosk has shown in his study of late twentieth-century surgery, such a strategy served the solidarity of the group, but it did so at some cost to patients and to the larger society.[40] The solidarity of early twentieth-century abdominal surgeons was informed by the beliefs and practices of their subculture. To gain a more rooted understanding of the cultural meaning of splenic anemia and its meaning for surgeons, we may turn to the exemplary American abdominal surgeon of this era, William Mayo, a man who shared with men of his time a belief in individualistic entrepreneurship in medicine, a sensibility echoed in other realms by presidents, industrialists, laborers, and explorers.[41]

The Mayo Clinic in Rochester, Minnesota, emerged during this period as a national exemplar of the lucrative cottage industry in abdominal surgery. It became a stage for playing out a public drama involving surgeons and bodily organs; patients were but minor characters in this drama. Hundreds of the newest operations—all kinds of "ectomies and ostomies"—were either invented or refined at the Mayo Clinic in the 1910s, and through the 1920s and 1930s the surgical findings of this small clinic in the American Midwest would be cited as gospel by doctors around the world. By the 1910s, the Mayos had become well known for innovations in gallbladder surgery, but they also perfected other novel abdominal operations, and William Mayo himself built an undisputed expertise in matters related to the spleen.[42] He and his associates performed hundreds of splenectomies, assigning an insidious identity to the organ. (In 1924 he suggested that, "of the organs of the reticula-endothelial system, the spleen is the most unstable.")[43] Through the 1910s and 1920s, the Mayo Clinic embodied an innovative and popular approach to healing, translating the image of "organic disease" into a viable specialty. Located in a small town in remote Minnesota, the clinic attracted thousands of faithful ill each year.

In his 1915 portrait of the Mayo phenomenon, a fellow doctor compared the clinic with the healing spas at Lourdes. "The character of the pilgrims to both places seems to sustain a striking resemblance."[44] In both cases, the faithful and the gullible traveled hundreds of miles to be saved from diseases that had baffled their local physicians.[45] In the case of the Mayo Clinic, it was as if all of the bodies arriving at its doors were destined to be operated upon. Organs of unknown function were casually removed. Broome observed that "many comments were made on the fact that in nearly every one of the abdominal cases . . . the surgeons remove the appendix whether apparently pathological or not."[46] What greeted patients at Rochester was a controversial, bold, and unapologetically surgical vision of patients and diseases.

Splenic anemia became associated with this popular surgical culture, in which the object of scrutiny was not the human being but the organic lesion. From 1908 through 1928, Mayo Clinic surgeons performed some five hundred splenectomies for an expanding range of diseases—not only for splenic anemia, but also for pernicious anemia and other "blood diseases" in which the spleen could be implicated in the disease process. As historian Peter English has noted of this era, "radical surgeons sought to extend their craft to a number of diseases traditionally outside their province."[47] Splenectomy and hematology provided the technical means of expanding this authority. Mayo readily acknowledged that this operational mind-set did not produce definite knowledge of pathology. Indeed, he carefully distinguished between the concepts of "pathology" and "clinical entity"—the former created from postmortem analysis, the latter created using clinical tools and observations. "While splenic anemia is, as pointed out by Osler, a clinical entity," Mayo wrote, "it cannot be said to have a definite pathological existence." Berkeley Moynihan—Mayo's friend and counterpart across the Atlantic—also admitted that splenic anemia was not a disease of unimpeachable existence, but he believed that it was "not unreasonable to hope that the removal of the offending organ may cut the progress of the disease."[48] Neither man suffered illusions about this so-called disease. Proof of the existence of splenic anemia depended upon the availability of patients for splenic surgery, surgical autonomy in diagnosis and therapy, and a favorable increase in the blood count and the patient's health after the splenectomy.[49] Published postoperative statistics were the best verification of the existence of the disease. Mayo knew that splenic anemia could exist only if surgeons remained free to engage in splenectomy and blood analysis.

In the years around World War I, as surgeons' freedom to use these tools expanded, many of them became unwilling to acknowledge the limitations of such operational thinking. The publications of the Mayo Clinic reports, Mayo's own writings, and Berkeley Moynihan's textbook on diseases of the spleen in the early 1920s solidified the sense that surgical knowledge was steadily accumulating, sweeping everything before it. As one editorialist saw it, "It has come to pass that the surgeon in his daily study and handling of living pathology has been able to illuminate many fields of internal medicine more successfully than many medical research workers of the past." Reviewers pointed to Moynihan and Mayo as pioneers. Since "the abdominal surgeon of large experience has the advantage over the internist that he can verify the diagnosis by direct, personal observation of the living pathology," it seemed doubtful that internists would be left with any role in medicine if surgeons continued to develop their skill, insight, and freedom of practice.[50] Advanced theories of the spleen's role in blood destruction were being generated by Mayo's surgical team and the hematologists working with them.[51] Most surgeons were convinced that, because of their unfettered practice, ignorance of the spleen was steadily receding, their autonomy was increasing, and the jurisdiction of internists was shrinking. However, by the 1930s they would see that precisely the opposite had occurred.

Critiques of Surgical Identity during the Progressive Era

While some surgeons looked forward to a future of expanding surgical practice, it was clear as early as 1900 that their expansion put surgeons into a difficult public spotlight. Their practices posed moral, medical, and legal problems for patients, legislators, and the profession at large. Moralists and muckrakers objected to their eagerness to operate—whether this enthusiasm was motivated by medical theory, scientific curiosity, or financial greed. A sustained critique of the surgical individualist was already under way by 1905. For some, the case of splenectomy was a case in point of surgical excess. Over the first two decades of the new century, legal controversy, moral outrage, and eventually institutional reform would circumscribe the surgeon's freedom of diagnostic and therapeutic movement, eroding his newfound independence and autonomy. The surgeon of the 1920s became more accountable to professional peers, hospital administrators, and others in the use of his tools. These developments redefined how hematology and splenectomy were to be used in medicine and led to the disappearance of splenic anemia.

Where surgeons focused on the sick organs (using splenectomy) and documented the lives they saved (using hematology and statistics), their critics focused on regulating the surgeon's hand and assailing his character. Was splenectomy an attempted rescue? Was it a necessary experiment? Or was it a premeditated murder? The aging W. W. Keen recalled that, even in the mid–nineteenth century, surgeons had been compelled to fend off objections to surgical innovation. He remembered how "surgeons who removed ovarian tumors were persecuted . . . As a student, I even heard them called murderers . . . because 'two out of three of their patients died.'" Keen brushed aside these accusations: "It ought to be worded 'one out of every three recovered,' for every recovery was a rescued life."[52] But in the eyes of some critics, semantics alone could not redeem the image of the surgeon.

In an extensive 1904 tract reminiscent of Lucretia Hubbell's 1878 article, Mary Dunham Hankinson-Jones stated flatly that splenectomy was murder. In *The Spleen; or the Human Battery*, Hankinson-Jones collected medical writing on the mysterious organ, arguing for the immorality of splenic surgery. Drawing attention to surgery's limited knowledge, Hankinson-Jones wrote, "We are told by the best authorities that 'the spleen has only an unimportant function, if any' . . . Some authors speak of it as 'not thoroughly understood,' which sounds as if it might be worth looking into."[53] Instead of assaulting the spleen, she insisted, physicians and surgeons should honestly admit their ignorance. Their envy of the divine body, she claimed, led these ambitious men to overrun what they could not master.[54] Splenectomy was no more than a carefully concealed act of murder. "Looking backward eight years, we can furnish living witness to prove that . . . to remove the spleen is simply murder."[55] In an age when many body parts—appendix, kidney, gallbladder, and spleen—seemed expendable, the wisest surgeons would refuse to undertake such operations.[56]

Other popular and medical commentaries echoed Hankinson-Jones's beliefs, urging the surgeon to stay his hand. According to muckraking journalist Samuel Hopkins Adams, "modern" surgeons were already adjusting their sensibilities by embracing principles of conservation, the same principles that informed the use of natural resources—minerals, water, forests, and wildlife. In a 1905 *McClure's Magazine*, Adams wrote that "where, twelve or fifteen years ago, the operator carried away with him a diseased organ, or all of it that he could get, to-day he excises the disease instead of the organ, performing not as much as he may, but as little as he can. This is the touchstone of modern surgery: to save not life alone, but the structure of the human body. Its watchword is conservation."[57]

Even ambitious surgeons like Weller Van Hook, writing in the pages of a 1906 issue of *Surgery, Obstetrics, and Gynecology*, endorsed these principles, but called for balance: "There are in abundance those who lay too much stress on the principle of cutting and tying whatever bleeds. On the other hand, there is a goodly array of those who scorn dexterity, . . . elegance and grace of manipulation, and—dare I say?—lessening mortality." Van Hook called for surgeons to police themselves using a few guiding ethical precepts. "It is morally wrong," he proclaimed, "for the surgeon to gratify curiosity as to morbid conditions by unduly prolonging anaesthesia, by making incisions too numerous or too long, or by manipulating tissues or organs too freely."[58] Van Hook challenged each practitioner to regulate his own practice (to control curiosity, restrict overcutting, and forgo extensive manipulation) and thereby to discipline his own exploratory zeal.

In the same years that Adams, Hankinson-Jones, and Van Hook questioned the autonomy of surgeons, a handful of clinicians and pathologists also sought to regulate surgical practice by using hematology to question the purported identity of splenic anemia. To be sure, their treatises were not muckraking exposes; they directed a subtler technical critique toward surgical practice and character. In their writings, bureaucratic oversight was substituted for Hankinson-Jones's moralism and Van Hook's self-discipline.[59] As early as 1904, Richard Cabot (author of the first American guide to the use of hematology) wrote, "I object to the term splenic anemia because it seems to suggest that the splenic enlargement is in some way the cause of the anemia, and for this there is no sufficient evidence."[60] Pathologists like Philadelphia's Alfred Stengel sought to temper surgical aggressiveness with a 1904 article pointing to the "varieties of splenic anemia." If this *were* a disease, he argued, it was not the same from one patient to the next. Analyzing the various hematological, clinical, and pathological findings in several cases where splenic anemia had been diagnosed and splenectomy had been performed, Stengel concluded that "there are very different sorts of cases that have more or less superficial resemblance, and I cannot share the view that all are probably instances of one disease . . . The ultimate solution of the matter must, seemingly, come from more careful clinical and pathological study."[61] More surgery, that is, would not solve the mystery of splenic anemia. It was up to the clinician and the pathologist to use hematology themselves to determine when splenectomy should be allowed and to evaluate the true character of this disease called splenic anemia.

Such attempts to regulate surgeons by using laboratory tools drew angry replies.[62] In a 1907 address to medical graduates, J. Chalmers DaCosta portrayed such efforts as part of the assault on individualism in an increasingly hostile, bureaucratic world. "A great peril of the present day," he warned, is "the decay of individualism . . . the possession of self-reliance, and of the power and courage to think and speak for one's self."[63] DaCosta turned his attention to the laboratories that had begun to proliferate in hospitals. They were the bane of surgical individualism.

> The world is ruled by the formulas of shallow men . . . They give implicit faith to every new theory from the laboratory, and every new theory from

a scientific dream book . . . All of us . . . give a great deal of attention to laboratory methods of supposed precision, and very little to absolute bedside
acquaintance with disease . . . But the microscope is not infallible; it is not
a supreme court . . . It is to be an aid, an assistant, an adjunct, a collabora-
tor, if you will; but not, as we are rapidly making it, a tyrant and a despot.[64]

Laboratory methods, called upon by surgeons to support splenectomy,
were also being turned against them by pathologists and internists intent
on regulating surgical excess. DaCosta, like other surgeons, saw this
oversight as an effort by "shallow men" and "despots" to limit individual autonomy and "bedside acquaintance with disease."

As if these assaults on surgical identity were not enough, splenectomy also became the focus of legal oversight and regulation. In his 1914
description of the Mayo Clinic, William Broome noted that many questionable operations were performed in the wake of surgery's expansion.
Some appendectomies were performed, for example, "for no other reason than a monetary consideration; some again are made by ambitious
surgeons merely to gratify their ambition." These developments brought
surgery under the scrutiny of reform-minded state legislators. Speaking
of unnecessary appendectomies, Broome suggested that "there should
be a ban put upon this kind of work, which is more or less a criminal practice." Yet he objected to certain legislative threats, such as those of the Col-
orado legislature, which considered forcing surgeons to "produce the defective appendices afterward or suffer imprisonment or fine . . . If such a
law were effective, up in Minnesota, for example, *all the surgeons at
Rochester would be subject to criminal prosecution.*"[65] Broome thought that
such legislative oversight was unnecessary and that surgeons should
work out a way to police themselves.

Court cases also reexposed the enduring gap between surgical
knowledge of the body and surgical practice. A 1912 New York state court
case aired in public the profession's confusion about the identity and purpose of the spleen. In August 1909, a machinist named Arthur Gallo won
$7,639 from the owner of a building where Gallo had been injured. Be-
cause of Gallo's internal injuries, Dr. Joseph Higgins had been compelled
to remove his spleen. But now Gallo, as plaintiff, sued the owner of the
building for the loss of his organ. Dr. Higgins testified that "it is a notori-
ous fact that the spleen is an unknown quantity to us medical men. We
do not know what its functions are. It is there, and the only reason we
have for assuming that it has any utility is assuming that the good Lord

intended it should have some."[66] Higgins was certain that the splenectomy would rob years from Gallo's life, noting that "the average length of life of a person after the removal of the spleen is five years." After Higgins's comments were published in the *New York Times*, however, they "aroused considerable comment among physicians." Two days later, several physicians denounced Higgins's statements.[67] An "eminent physiological researcher" responded that "about the only thing that medical science is sure of . . . is that [the spleen's] removal *does not have any effect on the life of the person* from whose body it is removed." In another court case from the same period, surgeons hastened to dispel the damaging popular belief that splenectomy reduced life expectancy.[68] Such accounts suggest that, despite surgical certainty, there remained considerable public and professional disagreement about the meaning of splenectomy and the proper technical documentation of its effects.

Far from quietly accepting the moral imperatives of abdominal surgery, observers of many stripes moved to reform the perceived excesses of the specialty. While Hankinson-Jones may have favored criminal prosecution of surgeons for murder, others suggested that surgeons could police themselves by containing their curiosity, and yet others stressed the need for peer oversight using the tools of hematology and pathological analysis. By the late 1910s, a variety of powerful medical organizations—the American Medical Association, the American College of Surgeons, and the American Hospital Association—had accepted the necessity of regulation, if for no other reason than to stave off reform from outsiders.[69] "Hospital standardization" became a watchword of medicine's self-reform in the late 1910s. Surgeons themselves saw the wisdom of moving toward "the adoption of a uniform surgical technic by surgeons in all general operative cases."[70] Standard methods of laboratory diagnosis—including the use of hematology by laboratory workers—were part of this hospital reform movement. Uniformity reassured anxious consumers and legislators, who were concerned not about technologies per se but about their proper use and regulation. Protocols for surgical practice constituted an administrative mechanism that necessarily limited the diagnostic and therapeutic autonomy of surgeons. Such reforms (as a natural consequence) threatened the existence of splenic anemia.

Even as the Mayo Clinic continued to thrive, surgeons embraced the benefits of incorporation and peer evaluation. By the mid-1910s, some had become reformers, themselves criticizing the dangers of surgical ambition and specialism. In his 1915 book on the "profit and loss account of modern medicine," Virginia surgeon Stuart McGuire admitted that individualists were often misguided by their own prejudices. Surgery's ambitious individualism had led to biases about the existence of diseases and created dangers for patients in the modern hospital. "The specialist, although an expert," noted McGuire, "is often narrow in his views and prejudiced in his opinions, so that he finds explanations for every symptom in the derangements of organs he treats . . . The modern hospital . . . has lived down its stigma of a death house . . . However, [it] is not without its dangers and disadvantages, as it offers opportunity and hence temptation to members of its staff, especially those of surgical ambition."[71] Despite such critiques, however, no new consensus on splenic anemia had yet emerged.

For the next decade, the proper interpretation of hematological evidence and its relation to the spleen became a central problem within medicine and surgery. Major books appeared on the subject, conferences were organized, and all of them subtly criticized the surgical construction of splenic anemia. In 1916, surgeon Beth Vincent of the Massachusetts General Hospital admitted that "the immediate effects of splenectomy are often strikingly favorable, but the longer the cases are followed the less encouraging they become . . . Remission may last 6 months but it rarely lasts a year."[72] Some physicians, relying on close hematological analysis, continued to defend a limited use of splenectomy but implied that the decision was the hematologist's to make—not the surgeon's.[73]

In a 1918 book, *The Spleen and Anaemia: Experimental and Clinical Studies*, two pathologists and a surgeon attempted to settle the question. None of the authors—Richard Mills Pearce, Edward Bell Krumbhaar, and Charles Harrison Frazier—was a strong advocate or opponent of surgery. The book devoted several sections to the spleen's role in anemia based on animal studies, and the final section turned to "its use as a therapeutic procedure in the treatment of diseases of man accompanied by anaemia," a practice that had gained "widely extended use during the last few years."[74]

Frazier—the surgeon—suggested that Osler's first provisional diagnosis of "splenic anemia" had been a mixed blessing. It represented an advance in medical thinking, but medicine was now ready to move on—to abandon splenic anemia: "It was not until 1900 that Osler's work familiarized the English-speaking world with the condition now generally known as splenic anemia," Frazier noted. "[Osler's writings] represented a distinct advance, in that they differentiated a new type of disease previously confounded with leukemia. The term 'splenic anemia' is now known, however, to include several distinct types, and its use should be restricted, if not, indeed, discarded entirely."[75] Because splenic anemia, in this view, incorporated a variety of other disorders, Frazier declared that "it has already become profitable to deal with them as independent affections." Those "independent affections" should be parceled out to their appropriate specialists, and the disease would cease to exist as such. Furthermore, Frazier noted, splenic anemia had never been a coherent disease to begin with, and so any statistical conclusions on the value of splenectomy in so-called splenic anemia were fundamentally unreliable.[76] Despite such treatises, through the World War I years the question of this disease's identity and existence remained unresolved.

The Decline of Splenic Anemia

By 1915, many surgeons themselves realized that, to maintain public confidence, they needed to reform their more ambitious, unskilled, and individualistic peers. It was another decade before this transformation would affect the epistemological status of splenic anemia. But one eventual by-product of the disciplining of the surgeon was the decline of splenic anemia as a legitimate disease. As surgeons were brought into a more corporate and bureaucratic practice, they released their grasp on the spleen, handed over the practice of hematology to laboratory-based pathologists and a growing number of hematological specialists, and thereby abandoned one of the disease concepts that had helped to endorse their modern identity.

Was "splenic anemia" a figment of surgical imagination, a loose collection of other diseases? Was it, like "chlorosis," a diagnostic artifact from a particular era and style of medicine? Or was it a true clinical entity? When Berkeley Moynihan, long established as an expert in abdominal surgery, was invited to give the Bradshaw Lecture at the Royal College of Surgeons in 1920, he chose the much-discussed topic of the spleen. A year later his lectures were published as *The Spleen and Its Diseases*. One American reviewer suggested that the treatise justified the continuing expansion of surgery, as "Sir Berkeley Moynihan . . . casts his eyes upon those last strongholds of the physician within the abdomen—the spleen and the cirrhotic liver." But Moynihan's message was quite ambiguous, and it was clear that he had come to celebrate progress in splenic surgery but also to mourn the passing of "splenic anemia."[77] Moynihan acknowledged that surgeons had lost their battle over the identity of splenic anemia.

Using a wartime analogy, Moynihan portrayed splenic anemia as a battleground that had been successfully seized by surgeons and then gradually lost in their ensuing struggles with internists and other specialists. "The truth appears to be that a large clinical group of cases, distinguished by enlargement of the spleen and anemia, is being gradually encroached upon by keener distinctions . . . than formerly existed." New techniques for the diagnosis of such diseases as syphilis, malaria, and kala-azar, deployed by other specialists, had caused many patients with anemia and splenic enlargement to be "withdrawn from the group of 'splenic anemia,'" robbing the disease of its coherence.[78] One Scottish physician echoed Moynihan's findings in 1922: "Splenic anemia . . . is probably not an entity. Cases usually become grouped under that heading by a process of exclusion and are found by the pathologist to present quite a variety of changes."[79] In truth, splenic anemia was an indefensible outpost—defended only by surgical autonomy and by the rhetoric of postoperative hematological and statistical evaluation.

Moynihan's book confirmed that splenic anemia was becoming a surgeon's ghost town. "The group is raided from every side," he wrote. "What remains? Only the forms of 'splenic anemia' the cause of which is unknown. Or as Mayo wisely and wittily says, 'Put in the form of an Hibernianism, *incomplete knowledge is essential for the diagnosis.*'" This was an ironic, self-mocking phrase indeed, for it acknowledged the limits of surgical knowledge, condensing this rediscovered ignorance into a "wise and witty" aphorism.[80] Beth Vincent surveyed the entire field in 1927, noting that "the majority of modern writers question whether we have in splenic anemia a disease entity."[81] Moynihan and his peers acknowledged that a new atmosphere of peer skepticism and corporate oversight now circumscribed surgical autonomy and thinking.[82]

Technologies, Specialism, and Disease Ownership

Medical pronouncements about the nature of disease have always played a role in shaping professional relations among specialists, and this was particularly true for surgeons in the late nineteenth and early twentieth centuries. The disease "splenic anemia" demarcated the terrain of surgery, drawing patients with particular complaints under a seemingly precise nosological rubric. At its discovery, splenic anemia was a new surgical outpost, defended by the tools of hematology, techniques of exploratory surgery, and methods of statistical analysis. Surgeons exerted autonomy in the deployment of these leading-edge technologies—and thus, in matters of diagnosis, therapy, and self-evaluation. But splenic anemia existed on vulnerable terrain. While surgeons were able to colonize the spleen for a time, competing specialists remained unconvinced of the legitimacy of their claim, and lay observers leveled their own criticisms at surgeons. By the 1920s, Moynihan wondered what remained.[83]

More and more, surgeons found themselves drawn into the cooperative world of the hospital, where diagnosis and therapy were no longer a matter of individual will, but cooperative, negotiated, and increasingly bureaucratic enterprises. Seeking the advantages of the new order, surgeons reaped the benefits of larger pools of patients but deferred to hematologists, internists, and pathologists in the interpretation of diagnostic tools. As a result they renegotiated the nature and "reality" of splenic anemia. In 1934, Chicago surgeon Franklin Martin reflected on the bygone era of exploration and autonomy in surgery: "We were indeed pioneers, struggling to escape from the jungle of an unknown and unexplored wilderness . . . Surgery was not standardized. Each of us had worked out his solutions alone. The wilderness with its jungle was being explored, and the most perplexing problems were being solved."[84] In their forays into the "jungles," the problem of splenic anemia was defined by the surgeon's ability to defend and legitimize it in diagnostic, administrative, and moral terms. As the individualistic craftsman entered the cooperative bureaucracy of the modern hospital, however, the reality of splenic anemia became a matter of institutional policy. "It is obvious to all of us," several physicians commented in 1940, "that the policy of removing spleens indiscriminately which was popular up to about fifteen years ago, has gradually given way."[85] This change in policy was itself the result of an effort to alter the identity of the surgeon, to discipline the explorer and specialist.

In his popular 1925 book, *The Pitfalls of Surgery,* Harold Burrows argued that the chief problem of modern surgery was the surgeon's failure to admit his own limitations to clients and colleagues. "The laity are too ignorant to protect themselves from the surgeon who overrates his own ability at their cost. And as far as for him, who shall administer the reproach?"[86] Since one could not trust surgeons to assess their own technical abilities, regulation and administration—watchwords of reformers—were necessary. Splenectomy in so-called splenic anemia and other diseases, noted Burrows, was one area where "the surgeon [was] . . . led astray by concentrating too small attention upon some individual symptom or physical sign, instead of taking a comprehensive survey of the whole pathological field."[87] By the 1930s, according to Isidore Cohn, "acceptance of cooperation in determining the meaning of enlarged spleens" had effectively reformed surgical sensibility. "In communities where such cooperation is not possible, a breadth of vision must characterize the attitude of the practitioner lest he become an enthusiast in one field and an obstructionist in another."[88] By the 1930s, bureaucracy, cooperation, and peer evaluation had replaced exploration as central surgical ideals.

The technologies that had sustained surgical practice and identity—hematology, splenectomy, and statistics—had themselves escaped the surgeon's control. Only with a hematologist to assist him could the surgeon of the 1920s determine the meaning of enlarged spleens. Blood analysis, once a tool to use as the surgeon desired, became the property of clinical pathologists and blood specialists. As we shall see in the following chapters, hematology took on new administrative and regulatory meanings in the modern hospital and in numerous other areas. It enabled pathologists to regulate relations among hospital specialists and to reconstruct themselves as scientific managers within the emerging bureaucratic order. In the fall of splenic anemia, clinical hematology robbed surgeons of a crucial self-justifying tool.

Surgeons never abandoned splenectomy, however, even though faced with persistent criticisms of the operation. For many, their faith in the technique remained strong. For one group in 1926, the admittedly temporary success of splenectomy in cases of anemia highlighted only that surgeons were not being allowed to go far enough. "Unfortunately," they concluded, "we have no means of removing the entire reticula-endothelial system from the body . . . therefore the danger of relapse is . . . not excluded by splenectomy."[89] In this thinking, the surgical focus was not misguided; it was overly regulated and constrained. Mayo Clinic studies continued to support the practice, which (these studies insisted) actually extended the life of patients.[90]

Throughout the twentieth century, splenectomy would linger—a therapy in search of a legitimating modern disease. In 1985, hematologist

William Crosby reflected on the topic of splenectomy, noting "that truth keeps going in and out of fashion. Splenectomy rides such a pendulum."[91] Indeed, when splenectomy is used today, it is often employed not as a therapy for a well-defined disease, but as a last desperate stab at a diagnosis. Modern discussions present splenectomy as a "diagnostic test." While splenectomy rides a pendulum, splenic anemia has never reappeared because the institutional oversight of surgical practice—created by the bureaucratic reforms of the 1910s and 1920s—has endured. The existence of the disease represents a brief moment of surgical autonomy before the modern surgeon and his favored technologies were incorporated into the bureaucratic enterprise of twentieth-century medicine. By the early 1930s, the spleen could be described once again as a "mysterious organ."

3

Blood Work

*The Scientific Management of Aplastic Anemia
and Industrial Poisoning*

On 10 July 1929, a *New York Times* article told the tragic story of George Mosher, a fifteen-year-old boy who had succumbed to a "strange malady" after months of medical care.[1] The plight of the boy had held the city's attention for several months. On the day young Mosher died, the newspaper's headlines read: "Disease Which Ravaged Patient for Three Months Called Organic, Originating Within Body." The disease was "idiopathic aplastic anemia," a rare and fatal blood disease "originating within the system of the victim rather than from any foreign source."[2] The postmortem evidence of the era indicated that the boy's bone marrow had simply stopped functioning. At the autopsy, the pathologist saw that there were few areas of healthy marrow remaining in George Mosher's body. These few existing sites of blood cell production were, as one physician noted of a similar case, "like the few men who remain in a factory when all others are on strike. They labor valiantly, but turn out a product [blood cells] which is incomplete and abnormal."[3] Young George had died because his own body (particularly the marrow, the factory of blood production) had failed him.

Among other students of disease, however, evidence had accumulated that "aplastic anemia" was not a failure of the body itself but a byproduct of labor conditions in industry. Beginning in 1910, a small number of Progressive era public health reformers argued that aplastic anemia was all too common in industrial workers exposed to benzol, a widely used industrial solvent. Aplastic anemia also seemed to be a growing problem as a side effect of medical chemotherapy. From the public health perspective, the disease was not an "organic malady," but the final stage of an insidious poisoning. The body's "valiant laborers" (the bone marrow) had not gone on strike of their own volition; they had been poisoned. The disease came unannounced, creeping over actual workers as they labored innocently in unventilated rooms of explosives, rubber, and can-making factories. Industrial health reformers portrayed aplastic anemia as a disease that had its origins in a corrupt industrial system— a system that had grown dramatically in the 1910s and 1920s and one that desperately needed reform.

Who would determine the true identity of this disease, aplastic anemia? Rising in institutional prominence was the hospital-based, laboratory-oriented physician concerned with the "scientific" management of disease. Also rising in the profession of public health was the industrial toxicologist, a medical scientist concerned with the social, political, and industrial profiles of human disease. Both looked to technologies of blood analysis to define the disease's true nature. Both saw themselves as "scientific managers," serving modern institutions—hospitals and factories—and bringing hematological expertise to bear on modern management. Some of these experts even defined themselves as "hematologists," linking their professional identity to the tools of blood analysis. In the 1920s, such laboratory skills enjoyed widening utility—in the regulation of industrial workplaces, in workmen's compensation rulings, and in the rationalization of scientific hospital management.

For several decades, hospital-based hematologists and industrial toxicologists pondered the following questions: What parts of the body—the spleen, the bone marrow, or the blood—were responsible for aplastic anemia, and which of the hospital's specialists should oversee patient management? Was this disease a by-product of industrial modernization and labor exploitation? Could hematological testing be a tool of enlightened patient management? And, in personnel management, did hematology provide methods for the identification of "susceptible" workers so they could be reassigned to safer tasks?

In the 1920s, hematology came into its own as a specialty practice. Scientific management of disease in clinics and factories became a prominent goal. Hospital-based physicians and public health reformers incorporated modern blood analysis into different sciences of "disease management." Blood studies, they insisted, had broad implications for patient management in the new hospital and for death prevention in the factory. Hematological evidence carried weight for factory managers, for insurance companies, and in workers' compensation hearings. As physicians and public health workers established expanded roles for their technologies in clinical and factory management, they crafted new identities for themselves and for the workers in expanding industrial enterprises. Just as discussions of chlorosis inevitably reflected attitudes toward American women, discussions of aplastic anemia (by the 1920s) reflected scientific attitudes toward the plight and character of American industrial workers. Aplastic anemia reveals much about the expansion, scope, and limitations of scientific management as a technology-based ideology in early twentieth-century America.

There are two distinct phases in the history of aplastic anemia—a pre–World War I history within the emerging hospital and a postwar history in the factory. The first phase traces the cultural ascent of the blood test, illuminating the evolving politics of knowledge production within the hospital. During the same era when blood analysis was transforming the ideas and identities of family doctors and abdominal surgeons (as we saw in previous chapters), it also reshaped the thought of pathologists. Traditionally, the science of pathology had focused on postmortem findings. In the case of aplastic anemia, pathologists had relied on bone marrow examinations at autopsy to diagnose the disease. Sawing through the large bones of deceased patients, they examined bone marrow cells microscopically in search of fatty deposits. Finding fatty cells in the bone marrow confirmed the diagnosis.[4] Although this kind of postmortem evidence produced authoritative diagnosis throughout the nineteenth century, in the early twentieth century the increasing availability of new tools of blood analysis challenged this orthodox view of "disease."

A new consumer-oriented logic in early twentieth-century hospitals placed high priority on diagnostic tools—such as the blood test—that could be used during the life of the patient.[5] These economic concerns nurtured subtle changes in pathologists' traditional practice and thought. As blood testing found a niche in hospital laboratories, medical practitioners began to produce definitions of aplastic anemia based on blood evidence. The increasing use of blood tests not only redefined the meaning of aplastic anemia (making it a disease of living patients), but also increased the prevalence of the disease's diagnosis. Clinicians and pathologists debated whether these two diagnostic practices—the postmortem exam and the hematological exam—uncovered two different diseases or whether they were merely two ways of describing the same disease. Initially, pathologists objected to the diagnostic trends of their day because they seemed to undermine an established medical science. Gradually, however, they embraced and promoted these developments. Furthermore, by the 1920s pathologists turned to the invention of other hematological tools, redefined themselves as scientific managers, and committed themselves to providing information to doctors that would facilitate the rational processing of patients.[6]

New tools, as I have suggested previously, recast professional work and identity—this was true for pathologists and for experts in scientific management, who were concerned not with consumers in the clinical realm, but with producers and laborers in the industrial world. Many public health reformers believed that "aplastic anemia" was in fact the final stage of "benzol poisoning" and that the modernization of hospitals would never bring true understanding of this disease. In Alice Hamilton's view, the expansion of hematological practice could become a tool of social reform and industrial regulation, a vehicle for attributing blame and responsibility not to organs but to the industrial interests. Hamilton's tools were often similar to those of the hospital workers, but her concerns were quite different. In a society where exposure to chemicals was increasingly a way of life for some industrial workers, she wondered, how would the ill effects of such chemicals be regulated?[7] Whether they believed that aplastic anemia originated in factory conditions or in the body of the victim himself, these experts used "aplastic anemia" to draw portraits of work and identity transformation in modernizing America.

Disease Born of a Poorhouse Science

Looking back at changes in diagnostic work during his career, one American practitioner wrote in 1931: "When I entered medicine [in 1895], diagnostic skill really meant . . . ability to designate accurately what would be found in the body if the patient died."[8] The discovery of "aplastic anemia" in the 1880s reflected this style of diagnosis. The disorder was first labeled in 1888 by Paul Ehrlich who, working in a Vienna clinic, analyzed the bone marrow of a patient who had complained of weakness and gradually lapsed into a bedridden state followed by death. The blood of this nameless man had shown signs of severe anemia—declining numbers of white and red blood corpuscles. After the patient's death, Ehrlich's postmortem located fatty, white deposits in the bone marrow.

This "aplastic" marrow, Ehrlich believed, defined a distinctive disease. Following this model of pathological science, any pathologist could search the large bones, sorting through the normal red areas of the marrow to locate "the disease," especially in patients who had suffered from anemia.[9]

Treatment was not the focus of this diagnostic science. Rather, this medical science—involving rigorous postmortem analysis correlated with previous clinical observations—sought to nurture a scientific sensibility among medical practitioners. The "clinical material" of large hospitals—most of them the poorest of the urban poor who ended up in places like Vienna's Allgemeines Krankenhaus—provided the tangible basis for producing knowledge of disease. To the nineteenth-century pathologist, such cases offered unparalleled opportunities for discoveries and insights. As one American recalled of his training in Vienna, "every patient was available for teaching purposes and the bodies of all deceased patients were examined post-mortem."[10] This context fostered the science of clinicopathological correlation. Organs and tissues were assumed to be the sites of disease. In the case of aplastic anemia, for example, the metaphor of the marrow as a factory and the blood as its product neatly encapsulated the pathologist's understanding. The quality, quantity, and morphological characteristics of the blood corpuscles held clues about the course of disease and indicated what might be found at autopsy.[11]

Many North American students studied in the hospitals of Vienna and other European cities, traveling there because of these opportunities for insight into disease. Returning home, some sought to reproduce this confluence of scientific practices by working in hospitals where they might gain access to patients and dead bodies. When William Osler published one of his first articles in 1877, on a case of "progressive pernicious anaemia," the paper highlighted the dissemination of this science and its assumptions. The marrow, he had learned during his travels and many autopsies, was the source of "the evil." Quoting German authors, Osler wrote, "'You will certainly agree with me in taking for granted that the . . . condition of the marrow stands in intimate connection with the fatal disease of the patients. . . . An important disease of the marrow must have a serious influence on the composition of the blood.'" Osler concurred with European pathologists, regarding the marrow as the "*fons et origo mali*"—the source and origin of the evil.[12] It took the rigorous practice of autopsy to see this evil, which manifested itself as blood degeneration and anemia.

Throughout the following decades, the diagnosis of aplastic anemia depended upon the pathologist's commitment to pathological science. In 1907, when a young physician training in pathology discussed a case of aplastic anemia, he spoke of it in these clinicopathological terms. The researcher, Ralph Lavenson, concluded that "in aplastic anemia we have a blood picture which is but a reflection of the condition of the bone-marrow."[13] Into the first decade of the twentieth century, the identity of aplastic anemia continued to reflect this admired scientific diagnostic tradition—with its assumptions of organic causation.[14]

For distinguished practitioners like William Osler, William Pepper, Alfred Stengel, and Frank Billings, pathology was respectable scientific work in medicine. Pathologists emphasized to their students that success as clinicians would depend upon their prior experience visualizing disease *after* death. "Let no opportunity pass to observe and record upon the tablet of memory the comparative appearances of diseased and healthy structures," wrote Michigan's Aldred Warthin. "Every advance in [this] direction . . . gives you an advantage . . . in the struggle for position, and widens the distance between you and the empiric." Memorizing the internal structures of the body provided an "objective" basis for sound clinical judgment. In his 1897 textbook *Practical Pathology for Physicians and Students,* Warthin suggested that "there is nothing so valuable as the pictures of disease conditions which every post-mortem reveals, . . . no physician can conduct a post-mortem without having his experience widened, his knowledge of disease increased, his tendency to subjectivity controlled, and his diagnostic faculties sharpened."[15] This was no mere abstract science, but a laborious method of disciplining professional sensibilities.

Yet it proved difficult to interest most doctors in this science of disease. Most practicing physicians had neither the time nor the inclination to create such pathological insights. Such objective knowledge was economically unrewarding for most practitioners and proved difficult to accumulate even for the experienced pathologist.[16] William Osler's commitment to pathology made him unique among his academic peers at the University of Pennsylvania. While many of these colleagues would take the afternoons to "engage actively in house-to-house practice," noted Osler's biographer, Osler's afternoons usually found him at Blockley— "the little two-story brick building which served in Osler's day as the half-way house to the Potter's Field . . . here almost every afternoon he was to be found . . . with his group of students accustomed to camp on his trail."[17] The work of diagnosis was easiest to pursue in these "half-way houses to the Potter's Field" where pathological "material" was easily obtained.

Despite their zeal for the science, such scientists often disagreed about the specific meaning of postmortem evidence. In one instance in 1894, Osler reported finding fatty cells in a few corpses and implied that such fatty cells were quite normal and not pathognomonic. Where Ehrlich had perceived abnormality, Osler saw normal cellular activity.[18] Thus, even when practiced pathologists like Osler located fatty marrow in their corpses, the finding did not guarantee a diagnosis of aplastic anemia. A rare disease, lacking uniformity of diagnosis and known to a tiny minority of medical practitioners, aplastic anemia did not gain quick and widespread recognition in American medicine. In his 1896 textbook on hematology, Richard Cabot did not mention aplastic anemia. Over the next thirty years, however, Ehrlich's discovery would become a better established disease—in part because of the changing practice of diagnosis. But at the turn of the century, few physicians knew or cared about its existence.

One reason for the early obscurity of Ehrlich's aplastic anemia was the significant public and medical distaste for pathological work, particularly for the autopsy.[19] Just as the very existence of splenic anemia (ch. 2) depended upon the freedom of surgeons to diagnose and treat as they desired, the existence of aplastic anemia depended upon the pathologist's freedom to do autopsies. But pathological investigation required individual conviction and in many cases secrecy in the face of religious and lay objections.[20] Warthin decried the many obstacles in the path of his science. "It would be well," he noted, "if the physician had legal right to make a post-mortem, but we [as a society] are not yet educated up to this point. On the contrary, an almost hopeless spirit of opposition to post-mortems seems to exist in this country." In the absence of state legislation making autopsies mandatory, Warthin asked every physician to use a "missionary spirit" to imbue the public with "a perception of the utilitarian aspect of the post-mortem."[21] Where diseases like aplastic anemia appeared at all in medical writing, it was because pathologists had gained access to a body in a poorhouse or in the county hospital and subjected that body to scientific investigation.

In the 1890s, the true aplastic anemic was not identified as a living patient. Such a diagnosis of aplastic anemia identified a disease process, a natural history of disease whereby a living patient had become a corpse.

One could never be sure that the disease existed in any particular patient until his or her death. The disease resided between the clinic and the dead house; its identity reflected the tools and professional commitments of pathologists. By the 1890s, however, the laboratory and its appeal to patients and practitioners was already beginning to alter this medical perception, as well as the prevalence of this obscure poorhouse disease.

Hematology: The Challenge to Established Science

Throughout the late nineteenth and early twentieth centuries, the hospital appealed to a small but growing clientele of paying customers.[22] As historian Owsei Temkin has noted, in this era medical consumers increasingly saw health as a "purchasable commodity." For consumers, the hospital's novel laboratory aids to diagnosis, surgical procedures, and new drug therapies seemed to be organized in a rational system—its appeal was not unlike the appeal of the modern department store. The proper management of diseases seemed to depend on efficient, cooperative organization, aided by the best new technologies—x-rays and a variety of laboratory tests.[23] New technologies in every new department of the hospital guided the conceptualization and treatment of disease. Thus, the laboratory represented one leading sector of scientific medicine. Already in 1903, Osler could write that "it is hard in this country to have the student see enough morbid anatomy . . . [because] the new pathology, so fascinating, and so time-absorbing, tends, I fear to grow away from the old morbid anatomy."[24] This "new pathology" was laboratory-based work.

The "new pathology" was nurtured by institutional developments and by medicine's changing social and economic relations. As hospitals grew and became increasingly cooperative and bureaucratic, physicians like Richard Cabot acknowledged that, "in the absence of a single dominating personality as an integrating factor in the hospital system, the best available substitute seems to be combined ward visits in which the pathologist, surgeon, chemist, and physiologist all work together."[25] Institutional medicine brought these experts together to "furnish all the data necessary for a modern diagnosis."[26]

In this milieu, biological data produced *during the life of the patient* took on higher value.[27] By 1900, laboratory-based analysis of sputum, urine, and blood seemed essential to good medical work. Private diagnostic laboratories flourished during these decades, providing services for hospitals and private practitioners. Such laboratory practice prompted a rethinking of diseases like aplastic anemia. In 1907, Ralph Lavenson (working under the guidance of pathologist Alfred Stengel in the newly founded William Pepper Laboratory of Clinical Medicine) read a paper before the Association of American Physicians (AAP), urging such a rethinking of disease.[28]

In the proper hands, Lavenson argued, blood analysis was a powerful diagnostic and prognostic tool that might *supplant* traditional pathological science. Did the confirmation of aplastic anemia have to wait for the pathologist's postmortem report? Lavenson believed not. He suggested that aplastic anemia was characterized by very specific blood changes and that "probably the most important [change], is the blood picture in which we find an almost complete absence . . . of nucleated red blood corpuscles and the total absence of megaloblasts."[29] By reading the blood, Lavenson claimed that the presence of two distinctive types of red blood cells—megaloblasts and nucleated cells—indicated marrow activity. Their absence in circulating blood, he asserted, identified a case of aplastic anemia. This determination could be made during the life of the patient. Using a simple blood test, doctors could now recognize when the marrow and blood-producing organs were failing and take appropriate measures. If his attempts to stimulate the marrow failed, at the postmortem the doctor could "expect to find, as we in fact do, a pale bone-marrow in which evidences of new blood formation are entirely wanting."[30] Lavenson displayed these postmortem findings. Richard Cabot casually suggested after Lavenson's presentation that "we might almost be prepared to report cases [of aplastic anemia] without the post-mortem findings."[31] A disease that one could formerly diagnose only after death could now be diagnosed during life, using hematological tools.

Blood work—counting corpuscles, measuring hemoglobin, and subjecting blood to a variety of chemical tests—posed an implicit but recognized challenge to the science of pathology. If a practitioner skilled in blood interpretation could predict what the marrow would look like after death, then what was the need for the postmortem? And couldn't this new diagnosis lead to treatments before patients died? The "new pathology" suggested that autopsies were not the only objective tool for diagnosing disease. The laboratory provided a practical guide to therapeutic decision making, whereas postmortem diagnosis merely promised benefits for future patients and practitioners. Writing in 1908, Richard Cabot pointed to two dilemmas of traditional pathological work—the problems of energy and opportunity. "Diagnosis," he wrote, "cannot be sure without an examination of the bone-marrow, which [will] show . . . the long bones . . . filled with fat from end to end. Of course, this describes the extreme case, and few pathologists have the energy or the opportunity to investigate all the bones of the body with such thoroughness as would be necessary . . . Ordinarily, the marrow of the femur is taken as a test."[32] Technical innovation and institutional demands for efficiency and convenience favored the new pathology.

As physicians and a handful of self-proclaimed "blood specialists" embraced these tools, they produced new knowledge of blood disease and spurred an increase in the number of cases of aplastic anemia. Between 1905 and 1925, American and English language medical journals published at least fifty papers on aplastic anemia.[33] While these authors acknowledged the importance of postmortem evidence for authentic diagnosis, they devoted great energy to describing the disease's subtle hematological features.[34] John Musser, in his 1914 study of aplastic anemia, noted that a good hematologist could virtually infer postmortem evidence from the blood picture. Such a statement reflected the ascendancy of laboratory work and its growing importance in clinical decision making. "Post-mortem examination of the bone-marrow is usually considered essential to an exact diagnosis," Musser wrote. "I believe, however, that the clinical course, the blood findings . . . are so typical and so unmistakable that the diagnosis can be readily made during the life of the patient, and I therefore have no hesitancy in reporting the following cases, although it lacks the final evidence acquired only by the postmortem examination."[35]

As he sat in the audience at Lavenson's 1907 presentation, pathologist Aldred Warthin bristled at Lavenson's use of the term *aplastic anemia*. Warthin suggested that by relying so heavily on laboratory data, Lavenson had confused two separate phenomena—the clinicopathological disease aplastic anemia and the purely hematological phenomenon defined by the absence of blood regeneration. These were not the same entity. Lavenson's mistake was his belief that blood pictures described actual diseases. As we saw in chapter 1, physicians like Frederick Forcheimer and Frederick Henry had similar doubts that chlorosis could be defined purely by hematological evidence.[36] The laboratory workers' use of hematological tools and other laboratory evidence raised episte-

mological problems for pathologists, as it had for family doctors in earlier decades, because they sensed that the identity of disease was changing as these new tools were deployed.

Leaning heavily on blood analysis, Lavenson claimed that each
anemia had a specific blood picture—aplastic type, pernicious type, and
so on. To Warthin, blood work was insufficient and unreliable as diagnosis. He believed that different disorders might show the same hematological profiles; despite these hematological similarities, they remained different diseases. Neither clinical evidence, nor pathological
evidence, nor hematological data by themselves defined true disease.
Disease depended upon clinicopathological correlation. Warthin concluded that one "should . . . not class [these cases] under the term aplastic anemia."[37] In response to Warthin's criticism, Stengel defended his
student by passing around the bone marrow specimen for his colleagues
to inspect. "I cannot agree with Dr. Warthin," he stated. "It is not necessary to have the bone-marrow universally affected . . . There is in this case
. . . an actual lack in the functional cells of the marrow; in other words,
there is a true aplastic condition."[38] By the end of the discussion, however, Stengel seemed to wonder whether it made any practical therapeutic difference whether the patient was diagnosed with one anemia or
another? Whatever one labeled the disease, wasn't the blood picture a
useful guide to medical decision making? Differences "in the pathology
of the cases," he suggested, "may not be clinically important nor of consequence so far as the outcome of the case is concerned."[39] In a modern
hospital environment (increasingly concerned with the outcome of clinical management), such clinicopathological precision seemed old-fashioned and irrelevant. These changing standards of diagnostic work provoked pathologists to speak of the "passing of morbid anatomy," as if
their science had come to the end of its natural life course.[40]

This hematological perspective of disease may have been "confused" from the standpoint of the traditional pathologist, but it was well
suited to the economic and cultural climate of the institution. In contrast
to the science of the dead house, the laboratory-based worker began to
develop a pragmatic hematological view of aplastic anemia geared to the
convenience of blood tests. It seemed obvious that bone marrow activity
could be inferred from the picture of the blood cells.[41] As pathologists
themselves became the directors of laboratories and leaders of laboratory medicine, they also embraced this convenient perspective.

Reflecting on this period from the 1970s, two pathologists characterized the time as a period of misguided hematological enthusiasm. Any sign of blood depletion came to stand for aplastic anemia, and confirmatory postmortem evidence was rarely sought. With the benefit of hindsight, these pathologists could see that "the terminology became confused, because 'aplastic anemia' became virtually synonymous with blood pancytopenia [general blood depletion]."[42] What these critics did not see, however, was the social forces driving the medical work and thought. In 1915, one author proclaimed that "the modern hospital is coming to be looked on as a laboratory . . . such an institution does its full duty only when it contributes . . . to the common fund of what may be termed 'hospital knowledge.'"[43] "There is no place to draw a line between what is apparatus and what is not," wrote William MacCarty of the Mayo Clinic. "Therefore, I say again that the entire hospital is the laboratory, or a series of laboratories."[44] In an era of increasing blood studies and proliferating blood specialists, the meaning of *diagnosis* itself was changing. The transformation of pathological work reflected changes occurring elsewhere in American business and institutional life. In factories and corporations, similar experts—engineers, scientific managers, and researchers—assumed new roles in rationalizing corporate production. In sharp contrast with the aplastic anemia that emerged as Osler moved between the clinic and the Blockley dead house, this new image of aplastic anemia was "hospital knowledge." It reflected the rising status of the laboratory worker in hospital culture.[45]

As a result of these social developments, the identity of aplastic anemia as a blood disease came into clear focus. And yet, the science of hematological interpretation proved no more dependable than the science it replaced. Different hematological specialists fixed their microscopes upon the blood cells, interpreting very different blood pictures as clear evidence of aplastic anemia. Where Harvard-trained George Minot designated decreased platelets as "purpura hemorrhagica," Hopkins-trained W. W. Duke saw a "classic blood picture of aplastic anemia."[46] Such specialists could not agree on any single best hematological definition of aplastic anemia, nor did they agree on appropriate therapies. They did not seek to create uniform rules of diagnostic work. They concurred on one fact—the bone marrow itself was only of theoretical importance in making the diagnosis. Even as some pathologists continued to complain about the decline of postmortems as a check on this kind of subjectivity, physicians and their institutions eagerly embraced hematological tools—the hemacytometer, the hemoglobinometer, staining methods, and chemical means of blood analysis—as a basis for defining disease.[47]

The Moral Economy of Blood Work

Why was this new image of disease so compelling? We might look beyond blood's functional value in hospital work, examining the cultural meaning of blood work for practitioners.[48] In the late nineteenth century, hospital-based physicians began to venture without apology into the laboratory, crafting new identities for themselves and for patients. One specialist observed in 1918 that "laboratory workers are becoming clinicians who are specializing in the utilization of certain apparatus for the purpose of preventing, curing, and ameliorating the ills of their fellow man. They are already an economic factor in the progress of mankind."[49] Less tentative than Lavenson or Stengel had been, laboratory workers of the 1910s were convinced that the laboratory blood test provided independent evidence of disease.

Self-styled "blood specialists" appeared in hospitals as well as in private practice. In 1910, Roger Lee became chief of one of the first "blood wards" in the country at the Massachusetts General Hospital (MGH). George Minot (just out of medical school and later to win a Nobel Prize for his work on pernicious anemia) gained his first experiences with blood diseases in Lee's ward.[50] Hypochromic anemia, discussed in chapter 1, rose into prominence in this context as blood specialists developed their techniques of staining and analyzing the features of various blood cells. The enthusiastic grouping of patients according to such blood classifications highlighted hematology as an independent clinical science.[51] As one physician noted, "On the basis of the blood examination, a diagnosis of aplastic anemia [could be] made and an unfavorable prognosis given." Despite the fact that his prediction was not fulfilled, this blood expert expressed continued faith in hematological evidence.[52]

George Minot's blood work is often portrayed as a symbol of the rise of an independent hematological sensibility. Minot's cousin and biographer, Francis Rackemann, wrote that "Minot saw in this hospital setting a rare opportunity to extend his interest into new areas of blood disease . . . He became impressed . . . with the relationship of polycythemia vera, a disease producing too many red blood corpuscles, and myelogenous leukemia, a form of cancer of the blood in which too many white cells formed."[53] As early as 1911, Minot began making sketches of reticulocytes—speculating that these immature red blood cells were indicators of bone marrow activity.[54] Minot came to believe that "confusion seems to arise from the lack of careful study of the blood," and at an early point he took it upon himself to expose the frequent "mistakes" and "confusions" of others.[55]

Popular writer Paul DeKruif explored the subtle tensions between Minot (the blood specialist) and James H. Wright (the elderly pathologist)—a tension that symbolized, for DeKruif, differences in their commitment to preserving life. Minot could be found "always working at blood, blood, blood. There was a smack of the one-track fanatic about the way he was always disappearing carrying blood from sick folks into his laboratory."[56] Wright, by contrast, was a curmudgeon wedded to medical convention: "'Dammit, Minot, can't you see it's the *bone marrow* that's sick?' Wright asked . . . Being a pathologist," DeKruif concluded, Wright "had this limitation: he was concerned with the way sickness killed humans, not about how to keep humans from dying."[57] The stories of blood and Minot dramatized the ways in which blood work represented (for DeKruif and others) the virtues of scientific management, and thus the preservation, of human life. DeKruif's characterization itself reflected the rise of the new hospital of the 1910s and 1920s and the purpose of its laboratory workers.[58] Laboratory science was a humane science, intimately concerned with life and its preservation, thoroughly rational and committed to rationalizing the production of patients.

While most older pathologists embraced these institutional changes, some continued to bemoan the passing of morbid anatomy. One advocate of the new pathology wrote that "the [older] pathological laboratory . . . was a kind of customs house where the last examination of earthly belongings was made . . . [it] remained some distance from the main hospital and always contained the morgue. It was a kind of gate between the physicians and the undertaker."[59] But another pathologist insisted that the work of autopsy should still be given a place in modern hospitals, noting that "sometimes one hears the flimsy remark that the field of the human necropsy has been worked over so thoroughly that there is nothing left to discover by this simple means."[60] The terrain of the hospital had changed, and with it the work of diagnosis. "Here and there throughout the hospital," William MacCarty wrote in 1919, "one finds today rooms equipped with various kinds of apparatus—apparatus for the purpose of studying the living, not the dead."[61]

This new professional role gave pathologists a clear managerial function; they performed valuable services for other physicians and for patients, but they were increasingly administratively anonymous. In this context the pathologist's ideas and practices could seem quite foreign, even to fellow doctors. One laboratory worker wrote to his medical colleagues in 1922 that "the laboratory worker is interested in your diagnostic difficulties, and in exchange for the efficient cooperation he is prepared to extend to you, in helping to solve your daily problems, he is entitled, I believe, to a degree of professional recognition befitting the character of the services he is able to perform."[62]

Writing in 1930, Morris Fishbein lampooned pathologists. "Behold the laboratory enthusiast. Secluded in his little cubby-hole at a magnificent salary . . . he has spent the last thirty years in a vain effort to prove that red cells are not really red." His ideas were portrayed as inventions. "The pathologist, who is the leader of the group, has been described as a doctor who invents diseases for other doctors to cure . . . To him the blood is a fluid which tells the ability of the patient to resist disease, the diseases which the patient has, and perhaps the diseases that the patient is going to have."[63] In his 1941 book *Doctors Anonymous,* pathologist William German reflected that, "as the hospital grew into a huge institution governed by administrators more concerned with management than with science, the pathologist became departmentalized, buried beneath the weight and complexity of administration, cut off from the privileges of his profession and from the public."[64] With administrative anonymity and seclusion came a certain degree of peer skepticism about the inventory of new diseases produced in the laboratory.[65]

Thus, even as hematology developed and expanded, physicians and other scientists continued to look skeptically upon this diagnostic work. Was hematology truly a centerpiece of modern diagnosis? Physiologist Alexander Maximow insisted that clinical blood experts incorrectly interpreted the relationship of blood to disease. The techniques of blood staining and analysis, Maximow believed, were "inadequate for solving the general problems of the *origins* of blood cells." Blood pictures revealed only a brief snapshot of a complex process, and diseases could not be inferred from those pictures. Such hematological concepts were "convenient, detailed, though somewhat arbitrary classifications."[66] The idea that the blood indicated pathological processes hidden deep within the bone marrow and the body was a convenient illusion.

In the case of aplastic anemia, clinical pathologists acknowledged these flaws as early as the 1920s, and they sought to invent corrective tools to remedy the inadequacies of blood work. In 1922, two investigators from a San Francisco hospital suggested that bone marrow puncture (a technique of drilling into the bone and removing samples of marrow) might provide compensatory diagnostic evidence during the patient's life, when blood tests proved to be inadequate. In promoting this new test, they acknowledged that "no reliance at all could be placed upon the study of the blood smear alone, for it might resemble any one of several of the severe anemias . . . If, however, marrow puncture will supply us with knowledge of the marrow pathology during life, it will be a distinct aid in differentiation [of diseases]." They hoped that "the method [will] be employed and data collected to determine whether it serves a place among recognized procedures."[67] Bone marrow puncture constituted a diagnostic compromise between the postmortem and blood analysis. It could be done during the life of the patient and still give direct evidence of the bone marrow. The puncture technique was a diagnostic tradeoff, however, in the sense that it was far less comprehensive than postmortem study, and it was also far more painful and invasive than blood analysis.

Amidst this multiplication of diagnostic tools, blood specialists became experts in clinical protocol. They became less interested in the world of disease outside the hospital and more concerned with the details of technology-based clinical decision making. Blood analysis was a key part of the moral economy of hospital work. Blood analysis could save a patient from unnecessary operations and from death at the hands of practitioners. "All the cases of aplastic anemia which have been splenectomized have died," noted James McElroy in 1926, "usually shortly after the operation." Timely blood analysis could prevent such tragedies. On the other hand, when the blood picture indicated "essential thrombocytopenia" (ETC), splenectomy had proved beneficial. Without actually defining these diseases in precise terms, McElroy asserted that whether patients lived or died depended on the hematologist. "We think it is extremely important to make this differentiation, especially since splenectomy has come so much into vogue in the treatment of hemorrhagic diathesis."[68] Blood analysis gained its legitimacy, in part, because of this role in the moral economy of clinical work.[69]

"Disastrous Innovation": Benzol and the Blood of Workers

These discussions about aplastic anemia inside the hospital seemed abstract and irrelevant to many observers. Consider the perspective of the industrial toxicologists. Just as the hospital was becoming more efficient and focused on process, so too was American industry. Many public health reformers of the era turned their attention to the health effects of modern factory work. Their perceptions of industrialization informed their own views of aplastic anemia, suggesting that what hospital workers thought of as an obscure pathology was in fact a widespread industrial hazard—benzol poisoning.

In public health's language, this was a better term than aplastic anemia. In 1910, a Maryland physician made this argument after examining several young women from a Baltimore tin can manufacturing plant, some of whom had died after suffering from bleeding gums, subcutaneous hemorrhages, and excessive depletion of blood cells. These cases had "occurred only in that room of the factory where benzol rubber solution was used"—indeed, "ten gallons of benzol a day were used and allowed to evaporate."[70] Hematological examinations revealed that "the most remarkable feature was the blood condition, and this can be best described as the picture of an aplastic anemia."[71] Autopsies showed a few signs of aplasia. Some European investigators had already linked exposure to benzol to headache, giddiness, difficulty walking, and death with signs of aplasia.[72] The 1910 case report suggested not only that benzol constituted a hazard in American industries, but that the pathology was essentially that of "aplastic anemia."

A changing industrial context helps to explain such cases, which rose steadily in number in the 1910s and 1920s. As the industrial factory had become a model of organized materials processing (Henry Ford's automobile plant being the most prominent example), workers and unions were challenged to adapt to new tools and materials, as well as new systems of "scientific management." The entry of the United States into World War I only accelerated these trends, increasing the demand for materials like steel, tin cans, rubber, paints, and explosives. War had severed America from foreign suppliers of major industrial materials and the chemicals used in their production. The manufacture of these materials depended upon chemical solvents like benzol. The surge in production in these industries exposed more and more workers to benzol. (In a similar fashion, as historians David Rosner and Gerald Markowitz have noted, the "introduction of all the power equipment that drove . . . mines, mills, and factories created vast quantities of dust that greatly altered the health experience of the millions of industrial workers.")[73] Scaling up of industry both created more aplastic anemia and allowed public health workers to put a human face on the disease. Within ten years of the first 1910 case report, the obscure hospital disease became the subject of extensive study outside the hospital.

Concerns with workplace efficiency guided much of the interest in benzol poisoning. Occupational disease was undoubtedly an important part of industrial policy. Writing in 1914 to a member of Missouri's state legislature, Frederick Hoffman (statistician for the Prudential Life Insurance Company and an influential advocate for industrial health) urged "the inclusion of occupational diseases . . . in any rational and well considered workmen's compensation act. Experience has shown that the borderland between industrial accidents and industrial diseases cannot be defined by law."[74] In the 1910s and 1920s, the worker's plight attracted the interest of men like Hoffman and of public health workers, labor organizers, and economists. Pathologists and physicians (with a few notable exceptions) reluctantly entered this public debate.

One of the exceptions was David Linn Edsall, who in 1914 established the Industrial Disease Clinic at the Massachusetts General Hospital and who acknowledged that most physicians were unwilling to validate the observations of factory managers and workers who witnessed the effects of industrial agents like benzol.[75] In 1918, Edsall had visited a leather-making factory and found out just how uninformed most physicians were about industrial poisoning. "The exposure to benzol was very severe and the ventilation very bad," he noted. "The manager called in the chemist and we went over the matter together . . . [The manager] told me that he had a man die some months before with hemorrhages, and though he did not know that benzol was seriously poisonous he had wondered whether the dope might not have had something to do with the man's death . . . He had asked the doctors in the town who had charge of the man . . . and they had said 'No.'"[76]

Most physicians (unfamiliar with factory conditions, wedded to laboratory work, and skeptical of worker testimony) wondered whether there was any proof at all of a causal relationship between benzol and aplastic anemia. In a somewhat defensive posture, they often sought to preserve the distinction between organic disease and industrial poisoning. Despite the hematological similarities between the two disorders, Harvard's George Minot insisted on segregating the clinical problem of aplastic anemia from the public health problem of benzol poisoning: "Such cases as those in which we recognize the etiology should be called by the name of the poison producing the disease condition."[77] All other cases would be labeled "idiopathic aplastic anemia." Others disagreed that clinical problems could be so easily distinguished from public health tragedies. A few, like "blood specialist" J. P. Schneider of Minnesota, argued that "proper emphasis should be placed upon the fact of toxic marrow destruction . . . a better term [than aplastic anemia] would be toxic paralytic anemia."[78] It seemed clear to Schneider that *toxic paralytic anemia* better captured the character and identity of this disease. Such a term implied, however, that (in fighting disease) doctors needed to focus not only on management in the hospital but also on management on the factory floor and on the human experience of disease.

Alice Hamilton: Constructing the "Susceptible Worker"

Of the public health workers of her era, Alice Hamilton was most ardent in her belief that "chronic benzene poisoning means aplastic anemia . . . and if the man survives that, it is impossible for us to say, in our present state of knowledge, that he can recover normal health."[79] In her writings in the 1910s and 1920s, Hamilton sought to draw a picture of aplastic anemia and benzol poisoning that evoked one singular problem—the plight of the American factory worker. While she was not a hematologist per se, her writings reflected the application of hematological tools in the industrial realm. For her, aplastic anemia was not a disease originating in the body; it started on the factory floor.[80]

Hamilton's writing originally cast aplastic anemia as the tragic end point of an industrial working-class drama—a story involving brave working men and women, the political economy of benzol use, and everyday exposure to insidious and lethal agents. In her early writings, she criticized the motives of industries. "To manufacturers," she stated, "the introduction of this cheap and powerful solvent may seem an advantage; to the physician, interested in the producer [i.e, the worker] more than the product, it can only seem a disastrous innovation."[81] But as Hamilton's own professional identity changed, so too did her analysis of benzol poisoning. After joining the faculty at Harvard Medical School in 1923, Hamilton avoided explicit critiques of the economics of benzol poisoning. She began using blood testing to identify men "at risk" for benzol poisoning, to determine the relationship of benzol to aplastic anemia, and to use such evidence to arbitrate compensation disputes between exposed workers and benzol-using industries.[82] By the mid-1920s, the identity of aplastic anemia had become less a by-product of industrial abuse and more a by-product of individual "susceptibility" and poor personnel management.

Hamilton's writings on benzol poisoning consistently criticized hospitals as well as industries. To clinicians the problem of benzol was minor when compared with other industrial hazards.[83] Working for the United States Public Health Service throughout the 1910s, Hamilton noted that, after the armistice, the existing surplus of benzol had prompted industries to seek new applications, increasing workers' exposure.[84] Hospitals, because of their clinical focus, seemed blind to such industrial maladies. "Not one hospital in 50 has records," she noted, "which yield the sort of information which the student of industrial toxicology craves and yet this is not elaborate."[85] Another industrial toxicologist wrote that "the information which is published [from hospital studies] is of comparatively little value to the statistician or to the student of industrial disease."[86] While industrial giants pursued efficiencies of scale and increased production, hospital specialists viewed disease with a characteristic myopia.

Hamilton believed that "in typical benzol poisoning the marrow is aplastic," but she also believed that bone marrow and blood specimens were insufficient for diagnosis. The "simple, unvarying picture of the pathology of chronic benzene poisoning as is found in our textbooks is certainly based on insufficient human material," she wrote.[87] Intimate knowledge of the factory floor, of changing patterns of materials processing, of exposure to chemical agents, and of the life of the American laborer was necessary for diagnosis.

Industrial managers agreed. One manager at DuPont, for example, clearly saw benzol use and anemia as management issues. In January 1923, Joseph Moosman (a production manager) looked over a bulletin from his Safety Division documenting two cases of fatal chronic benzene poisoning in "vigorous and young" employees. The medical officers acknowledged that the use of benzene in the rubber and tire industries had resulted in "a considerable number of similar cases." In the DuPont incidents, after prolonged anemia "the first died two weeks after being taken to the hospital, and the second in about three weeks."[88] Improvements in plant ventilation had failed to prevent the poisoning, and blood transfusions had been futile.[89] Scientific management had failed to control this disease on the factory floor and in the hospital, yet physicians and managers continued to believe that the tools of scientific management offered their best means of further intervention.

Hamilton too came to perceive these as problems of personnel management, rather than of industrial greed. An exchange of letters with a large distributor of benzol in January 1924 illuminates this shift toward investigating the worker rather than industry. In the Barrett Company's effort to enable their benzol customers "to handle various coal tar solvents efficiently and with perfect safety," one of its managers asked Hamilton for advice on benzol's proper handling.[90] "Those of us here at Harvard," she replied, "who have paid special attention to this subject feel that . . . the problem of protection of the men and women engaged in industrial processes which involve the use of benzol can be solved only after careful scientific study."[91] Hamilton's ideal studies used hematological investigation with urine, air, and materials analysis to examine individual workers and their immediate environments. Hamilton suggested looking for "the earliest symptom or change in blood or urine which can be depended upon to give warning that the individual . . . is susceptible to benzol *in time to shift that person to other work and so avoid real poisoning*" (emphasis added).[92] In shifting away from a critique of corporate excesses, Hamilton identified aplastic anemia as a by-product of poor management strategies.[93] Hematological testing could become one basis for rational industrial management.

Laboratory methods offered a key to identifying "susceptible" workers and moving them to safer work stations. Environmental studies could determine the "safe limits" of benzol use. In 1923, the National Safety Council began its own study of benzol in American industries. Their findings further expanded the role of blood studies in industrial policy. The council found "that out of 84 men employed in processes involving more or less continuous exposure to benzene fumes, 13 or about 15 percent, have shown a blood picture strongly suggestive of benzene poisoning."[94] Despite such "suggestive" findings linking benzene to blood degeneration, the relation of benzene to the disease aplastic anemia remained unclear.

Seeking a sympathetic hearing, one California doctor wrote to Hamilton in 1930 concerning one of his patients with aplastic anemia, about whom there "was considerable discussion and diversity of opinion regarding the etiology of the case." The physician complained that, despite exposure and blood degeneration, the patient "was denied compensation by the industrial commission. The only tenable diagnosis in the case, however, are either idiopathic aplastic anemia or one secondary to the benzol in the gasoline. The occurrence of his symptoms in connection with his type of work personally is convincing to me of the etiology of the case."[95] Personal conviction and strong suggestion, however, did not convince physicians on such commissions. They saw aplastic anemia as distinct from any mode of production. To include "exposure to benzol" in the etiology of aplastic anemia would have constituted an expansive critique of industrial practices. Numerous physicians, lawyers, and public health officials turned to Hamilton, seeking her authentication of these sufferers.

In response to the ebb and flow of such cases, physicians and experts like Hamilton spoke of monitoring the "personal idiosyncrasies" of workers. The 1923 DuPont bulletin had suggested that "employees, both salaried and payroll, should be watched carefully and any prolonged absence from work on account of 'sickness' should be promptly investigated and if conditions are suspicious, the plant doctor and the Medical Division should be advised at once."[96] Various air-monitoring methods were suggested, including a variation on placing canaries in coal mines: "If such work [with benzol] has to be performed constantly, a cage of white mice should be kept for use as 'detectors.'"[97] In a letter to L. M. Foss of General Motors, DuPont's Moosman suggested that "occasionally a person will be found who is more susceptible to these vapors than the average, generally due to personal idiosyncrasies." He advocated prompt identification of such susceptible workers. "When these exceptional cases are encountered they should not be permitted to continue in this kind of work. Cases of this kind will generally complain to not feeling well after working with material several days, and can be verified by a skin eruption or a blood examination."[98] In her 1925 book, Alice Hamilton acknowledged that blood tests could be used to distinguish the defective worker from his hardy counterpart. She noted that "certain constitutional defects are generally regarded as rendering a person unfit for employment in poisonous trades . . . [the previous existence of] anemia will add to the danger of benzene poisoning, and of plumbism, anilinism, etc. which might involve loss of red cells."[99] Regular blood tests were integral to the detection of these weak workers and therefore were a useful tool in managing the workforce.[100]

In time, Hamilton and other public health advocates would settle into this management stance. As Harvard professor and hematological expert, she was regarded as an expert witness and a legal arbiter on benzol poisoning and aplastic anemia.[101] Through the 1920s and 1930s, she advised medical practitioners, benzol producers, benzol users, and workmen's compensation commissions. In April 1932, for example, she accepted "a retainer on behalf of . . . the Davol Rubber Company, and [was] therefore not in a position to give my services to the defendant side." In her service to the company's law firm, Hamilton confirmed that "there is no evidence aside from animal experiments that poisoning by benzol predisposes to tuberculosis."[102] In another case that same year, she supported the claim of "a leather worker, Fred B., who died November 17, 1932, the diagnosis of the attending physicians being benzol poisoning . . . There is," Hamilton wrote, "I believe, no dispute as to the correctness of this diagnosis." She speculated that the man may have had a higher susceptibility than most.[103]

Despite much evidence to the contrary, Hamilton believed that early blood testing might have saved his life. "Had a blood examination been made at the time it would doubtless have revealed this condition." Failure to scrutinize the workforce closely, she concluded, resulted in tragedy. "By the time the first blood was noticed in the saliva this damage to the bone marrow had reached a serious stage, the man was already profoundly poisoned. Had he then quit work and received appropriate medical care, it may be that he would have been saved, it may be also that the disease would have gone on to a fatal termination."[104] As she wrote later, "It is well to remember that a correct diagnosis of benzol poisoning is important, not only because of the scientific interest, but because life and death often hinge on the physician's decision whether or not the victim shall return to his old job."[105] Hamilton promoted the value of hematology in managing the continuing problem of benzol poisoning and aplastic anemia on the factory floor.

The role of hematological specialists expanded into new realms, and they endorsed prevalent managerial ideals of this period in American history. Blood tests for aplastic anemia would be carried out in hospitals, in courtrooms, in compensation hearings, and on factory floors. The disease's proper identification was an issue of ongoing debate. What tools were necessary for true "diagnosis"? Was bone marrow evidence after death the only true diagnosis? Were hematological signs of blood depletion sufficient for diagnosis? What kinds of blood picture mattered? Was exposure to benzol alone dependable for diagnosis? Or were personal idiosyncrasies causative? In the 1920s, aplastic anemia had multiple identities. Its diagnosis encoded beliefs about the identity of workers, personal versus corporate responsibility, industrial innovation and its consequences, the regulation of work, and social relations in industrial America. During this period, the identity of aplastic anemia was significantly reshaped by the expansion of industrial America, by working-class concerns, and (most significantly) by ideals of scientific disease management. Just as hematology had reinforced moral management in the 1890s, by the 1920s and 1930s hematology reflected both the scope and the limitations of scientific management.

Hematology as Scientific Management circa 1927

What had been an obscure abnormality in the 1880s had become a well-known disorder in the 1920s, its identity linked to issues of work in modernizing America. By the late 1920s and early 1930s, most physicians could not ignore the role of large-scale manufacturing processes in the production of aplastic anemia. The use of benzol in the industrial production of rubber, tin cans, and explosives had helped to create a vivid portrait of aplastic anemia as a disease of industrial workers.[106] Nor could physicians ignore the limitations inherent in their various diagnostic tools and sciences, all of which provided selective and incomplete portraits of disease. Postmortem evidence revealed one disease; hematological analysis revealed another, perhaps related disorder; bone marrow biopsy revealed yet another. Exposure to benzol suggested another diagnostic science, and notions of susceptibility suggested another diagnostic style. Laboratory-based blood analysis played an increasing role in the identification of disease because blood analysis fit neatly into an emerging management-oriented system. From the vantage point of later decades, this hematological vision provided an arbitrary basis for diagnosis. Despite its diagnostic flaws, hematology played a crucial role in the identification and control of disease, in the regulation of the hospital and the factory, and in the arbitration of blame in disputes over worker compensation.

The case of a "Russian Jewish furniture finisher" sheds light on the fallacies of scientific disease management and on the negotiated identity of aplastic anemia. The case, as reported in a 1927 *Boston Medical and Surgical Journal,* framed for medical readers the continuing tensions between medicine and public health over a vision of disease and the limitations of scientific management.[107]

The furniture finisher had died after two difficult months in the hospital, his stay complicated by a lack of medical consensus. One staff member lamented that "there was much difference of opinion as to the diagnosis." Another confirmed that "no one could agree upon the actual findings in the blood." Richard Cabot himself reflected that many clinicians did not trust the blood analysis unless they had done it themselves.[108] Different members of the staff interpreted the man's declining numbers of white and red blood cells differently, advocating different forms of management—blood transfusion, liver diet, and finally surgical removal of the spleen. One month after the splenectomy was performed, the furniture finisher became comatose and died. Publication provided an opportunity for a collective reevaluation of the patient's management.

The discussion revealed the limits of scientific disease management, when an anonymous student pointedly asked whether "the operation [splenectomy] was justified." The operating surgeon resented the student's implication, insisting that the patient "did not die from the splenectomy at all. He died from the disease."[109] But what *was* the disease? Cabot called on his associate in pathology James Wright to perform a postmortem examination. The bone marrow, Wright noted, revealed a yellow, fatty material, which proved that the patient died of "aplastic anemia." Cabot disagreed, and Wright inquired, "What are your objections to its being aplastic anemia?" Cabot then responded that "there is too much evidence of [blood] regeneration." This chorus of experts reached no conclusion, as they inquired into the meaning of the blood, the origins of this disease, and the explanation of one man's death.

The anonymous student opened another line of inquiry, asking if there was any "evidence that [the patient] had close contact with benzol." Cabot discounted this explanation, however, on the grounds that, while the man was known to work with benzol in the furniture finishing shop, "none of the other men on the job had any benzol poisoning."[110] If all of these men were not affected, then could benzol be blamed? Perhaps, Cabot suggested, this man had a special vulnerability to benzol, concluding "This, I think, is questionable territory." Here the clinical discussion ended. It remained for those outside the confines of this institution to explore other options—to criticize the hospital's diagnostic assumptions and limitations, to explore the industrial origins of aplastic anemia, and to suggest that there might be social and economic origins of this modern disease.

In the 1920s and 1930s, physicians placed enormous faith (indeed, too much faith) in blood reading and modern scientific management. Laboratory specialists were invested with the authority to determine hazardous chemical levels, to test the blood of employees, to recommend shifting workers to other roles in production processes, to arbitrate compensation disputes, and to suggest reforms in the manufacturing processes. Finding (or rather constructing) "susceptible" employees—those with weak blood—was also a vital function of hematology as its role expanded. In court cases, "evidence" of susceptibility placed the burden of guilt on workers. Susceptibility played a critical role in determining whether workers should be compensated for illness or disease. Alice Hamilton acknowledged that, although compensation cases were often decided on the basis of blood studies, "diagnosis" was a more complex enterprise—entangled with bureaucratic and specialty assumptions, with work relations, and with the politics of benzol use and labor relations.[111] "Susceptibility," however, was a convenient rationalization of hematological ignorance, a subtle managerial gesture shifting attention away from professional ignorance and toward a tainted identity and the expert's role in locating it.

Blood work in both factory and hospital represented a conceptual and administrative system for managing bodies. Terms like *chronic benzol poisoning, aplastic anemia, benzol susceptibility,* and *toxic paralytic anemia* implied different visions of disease identity and vastly different conceptual constructions of responsibility for disease. In a society dedicated to industrial innovation, in which exposure to new chemical agents was becoming a way of life and in which bureaucratic growth was widely embraced, the interpretation of blood became a vital administrative tool. Scientific management itself had little effect on the decline of aplastic anemia; indeed, the gradual decrease in industrial benzol use precipitated the disease's decline. The goal of hematology was to *manage* disease, and much of this blood work involved the packaging of disease identity for wider cultural consumption. (This theme is explored further in chs. 4 and 5.)

The 1920s inaugurated modern managerial roles and identities for hematologists, roles that have since grown and evolved with the changing relationship of hematology to policy making and regulation. (Ch. 6 examines the evolution of this regulatory role in the 1950s and 1960s by examining the controversy surrounding the resurgence of aplastic anemia and its links to the antibiotic chloramphenicol.)

4

The Corporate "Conquest" of Pernicious Anemia

Technology, Blood Researchers, and the Consumer

"The saga of pernicious anemia," wrote one recent medical observer, "remains one of the most compelling accounts of man's conquest and understanding of disease."[1] Contemporaries regarded the discovery of a cure by two Harvard researchers as an "epoch-making" event for medicine and hematology, surpassing in importance the discovery of insulin in 1922.[2]

According to the now conventional story, after decades of mistaken descriptions and thousands of deaths from this insidious depletion of the blood, the disease's correct definition emerged from the work of two clinical researchers—George Minot and William Murphy.[3] Since the 1880s, the mysterious decline of red blood cells had been regarded as the central event of the disease. With the rise of modern methods of clinical investigation, however, these physicians could see that patients were dying from a more complex disease. Blood depletion combined with gastric, dietary, and other symptoms characterized the disease. Clinical researchers like Minot, although committed hematologists, were developing an integrative multidimensional view of disease.

Prompted by pathologist George Whipple's research on the feeding of liver to anemic dogs, Minot and Murphy fed liver to their patients. In a now famous 1926 paper, they announced its miraculous benefits for forty-five otherwise doomed souls.[4] By 1928 (with the assistance of Minot and his associates), the Eli Lilly pharmaceutical company produced a liver extract that became widely available to researchers, clinicians, and general practitioners as "Liver Extract No. 343." Popular and professional acclaim soon followed. In 1931, the popular journal *Scientific Monthly* awarded the researchers its $10,000 prize for scientific excellence and proclaimed a cure of this "dread disease which . . . baffled physicians for generations."[5] International scientific acclaim for Minot, Murphy, and Whipple came in the early years of the Great Depression, when the three researchers traveled to Stockholm, Sweden, to receive the 1934 Nobel Prize in Medicine or Physiology.

This dramatic story of the conquest of pernicious anemia has a crucial place in the collective historical consciousness of modern medicine and hematology, highlighting the place of modern technologies in diagnosis, in clinical research, and in the production and evaluation of effective therapies.[6] The use of the liver extract itself became a research tool. Administered to patients, it helped to produce new knowledge about the hematological mechanisms of this disease. The fact that liver provoked a "reticulocyte response" in sick patients became a clear indication of the curative effects of liver, liver diet, and liver extract. For all of these reasons, one British observer in 1955 reflected that Minot's 1926 paper resembled "the gentle opening bars of a great unfinished symphony, of which some movements have even now not yet been composed, much less played."[7] In this conventional outline, the story of this disease's "conquest" was a powerful validation of the maturation of hematology and of technology-based clinical research. Hematological investigation, undertaken in a broad-minded research setting, had revealed the essence of the disease process.

Minot and Murphy were themselves aware of one problem in this "conquest of pernicious anemia." Liver extract was being used increasingly as a diagnostic test, and pernicious anemics who did not recover or who did not show a reticulocyte response after liver treatment posed a dilemma of disease classification. In a 1929 letter to a fellow physician whose patient had gained no relief from liver extract, Minot suggested that the patient must have been misdiagnosed. In such a failure of liver extract to bring relief, Minot wondered whether the case was really pernicious anemia: "[There is] no way of being certain in a brief test period that a patient with such a high initial red blood cell count . . . actually has the disease," he wrote.[8] Throughout the late 1920s and into the 1930s, many of these patients died while showing unrelieved, familiar symptoms of pernicious anemia. In his Nobel Prize address in 1934, Minot explained nonetheless that "failure of liver therapy in a case diagnosed as pernicious anemia implies inadequate treatment, an incorrect diagnosis, or the existence of complication."[9] Throughout this period, physicians debated the status of these anomalous patients—about 20 percent of the pernicious anemic population.[10] Were they truly pernicious anemics, or sufferers from another, related disease? A key development during this decade was the way the patient's response to Eli Lilly's liver extract was interpreted as a kind of bioassay, a diagnostic technology in its own right retrospectively constituting "the disease." Rather than curing *all* of the patients ordinarily diagnosed with pernicious anemia, the disease *became*, by definition, that entity which was cured by a new consumable and de facto diagnostic technology—liver extract.

To understand the changing identity of this disease, we must examine the changing identity of the academic clinical researcher and his relationship with the pharmaceutical industry. In his 1956 autobiography, Roger Lee—a Boston hematologist who had participated in this unfolding drama—reflected on how academic medicine's commercial ties had transformed medical writers into spokesmen for the drug industry. "To be sure," Lee wrote, "one may read in a modern text, although never in Osler's writings, such a crime against logic as the statement that pernicious . . . anemia is controlled by the administration of liver—and also that the administration of liver is an absolute therapeutic diagnostic test for pernicious anemia. Of course, neither of these two statements is true, and it should not require a professor of logic to point that out."[11] Lee believed that the modern definition of pernicious anemia conformed to a false drug-centered thinking that was unfortunately all too pervasive during the antibiotic era. (In ch. 1, we saw how physicians in the same era similarly reconstructed "chlorosis" to conform to this drug-centered thinking.) Lee was "reasonably certain that the heads of pharmaceutical houses must experience a feeling of satisfaction on seeing how articles of medical men in the medical press often take on the flavor of advertisements for commercial nostrums."[12] The modern view of pernicious anemia did not reflect thoughtful, scientific analysis, Lee suggested, but a "trend toward careless, casual, and . . . optimistic thinking" and an uncomfortably close alliance between medical thinkers and commercial interests.

What then are historians to make of the conquest of pernicious anemia? How did the drug-centered vision of the disease differ from Osler's? Undoubtedly, the modern definition was "real" for many doctors and for at least 80 percent of pernicious anemia patients who seemed to benefit from liver extract. Like Lee, many contemporary physicians both embraced these therapeutic findings, but at the same time rejected their purported implications for disease definition. For others, however, blood analysis technology and the new drug became key tools cementing a modern corporate relationship between clinical researchers and the pharmaceutical industry and confirming this view of disease.

In this chapter, I will argue that the debate about the true identity of pernicious anemia reflected cultural anxieties about corporate relationships and about medicine's social structure. Between 1900 and 1930, fundamental economic changes had occurred in American research medicine, as in other areas of medicine and American society. As we have seen in previous chapters, the family doctor, the surgeon, and the pathologist all saw their medical practices transformed during these years. Robert Weibe and other historians, and more recently T. J. Jackson Lears, have commented on the sweeping corporate transformation in American society and culture between the 1880s and the 1920s. "The old culture," Lears wrote, "was suited to a production-oriented society of small entrepreneurs; the newer culture epitomized a consumer-oriented society dominated by bureaucratic corporations."[13] How people thought about disease reflected and reinforced these social trends. Splenic anemia, for example, a favorite disease of the individualistic surgeon, found no legitimate place in the modern corporate hospital. The new pernicious anemia was likewise an artifact of the emerging corporate medical order. The use of a mass-produced drug to redefine a disease may seem natural to us in the late twentieth century, but in the 1920s this reflected a profound and much-debated shift in medical thought, practice, and culture.[14]

Pernicious anemia was never a stable, well-defined disease entity, even after its supposed conquest. Beginning in the 1890s and continuing to the present, physicians have debated its correct identity and symptoms. Today, physicians would assert that liver feeding addressed only one of the many mechanisms of pernicious anemia. In the early twentieth century, however, physicians debated a narrower range of questions which spoke to their own social context and intellectual preoccupations. Was the blood picture the most important aspect of the disease? If so, at what red cell count could a patient be said to have "pernicious anemia"? What role did nonhematological symptoms—gastric disturbances, splenic enlargement, or spinal cord degeneration—play in the disease? What status should liver diet be accorded in the conceptualization of this disease? In the years from the disease's discovery in the nineteenth century to its "cure" in 1926, different specialists vied to define and thus own and control this disease. By the early 1930s, Minot's hematological perspective emerged triumphant. Once, pernicious anemia had been as obscure as aplastic anemia and splenic anemia. The pernicious anemia that emerged in the early 1930s was a well-known disorder. It was also a different disease from that of the previous generations. Its new popular identity was sustained by a new culture—that is, by evolving institutional arrangements, technologies, and economic relations of academic medicine.

Disease Identity and Therapeutic Humility in Osler's Decade

Pernicious anemia first came into prominence in America within a small circle of research-minded medical practitioners including William Osler, George Dock, and William Pepper. Pernicious anemia attracted their attention not because it was a prevalent disease, for it was not. It was, however, scientifically interesting. Osler, Dock, and Pepper published frequently on the disease in the pages of the *American Journal of Medical Sciences,* translating and abstracting many articles from European and British publications.[15] The problem of pernicious anemia—its natural course, its proper diagnosis, and its treatment—presented a compelling puzzle, and it was a useful vehicle for educating uninformed medical practitioners about standards of disease research abroad. By the 1880s and 1890s, this particular disease exemplified many of the scientific aspirations of this coterie of American practitioners. They saw in the diminution of red blood cells and in the appearance of unusual forms of the blood cells (megaloblasts) a remarkable new illness, an educational opportunity, and a chance to contribute to international medical knowledge.

In the 1880s, pernicious anemia was not well known to physicians or laymen. Few Americans would have found cause to complain of "pernicious anemia." With this state of widespread professional and popular ignorance, Osler and his compatriots sought to make such diseases better known. It had been first described, some claimed, by Addison in England in 1849 and could be recognized by a clinical course quite distinct from that of any other disease.[16] A healthy businessman without obvious vices or dissipations might call on your services one day, and he would tell of having been beset without warning by a profound lethargy. His complaint might follow Addison's classic 1849 description: "It makes its approach in so slow and insidious a manner that the patient can hardly fix a date to the earliest feelings of that languor . . . The countenance gets pale, the whites of the eyes become pearly, the general frame flabby rather than wasted . . . There is an increasing indisposition to exertion, with an uncomfortable feeling of faintness or breathlessness in attempting it . . . [In time] the appetite fails . . . the debility becomes extreme—the patient can no longer rise from his bed."[17]

Unlike tuberculosis, the much feared "wasting disease," pernicious anemia left its patients plump, but flabby and debilitated, and eventually dead. In Addison's description, the patient "falls into a prostrate and half-torpid state, and at length expires: nevertheless, to the very last, and after a sickness of several months' duration, the bulkiness of the general frame and the amount of obesity often present a most striking contrast to the failure and exhaustion observable in every other respect."[18] The disease presented a paradox—a striking contrast between outward physical appearances and inward health. Temporary improvement was another deceptive feature, but physical incapacity eventually took over. The disease was, thus, very often an extended and tragic affair. "The average course of the affection," commented Osler, "is from six to twelve months." There was often no extreme pain, no emaciation or wasting away, only this characteristic decline where lethargy led eventually to death. There was also a distinctive picture of declining blood elements.[19]

To Osler and his peers, morality, lifestyle, and fidelity to the doctor's wishes could all affect the disease's natural course. An 1890 editorial in the *Boston Medical and Surgical Journal* noted that "there are several factors which may be regarded as predisposing to its development, such as insufficient food, bad hygienic surroundings, depressing moral influences."[20] In 1901, Frank Billings told of an aging lawyer in whom overwork and financial anxiety preceded pernicious anemia. "The last few years he had been at work upon a patent which he believed was worth a fortune, and recently arrangements were made for its adoption . . . which has brought him increasing care and anxiety . . . Three months ago he noticed that he was not as strong as usual."[21] Another Philadelphia physician recalled two exemplary cases—one in an idle gentleman, the other in a careless sailor. In the latter case, he wrote, the sailor was "in my ward at the Pennsylvania Hospital for four or five months, then went back to sea, having apparently recovered; he took no medicine while at sea, and remained well, but he came back to the hospital in about seven months, the symptoms having returned, and he died in the hospital."[22]

Pernicious anemia was a disease lying in wait to manifest itself after any moral failing. Noted Alexander McPhedran, "The recovery may be almost complete and remain unchanged for a year or more; but examination of the blood always shows some characteristic deviation and a relapse may be confidently expected sooner or later."[23] The blood picture was one of many moral indicators. For this generation of academics and nonacademics alike, it constituted a moral sign of the biological consequences of overwork, impulsiveness, indolence, or immorality. In young girls with chlorosis, as we saw in chapter 1, the blood picture indicated overwork, capriciousness, and the cultural stresses of modern womanhood. In men, the blood picture (intersecting as it did with the moral life course) could reflect the ways in which excessive drinking, dissipation, or overwork made manifest latent diseases like pernicious anemia.[24]

The primary concern of these physicians was to promote a clinical science of disease, a science that involved the careful analysis of blood and chronicling of clinical events. Their science often focused on the natural history of disease. In pernicious anemia, patients showed no distinctive lesions at autopsy.[25] Rather, the disease was most interesting as an unfolding clinical drama, a natural "process" revealed by a chart of the blood counts and chronicled by clinical observation. The characterization of this disease became a prominent focus, especially for members of the Association of American Physicians, an elite national group striving to raise themselves above common practitioners through attention to clinical science.[26] In their writings, AAP physicians stressed that, on its surface, pernicious anemia might *seem* like just a simple anemia or chlorosis, but it was not. Following the debate abroad, its members devoted much time to the problem of pernicious anemia, and by the 1880s and 1890s the disease was well known as a separate clinical entity among the society's readership.[27]

What was the identity of pernicious anemia according to these physicians? A key characteristic was its stubborn unresponsiveness to drug therapy. In their therapeutic skepticism, these physicians distinguished themselves clearly from those of the later era of liver extract. In a period when special claims about miraculous new drugs abounded in public and medical discourse, the typical AAP physician held himself above crass commercialism. Therapeutic optimism was commercial folly. In 1902, Osler chastened his peers that, "in the fight which we have to wage incessantly against ignorance and quackery among the masses and follies of all sorts among the classes, diagnosis, not drugging, is our chief weapon of offense."[28] In many ways, their views of pernicious anemia echoed their professional commitments to a noncommercial medical science. In 1889, for example, Francis Delafield pointed out that "a very little experience will show you . . . that the case of simple anaemia will get well under a certain plan of treatment, and that the cases of pernicious anaemia never do anything better than improve somewhat and then get worse again; and each time they get worse they are worse than they were the time before."[29] Only the most crass and optimistic physicians would insist that arsenic or some other drug cured pernicious anemia.[30] For thoughtful observers, this was but an illusion. Such tonics, at best, only delayed decline and death.

The unpredictable remissions and relapses of pernicious anemia made the evaluation of drugs even more difficult, if not impossible. Physicians were often fooled by spontaneous remissions into thinking that their treatments had worked. Frank Billings would not be so presumptuous as to second guess nature. In one case, he noted, "the improvement wave . . . occurred coincidental with the restorative tonic treatment, and at first sight it would seem that the treatment had something to do with the great improvement; but . . . improvement may take place in these cases without the aid of restorative tonics, and . . . in some instances at least remedies have received credit in pernicious anemia, when in all probability it was the natural course of the disease which brought about the improvement, and not the drugs used."[31] Alexander McPhedran repeated this dictum in 1900. "In estimating the value of the treatment in any disease," he warned, "it is necessary to take due account of its natural course. This is especially true in pernicious anemia, whose course is subject to such sudden and extreme changes."[32] For these physicians, then, a commitment to science, an aversion to commercialism, and a cultivated research identity meant that any dramatic claim of a cure of pernicious anemia would be difficult, if not impossible, to defend.

One thing was certain: the disease, by definition, ended fatally. While the patient was still alive, Osler noted in the 1880s, the best diagnostic term to use was *idiopathic anemia*. But, "if the case goes on to a fatal termination, the designation of pernicious anemia is appropriate."[33] The term *pernicious anemia* was (like aplastic anemia) a postmortem label, a starting point for academic discussion. A physician may have used iron treatment, arsenic, and various tonics and diets. But when all was

done, it was the natural course—the insidious onset, the pattern of physical decline, the peculiar features of the blood, the remissions and relapses, and the inevitability of death—that defined pernicious anemia.
As Richard Cabot and F. C. Shattuck wrote in 1896, "fatality is not in itself the distinguishing mark of the disease . . . Yet in this country and with
our present ignorance of its cause it *is* a fatal disease."[34]

AAP physicians had devoted much attention to blood examination
to buttress their claims. Osler stressed that "the reduction in the number
of red corpuscles is the special feature of the disease . . . Instead of a cor-
puscular richness of 5,000,000 per cubic millimeter, the number may be
reduced to one-quarter, or even one-tenth."[35] In addition to the reduction in numbers of cells, Osler noted, "the corpuscles show a remarkable
irregularity in form—an irregularity which, so far as my observation
goes, is *never met with to the same extent in other conditions.*"[36] Osler adopted *poikilocytosis,* the term of the German pathologist Quinke (and later
Ehrlich's term *gigantoblasts*), to describe what he saw as characteristic
blood evidence in pernicious anemia.[37] Others searched for telltale
megalocytes and megaloblasts in the blood. Yet others scanned merely
for low numbers of red blood cells. Into the last decade of the nineteenth
century, AAP physicians embraced hematology in highly individualized
ways to give identity to pernicious anemia.

The proliferation of hematological techniques conflicted in several
ways with older traditions of scientific diagnosis, as we saw in previous
chapters. We saw how men like Frederick Henry objected strenuously to
the growing reliance on hematological reductionism in diagnosis.[38] Writing in 1889, Francis Delafield argued that "there are a good many physicians who believe that pernicious anaemia is practically nothing but a
bad simple anaemia; that if you have a simple anaemia bad enough, you
can be said to have pernicious anaemia. This I do not think is true. I think
the two conditions are absolutely separate and have nothing to do with
each other."[39] At the 1889 AAP annual meeting, however, Henry responded that pernicious anemia was an arbitrary construction. Its status
as an "independent entity" was not based on any traditional diagnostic
criteria.[40] "It is admitted by all," Henry wrote, "that the clinical features
of this disease are common to a number of affections, especially cancer
and atrophy of the gastric glands; but those who argue most forcibly in
favor of its independent nature exclude from the category of pernicious
anaemia all cases in which an anatomical lesion of any organ is found.
This appears to me unscientific."[41] Henry concluded that "pernicious

anaemia is a process, not a disease . . . [and] it is closely related to chlorosis."[42] But Henry was in the minority among AAP members, many of whom had invested energy in establishing the independent existence of this disease.[43]

By 1900, the laboratory had become even more central to medical thinking about blood diseases, and a spectrum of voices engaged in this heated debate. As numerous historians of medicine have argued, the use of laboratory-based tools gave rise to sharp divisions within the medical profession.[44] In 1901, physician Henry Hewes recalled that, "among the special methods of the study of disease which have been developed in this recent era of laboratory methods, one of the most important and practical . . . is that of the examination of the blood."[45] With these developments, doctors wondered whether it was moral influences and clinical events that defined pernicious anemia or whether the discrete appearance of "megaloblasts" in the circulating blood could define the disease. Hematological diagnostic practice was easy enough; megaloblasts were recognizable to any physician trained in microscopy.[46] By the early years of the century, more and more clinicians began to suggest that the sighting of large-sized red cells—"megaloblasts"—was central to the disease's definition.

When Richard Cabot presented a report on 110 cases of pernicious anemia in 1900, for example, he argued that "there are undoubtedly periods in the course of most cases of pernicious anaemia in which the diagnosis cannot be made by the blood examination alone." Yet he believed that great vigilance in blood examination would always uncover distinctive hematological signs.[47] Frank Billings agreed, noting that "the proportion of megaloblasts varied with the severity and stage of the disease, usually gaining a numerical ascendancy over the normoblasts when the disease was advanced."[48] At the turn of the century, George Dock assessed the situation best. He lectured to his students in 1899: "We have two different conceptions of pernicious anemia; one that is dependent on the condition of the blood and the other on the history of the disease."[49] In one conception, the doctor's knowledge of the clinical and moral history of the patient played a prominent role in disease identification. In the other, hematological technology played the dominant role.

Frederick Henry continued to stand firm against such diagnostic fads, refusing to accept that pernicious anemia could be so neatly defined by laboratory evidence. The diagnosis of pernicious anemia was not the exclusive right of laboratory experts.[50] Henry accused men like Richard Cabot of elevating laboratory evidence to a false and exalted status. When questioned about whether a previously reported case of his own was "true" pernicious anemia, Henry became angry and restated the facts of his case. "I presume no member of the Association has now any doubt that this is a typical case of pernicious anemia, although, in my opinion, there never should have been the slightest question concerning the diagnosis," Henry argued. "The demonstration of megaloblasts in the blood was not at all necessary to confirm it. There is a tendency at the present time to regard the presence of these cells in the blood as the sole criterion of pernicious anemia." He heatedly rejected this specious and faddish belief. "According to this view," he stated, "if megaloblasts are not detected in the blood the diagnosis of pernicious anemia is unwarranted. Such a doctrine appears to me as pernicious as the disease to which it is applied."[51]

The "pernicious doctrines" of laboratory enthusiasts stirred Henry to his final point—that doctors owned diagnosis, not laboratory workers. "If the presence of megaloblasts in the blood were pathognomonic of pernicious anemia, the diagnosis of the disease could be made more accurately in the laboratory than at the bedside. Now, this is by no means the case." This would be the tail wagging the dog. "The diagnosis," Henry concluded, "is most firmly based upon the tout ensemble of signs and symptoms, both positive and negative."[52] Microscopic interpretation, it seemed to Henry, was nothing more than a veiled attempt to shift diagnostic authority to the laboratory. For this breach in the diagnostic hierarchy—and this breach alone—Henry rejected the new dictum.

Other physicians objected, although less emphatically, to diagnostic rule by laboratory enthusiasts. In 1902, John Morse, writing about "some cases which were not pernicious anemia," insisted that many anemias showed the so-called blood picture of pernicious anemia. Morse reported these cases "with the object of emphasizing the writer's belief that the diagnosis of pernicious anemia cannot be made with certainty on the basis of the condition of the blood alone."[53] Others, like Chicago's James Herrick, continued to speak out against the false faith that too many physicians placed in the laboratory tools of hematology. "The laboratory," Herrick suggested, "is viewed as a sanctum sanctorum pervaded by a purer light than the wards of the hospital." But this was a false piety. "Often, we have seen the positive diagnosis of pernicious anemia made from the blood smear, sent into the laboratory. We know this is possible, but it is risky."[54] Such disagreements reflected deepening divisions among hospital-based specialists.

By the early years of the twentieth century, the debate about the identity of pernicious anemia had spilled over from the narrow circle of AAP physicians into wider medical circles. The fate of pernicious anemia would be decided, not within the elite clique of AAP doctors, but by the expanding numbers of hospital-based specialists.[55] British physician Sidney Coupland admitted that, based on the expanding variety of contemporary medical opinions, pernicious anemia must be said to have no discernibly consistent identity—neither the clinical course, nor the blood picture, nor the postmortem appearances presented constant features. "It is difficult," he wrote, "even in light of modern research, to frame a satisfactory definition of this affection—one which shall not be too wide, nor, on the other hand, too narrow to embrace the varied conditions under which this severe form of anaemia is known to arise . . . The difficulty is enhanced by the fact that the clinical phenomena are not in themselves distinctive, not even the characters of the blood." Perhaps, Coupland suggested, within the spectrum of cases commonly labeled pernicious anemia there existed a residual group that was "true" pernicious anemia: "There is good ground for believing that . . . there remains a residue of cases of progressive anaemia, to which the term 'primary' may be assigned; and it is to this class that we may assign, at least provisionally, the name pernicious."[56] This was the same contingent view of diagnosis, of course, that led William Osler to grant a "provisional" existence to splenic anemia. "The diagnosis of pernicious anemia," Coupland concluded, "does not rest on any very certain basis."[57] With the rise of the hospital as a site of knowledge production, the use of discrete clinical tools and procedures on living patients would now play a crucial role in reconstructing this disease.

The Fragmentation of Pernicious Anemia, 1900–1925

The early twentieth-century hospital provided American physicians with a novel workplace. The hospital was becoming a site where middle-class consumers—clerks, professionals, secretaries, and even the well-to-do—sought access to a wealth of new diagnostic tools and, presumably, improvements in health. Specialists in a variety of fields resided there, finding this a stimulating place for medical casework. In the case of pernicious anemia, each symptom attracted its own specialist. And each specialist brought specific rules of conduct and diagnostic criteria to reify the connection between symptom and pathology. From 1900 to 1920, gastroenterologists, neurologists, surgeons, laboratory-based physicians, and clinicians offered new insights into the biological identity of this pathology. Because of their work, by the 1910s pernicious anemia was an unpredictable, varied, and multifaceted syndrome—defined by different specialists according to the symptoms each group thought to be central. The confusion of the time only reflected the way in which specialists were carving up the problem according to their specialty and defining their place in an emerging hospital system.

Pernicious anemia entered a distinctly bureaucratic phase, leaving behind its former identity as a single disease with a natural, enigmatic clinical history. The diagnostic laboratory offered the most compelling revision of the classical picture of disease. As late as 1917, Ralph Larrabee acknowledged that many physicians had come to depend entirely upon the blood picture to define pernicious anemia. He objected, however, that there was "considerable confusion as to the points of difference between the blood of pernicious anemia and that of the benign or secondary forms." Larrabee, like many others, thought that blood had been granted an inflated importance in diagnosis. "The blood picture," he wrote, "is not pathognomonic . . . I have seen the pernicious type of blood in syphilis, in cirrhosis of the liver, in lead poisoning and in a small cancer of the intestine."[58] Although this recalled Frederick Henry's concerns, such objections in the 1910s occurred amidst increasing specialty development. A variety of other specialists—abdominal surgeons, neurologists, and gastroenterologists—had by now also rethought pernicious anemia from their own specialized understandings and debated the true location (both institutionally and corporeally) of this disease.[59] It becomes difficult for the historian to distinguish the identity of the disease from the identity of the practitioner.

Abdominal surgeons, relying heavily on the hematologists for support, suggested one interpretation. William Mayo saw pernicious anemia as a disease of the spleen and concluded that "in pernicious anemia there is increased hemolytic [blood destruction] activity of the spleen." "Most of the cases," Mayo claimed, "were reported as improved after splenectomy."[60] Mayo and other abdominal surgeons frequently reminded their nonsurgeon peers of the immense value of splenectomy in such cases. The disease, they argued, was no more than a variation on "splenic anemia," the enlarged spleen being the "agent of destruction" of the blood.[61] After operation, patients experienced increases in red blood cells and decreases in the number of megaloblasts—hematological proof of surgical benefit. But as with splenic anemia, nonsurgical practitioners remained skeptical—perhaps more so in the case of pernicious anemia. Whereas splenic anemia was a disease without a well-established identity in the nonsurgical context, pernicious anemia had become well established as an enigmatic clinical disorder, a sophisticated deceiver of therapeutic optimists of many stripes.

Surgeons like Mayo did not dispute that pernicious anemia was a blood disease; rather, they depended upon hematology to legitimate the surgical argument. The disappearance of megaloblasts became for them a crucial postoperative indicator, a bellwether of surgical efficacy. Mayo recognized the value of this evidence to the surgical enterprise. His enthusiasm was also tempered by the knowledge that pernicious anemia, as previously defined, ran an unpredictable course. "It is of course, too early to pass critical judgement," he wrote, "on any therapeutic measure in a disease that runs such a bizarre course as pernicious anemia."[62] Nonetheless, surgical experiments continued. Abdominal surgeons sought to introduce a new operational thinking into disease definition, to expand their realm of medical practice, and to usurp areas of expertise previously demarcated as "medical." (See ch. 2.) Surgery's bold and precise view of disease appealed within medical circles and in popular venues.

Some experts on pernicious anemia, however, were not convinced of the effectiveness of splenectomy. Philadelphia pathologist E. B. Krumbhaar noted in 1916 that a long-term analysis of postsplenectomy patients showed that "of the individuals who showed improvement shortly after operation [64.7 percent of 153 patients] . . . a large number have failed to maintain this improvement, and have since died in a relapse or from intercurrent illness."[63] Such findings refuted surgery's optimistic claims. In similar reviews, George Minot and Roger Lee noted in 1917 that, while splenectomies had been increasing in the past four years, "the results from splenectomy have not been as great as was first expected." To be sure, removal of the spleen showed that "definite improvement follows splenectomy more consistently and uniformly than after any other form of treatment." But these authors concluded that "splenectomy is in no sense curative, though a more profound change in the blood occurs after splenectomy than by [any] other means. The eventual progress of the disease is not essentially changed by splenectomy."[64]

Thus, the image of a distinctive enigmatic clinical course of pernicious anemia remained a formidable foe for the therapeutic optimist—splenectomy offered, at best, temporary relief.[65] At worst, relief was a surgical illusion. Despite their skepticism, many experts embraced abdominal surgery, if not as a radical cure of this disease, then as a desperate last measure. One of the harshest critics of splenectomy noted that "a total of 50 patients were operated on in the Mayo Clinic between January 1, 1910 and April 1, 1917; $\frac{1}{2}$ of these patients are now dead; 3 deaths were operative."[66]

Other specialists tackled the problem of pernicious anemia from their own perspectives, arguing less emphatically than the surgeons, but no less persistently, that the disease's traditional identity be reconstructed. In 1923, Thomas Buckman of Boston acknowledged that "in recent years it has become the fashion, and with much justification, more and more to regard factors other than the blood in making the diagnosis of pernicious anemia. Attention is especially directed to the nervous system and the gastrointestinal tract."[67] Gastroenterologists and neurologists elevated what had previously been regarded as secondary symptoms to the level of primary features. Some regarded these symptoms as possible causes of the abnormality. These new fashions in diagnosis reflected the ways in which emerging specialists seized upon key symptoms both to redefine the identity of pernicious anemia and to craft a role for themselves in its management.

As early as 1910, Julius Friedenwald of Baltimore took a lead in defining the new specialty of gastroenterology and its disease concerns. He did so, in part, by arguing that "gastro-intestinal disturbance" had a long, but generally understated, presence within historical characterizations of pernicious anemia.[68] Friedenwald uncovered distinguished predecessors to support his view of the disease. The mid–nineteenth-century American physician Austin Flint had documented "degenerative changes in the gastric mucosa," and a few subsequent observers in the late nineteenth century had tried in vain to elevate this symptom to primary importance.[69] Friedenwald adopted their struggle. Based on his study of 58 cases, he concluded that it was impossible to state categorically that gastric problems "caused" pernicious anemia.[70] However, the coincidence of gastric and hematological symptoms implied at least a common origin.[71] In Friedenwald's view, gastric symptoms were as central as blood symptoms in defining the disease, and these gastric symptoms warranted closer attention from gastroenterologists and from clinicians.

This argument merely exemplified the ways in which specialists sprung up in early twentieth-century hospital medicine, mediating the epistemological terrain among surgeons, laboratory men, and other internists. At the time gastroenterologists were themselves at the center of debates about the proper management of the ulcer (surgical operation versus medical therapy). Their involvement in the management of pernicious anemia was relatively minor, but they did carve out a coequal therapeutic role for the fledgling specialty.[72] Some physicians had previously touted the benefits of hydrochloric acid therapy. In 1899, for example, George Dock suggested that in pernicious anemia "there is a lack of hydrochloric acid . . . [and] Of course if the patient can't digest well recovery from his anemia is out of the question. So evidently the treatment of the stomach is the most important thing . . . We give him hydrochloric acid, and in addition to that we give him nutritious food in as large quantities as he can digest."[73] Despite Friedenwald's reminders, only a few physicians agreed that gastric disturbance, hydrochloric anacidity, and nutritional problems defined the disease. It would be another ten years before two researchers at the Peter Bent Brigham Hospital in Boston observed that, of 105 patients with pernicious anemia, "gastric anacidity" occurred in 104.[74] By the mid-1920s, some gastroenterologists believed their time had arrived. In 1926, A. F. Durst observed that "twenty five years ago pernicious anemia was almost universally considered to be entirely a 'blood disease.'" But, he continued, "we have come to feel that the blood changes do not constitute the entire picture but that they bear much the same relation to the disease as does the blood picture to the entire syndrome of lead poisoning."[75] Blood pictures were clues rather than diseases themselves, revealing poisonings or the workings of extrahematological processes. For Durst, a valuable understanding of the "entire picture" emerged from the study of gastroenterology. "Can the development of pernicious anemia be prevented by administration of hydrochloric acid? Is similar therapy of value in the early stages of the disease?"[76] Durst concluded that these questions could be answered only with more careful studies of the gastric system.

Yet another perspective was added to this symptomalogical politics by the neurologists. Their assertions—that neurological problems lay at the core of pernicious anemia—developed quite slowly in the 1910s, a by-product of budding specialism and clinical experiences. In 1918, H. W. Woltmann, a neurological specialist employed by the Mayo Clinic, reviewed the previous two decades of pernicious anemia scholarship, noting how frequently physicians had mentioned spinal cord symptoms among the standard symptom complex. On the basis of some 150 cases reviewed, Woltmann concluded that "in 80.6 percent of moderately advanced cases of pernicious anemia, there is indisputable evidence of nervous-tissue disintegration." Such statements were a declaration of the neurologists' right to be involved in disease management. Not surprisingly, neurologists urged that diagnostic examination of the nervous system was a valuable way of "differentiating pernicious anemia from other anemias."[77] Neurology, like gastroenterology, added another dimension to the increasingly complex bureaucratic identity of pernicious anemia.

Was it a blood disease, a gastric disorder, a splenic pathology, or a neurological disorder? While the most aggressive claims about the management of pernicious anemia came in surgical practice, neurologists and gastroenterologists suggested significant diagnostic refinements, advocating for their involvement in management and even suggesting subtle changes in the disease's name and identity. In a 1922 report entitled "Combined System Disease," neurologist Richard Harvey noted the merging of pernicious anemia into existing neurological classifications, a blurring that suggested neurological "ownership" of the disease. Woltmann's 1918 findings provided a starting point for Harvey's analysis.[78] But Harvey went further than Woltmann, insisting that serious attention be given to the relationship between these two diseases.[79] Other neurologists asserted that "no definite line can be drawn between pernicious anemia accompanied by spinal-cord changes and subacute combined degeneration of the spinal cord accompanied by anemia." If clear lines could not be drawn between diseases, could clear statements be made about their identity, proper ownership, or proper management?

Bureaucratic specialism in the 1910s brought new aspects of the disease into view, simultaneously blurring the "true identity" of the once coherent clinical construct. How might this have impinged upon a hypothetical patient with pernicious anemia in the year 1915? Consider a forty-seven-year-old Boston man concerned about weakness, lethargy, and a barely perceptible tingling in his fingers. His acquaintances may have told him he was pale, and his family doctor may have suggested a visit to the newly opened "blood ward" at the Massachusetts General Hospital. There the work of diagnosis might have included a blood count, revealing a paucity of red blood cells. Was it very low? Were megaloblasts present? A regime with "blood building" tonics might be suggested, and if this man's blood count continued to decline, a blood transfusion might be attempted using most likely the blood of a family member. The more neurologically inclined specialist, however, might note the tingling as evidence of combined system disease. An internist, on the other hand, might suggest that attention be given to a regime of hydrochloric acid therapy and a nutritious diet. If, by chance, the man's spleen was enlarged, the option of splenectomy would be raised. Technological development, diagnostic advance, and therapeutic specialism brought increasing complexity and uncertainty to the once individualistic practice of diagnosis, therapy, and outcome evaluation. This diversity of disease perspectives reveals that the modern hospital was truly an embarrassment of riches, in search of organization and vision.

In the midst of these advances, many physicians clung to a scientific tradition free of commercial folly, believing that a natural, unpredictable, progressive, degenerative, and fatal clinical trajectory defined pernicious anemia. At their most traditional, such believers voiced staunch skepticism about all of these newfangled treatments, cures, and diagnostic innovations. In 1917, Ralph Larrabee referred with irritation to those who forgot that pernicious anemia was by nature an enigmatic disease: "[A] fact which renders difficult an estimation of the value of treatment in this disease is its proneness to undergo remissions—periods during which the patient is much relieved, or even apparently well."[80] So constructed, the disease was designed to reveal the folly of modern therapeutic arrogance. To Larrabee, this disease necessarily implied a therapeutic modesty that few of his medical peers embodied. Larrabee remained perplexed at some physicians' grand claims about curing pernicious anemia. He wrote that the disease's tendency toward remissions, "is perfectly well known to all students of the disease and yet we see, again and again, cases reported as 'apparently cured' or even as 'cured' without qualification, two or three months after some new method of treatment. As remissions lasting over a year are common under any form of treatment, the absurdity of such words is obvious."[81] This mixture of humility and skepticism was evident even in George Minot's thinking when he wrote in 1917 that "judgement about the results of therapy are difficult on account of the natural tendency for remission in the disease."[82]

From 1900 to 1925, hospital bureaucracy, specialization, and an enduring therapeutic humility had left their marks on medical constructions of pernicious anemia. Most of the specialists of the 1910s envisioned *dis-*

ease as the functional failure of particular organ systems. Whether gastric, splenic, neurological, or hematological symptoms were primary or secondary, causal or subsidiary, reflected professional tensions and commitments concerning the hierarchy among specialties. General practitioners of the era, however, believed that pernicious anemia was a complex amalgam. A few held to traditional views of this disease as an enigmatic natural entity. Unlike the generation of academic doctors who had brought pernicious anemia into American medical literature, few among the new breed of specialists wondered how moral influences or lifestyle affected the course of relapses and remissions. The new specialists consciously sought to abstract the disease from the moral matrix of patients' lives. The disease possessed a clinically fragmented, organic identity that reinforced specialization and the search for organic causation.

In reviews of literature, small conferences of experts, and books published on the spleen, the blood, and the stomach, specialists brought their preferred order and regularity to a fractured diagnostic and therapeutic situation.[83] How they thought about disease depended upon the technologies deployed within the hospital and on the social relations of hospital practice. Diagnostic tools and therapies constituted selection principles that, specialists believed, would sediment out the true disease from amorphous complexes of symptoms. Thus, pathologist E. B. Krumbhaar suggested that "the term pernicious anemia may later be found to include more than one clinical entity . . . If this were found to be true, it might well be that some of the discordant results that have been observed after splenectomy are due to the fact that the operation was of value in one or more types and contraindicated in others."[84] As Krumbhaar's thoughts reveal, some physicians were well aware of the ways in which available technologies were rewriting the disease's identity. Most specialists had faith that somewhere amidst this complexity lay a simple answer. Yet, as I've pointed out in previous chapters, by the late 1910s and early 1920s, the problems of specialization and therapeutic individualism were clear. Against this backdrop, it is not surprising that the need for standardization, the regulation of diagnostic techniques and therapeutic practices, and the management of clinical work relationships were underlying themes in the review literature, in conferences, and in disease treatises of the period.

In 1916, Harvard-associated physicians organized a conference of specialists from across the country to discuss the various rationales for defining and managing pernicious anemia. Most of those present concerned themselves with the proper relationship between key symptoms. Did spinal cord changes disappear with improvements in the blood picture? Should transfusion always precede splenectomy? Will the neurological aspects of the disease disappear with the administration of HCl or with blood transfusion? How was one to define "improvement" in pernicious anemia patients—by observing their blood, their neurological symptoms, or the overall appearance of the sick person? Opinions varied, depending on the specialist's frame of reference.[85]

George Minot, Harvard Research, and the New Pernicious Anemia

A few of these specialists were also university-based physicians, undertaking their own search for order, situating themselves in newly created research clinics. Such centers claimed to be removed from narrow specialty debates about diagnostic and therapeutic rules of conduct.[86] In 1911, William Osler suggested that more hospitals should be taken over by such university men: "We need an invasion of the hospitals by the universities . . . The men in charge of the units must be paid salaries sufficient . . . to give it the first place in their lives . . . In the United States," Osler noted, "these changes are rapidly progressing."[87] George Minot's own career reflected these trends. In the early 1910s, Minot began at the Massachusetts General Hospital and worked for a time in Roger Lee's "blood ward." New research facilities such as the Collis P. Huntington Hospital and the Peter Bent Brigham Hospital sprang up around the medical campus, created by philanthropic endowment and geared to the study of specific diseases. In 1923, Minot became chief of the Huntington's medical service. In the same year, the research culture spread to Boston City Hospital, which created the Thorndike Memorial Laboratory—the nation's first research facility associated with a municipal hospital.[88] Such dedicated research sites established a new context for the selective deployment of medical tools and fostered new modes of knowledge production.

New institutional arrangements placed researchers far from crowds of clinicians and competing specialists. The by-product was reordered thinking about such diseases as cancer and pernicious anemia.[89] Like many of his peers, Minot searched throughout the 1910s and early 1920s for a simple principle for defining true pernicious anemia. Working closely with surgeon Beth Vincent, blood specialists Roger Lee and Ralph Larrabee, and pathologist J. H. Wright, Minot also came to appreciate the multidimensional character of pernicious anemia. But as a blood specialist himself, Minot appreciated the special role of blood in pernicious anemia. As early as 1911, he suggested that the "reticulocyte count" could be taken as a key measure of marrow activity in pernicious anemia. Eight years later, having accumulated experience using hemacytometers and staining methods in reading blood, Minot began to criticize the "mistakes" and "confusions" in general discussions of blood disease.[90]

This cooperative environment (in which Minot interacted with colleagues, yet developed his hematological convictions) nurtured a flexible research ethos. Isolated from clinical politics, researchers focused on the study of specific physiological mechanisms to establish the legitimacy of one disease perspective over another. They sat in judgment of clinical practice. Between 1920 and 1926, George Minot and William Murphy were given institutional freedom that few clinicians enjoyed. They enjoyed enormous freedom to observe, triage, treat, manage, and reclassify patients with pernicious anemia. Minot was quite secretive about their work—a privilege that few ordinary clinicians could obtain.

From their studies, they defined "true pernicious anemia" on the basis of hematological symptoms, other symptoms becoming secondary. Diagnosis was never made in haste or to satisfy the needs of patients, and only one therapeutic modality was tested at a time.[91] Delayed diagnosis, therapeutic focus, and long-term supervision were not privileges easily obtained in routine medical practice; they were, however, privileges of university-based medicine. In 1926, Minot and Murphy published a brief statement in the *Journal of the American Medical Association (JAMA)*, announcing that a regimen of liver feeding had restored a large number pernicious anemics to apparently normal health. This finding emerged from a new research context and depended heavily on their ability to use technologies of diagnosis and therapy free from the bureaucracy and day-to-day moral economies of clinical work.

Two anecdotes illustrate the stark contrast between research culture and hospital culture, between the values, assumptions, and practices of the researcher and the physician during this era. Well before 1926, pathologist George Whipple had worked on producing a kind of pernicious anemia in dogs and experimenting with various dietary treatments. (Whipple would later receive the Nobel Prize, along with Murphy and Minot, for this work.) In a paper published after the Minot and

Murphy paper, Whipple suggested that liver treatment might have been discovered earlier but for entrenched clinical prejudices. Whipple recalled that in 1918 he had convinced a young clinician in a San Francisco hospital to treat pernicious anemics with a liver extract. "About ten years ago," noted Whipple, "Dr. Hooper, who was associated with me then, made an alcoholic extract of liver and got permission from the medical clinic to use it in several cases. In two of those cases there was remission." These findings had been rejected because of ingrained clinical beliefs that the disease had a natural course of relapses and remissions. "Dr. Hooper received so many amused and critical comments from the medical staff [who claimed that the remissions were spontaneous] that he discontinued the work, much to our regret."[92] For Whipple, the anecdote highlighted how a valuable discovery had been ignored because of entrenched clinical beliefs. Research units, by contrast, provided a liberating environment for the Dr. Hopper's of American medicine. Clinical research placed decision making into the hands of the inquisitive individual researcher, placing knowledge production above patient care per se.

Research institutions constructed a new ethic concerning the use of technologies, and they endorsed a new identity for physician and disease. William Murphy recalled a story from his days at the Brigham hospital, which further exemplifies this trend. By the early 1900s, blood transfusions—admittedly temporary "blood-building" measures—had become a common treatment for pernicious anemia, particularly for patients in severe decline. In 1917, Minot had insisted that, despite its limitations, "No case is too sick for transfusion. Transfusion can give rapidly symptomatic benefit."[93] After early, promising indications about the value of liver feeding, the Brigham's director continued to lay down a conservative research policy. As Murphy recalled, "[He] knew the benefits of transfusion lasted only a few weeks, [and] he was not willing to compromise the patient's condition in any way." But in order to establish the efficacy of liver therapy in its own right, Murphy later recalled, "it was important not to complicate the liver treatment with transfusion. [In one case] I stayed up very late trying to decide whether to give him the transfusion or give him the liver."[94] Murphy wanted to deny transfusion and continue the liver diet, especially in the dying patient. Contrary to the director's policy, he suspended the transfusions. Day after day, according to his story, the patient's blood levels fell, he became weaker, and he seemed to be heading for certain death. But one morning, he made a

miraculous recovery.[95] The inquisitive research ethos enabled this conduct in diagnosis, therapeutics, and therapeutic evaluation.

Minot and Murphy's work signaled only the opening stages of the
redefinition and conquest of the disease, the start of a complex shift in
academic medical practices, research values, and assumptions about the
blood, liver diet, and disease. Moreover, these researchers promoted the
disease's subtle reconstruction. Even as they announced the benefits of
liver, Minot and Murphy excluded many patients traditionally characterized as pernicious anemics from their studies.[96] They chose not to
dwell on any problems of disease classification, noting only that their observations were made on "forty-five patients with *typical* pernicious anemia" (472). Nor did they describe the spinal cord problems, gastrointestinal disturbance, splenic symptoms, or subtleties in the differential
administration of liver and blood transfusions. Their primary focus was
on the diet and blood. "While the problem of diet in the treatment of pernicious anemia is by no means new," they wrote, "in our opinion its possible importance has not heretofore been generally recognized." The relationship between diet and the blood, they noted, was a classic concern,
for "even Shakespeare recognized that improper food might impair the
state of the blood" (470). The study was also current in its appeal. Citing
the popular 1923 book, E. V. McCollum's *Newer Knowledge of Nutrition,*
the authors pointed to the general rise of popular interest in vitamins
and the other components of a healthy diet.

In medical memory, the story of these forty-five patients exemplified the triumph of modern academic medicine and its new experimental tools, but the story, as told at the time, started and ended ambiguously. In their study, neither liver treatments nor hematological responses
were uniform. Minot and Murphy noted that "our data strongly suggest
that the patients who commenced treatment in the hospital and those few
able to have a trained nurse at home have improved on average rather
faster and to an even better degree than the others." The diets made patients "much better," but were not uniformly curative. "All except one,
who has recently omitted her diet, are now at the least in a very fair state
of health, and if it were not for disorders in some due to spinal cord lesions, would have an appearance to a layman of being essentially well"
(471). The authors did not attempt to explain these "spinal cord lesions,"
nor did they see these symptoms (as might a neurologist) as essential to
the disorder. Indeed, they were more concerned with the influence of diet
on hematological improvement. "Following the diet," they wrote, "all

the patients showed a prompt, rapid and distinct remission of *their anemia*, coincident with at least a marked symptomatic improvement, except for pronounced disorders due to spinal cord degeneration" (emphasis added). Hematological improvement "was heralded in the peripheral blood . . . by the beginning of a most definite rise of the reticulocytes (young red blood corpuscles)." Between 1926 and 1934, a new dietary and hematological definition of pernicious anemia would emerge. Its initial discovery owed much to institutional changes and changes in the deployment of tools in this emerging research culture; its appeal and acceptance, however, can only be explained by exploring an emerging American consumerism, the culture of routine medical practice, and dramatic changes in medical-pharmaceutical relations in the 1920s.

The Pharmaceutical Construction of Disease, 1926–1934

The definition of pernicious anemia was still in flux, and its consolidation around the Harvard researchers' model depended upon the changing relationship between these researchers and the Eli Lilly pharmaceutical firm. The "truth" of their claim depended on advertising, marketing, and the patterns of drug prescription by physicians and drug consumption by patients. The immediate responses of physicians to the study by Minot and Murphy ranged from elation at a cure for pernicious anemia to entrenched skepticism. In time, however, the ways in which physicians and researchers used liver products led to a pragmatic redefinition of the disease along pharmaceutical lines.

After World War I, pharmaceutical companies and many medical researchers created new business relationships. While earlier academic physicians like William Osler had viewed the claims of the drug houses with great skepticism, after the war a mutual interest in research and cooperative enterprises brought academic physicians and drug companies closer together. As historian John Swann has noted, many new forms of collaboration emerged in the 1920s—industrial fellowships, grants, and consultantships to individual researchers. Exchanges of ideas between industrial and academic researchers occurred at annual medical meetings and through arranged lectures. A growing number of drug innovations resulted in university-corporate patents and production contracts.[97] By 1927, Eli Lilly began working with Harvard's Pernicious Anemia Commission to orchestrate the isolation and mass production of a marketable liver extract. The Eli Lilly–Harvard collaboration exemplified the corporate ideal of the 1920s. (Eli Lilly had also forged research agreements with the University of Toronto group on the production of insulin.) By 1928, Eli Lilly's "Liver Extract No. 343" was available for market, advertised as the "only product that had the unqualified approval of the Harvard Pernicious Anemia Commission."[98] The production and availability of this liver extract helped ensure that Minot's definition of pernicious anemia would become, for this crucial period, *the* definition of pernicious anemia.

Physicians had responded quickly (and for the most part, enthusiastically) to the 1926 Minot-Murphy announcement in *JAMA*. When Lilly's liver extract appeared, they seized the opportunity to perform a study of their own, report a case successfully cured, or offer their own assessment of the drug. Some, like J. H. Means and Wyman Richardson, reported that "the change in the physiological picture that occurs in some of these people [was] a little short of miraculous."[99] One physician at the Massachusetts General Hospital mocked the use of splenectomy as a supposed "surgical cure" of pernicious anemia. "It seems to me that temporarily, at least, any question of splenectomy in pernicious anemia is absolutely relegated to the dump heap," he pronounced. "There is no doubt whatever that anybody would rather eat liver than have his spleen removed."[100] Liver therapy and liver extract provided a simple dietary intervention that was quick and noninvasive, and in the late 1920s many physicians published reports of their dramatic benefits.[101]

Other physicians reported mixed results. Armand Cohen of Louisville, Kentucky, found that in one of his cases, although Eli Lilly's Liver Extract No. 343 had reduced the anemia, there was "no marked improvement in symptoms referable to the central nervous system."[102] At one 1928 medical conference, a group of researchers from Michigan's Henry Simpson Memorial Institute confirmed that, "while a great majority of our patients with pernicious anemia have shown an immediate and gratifying response to treatment with liver, there has been a small group in whom the results were less satisfactory. The patients who have not responded in a satisfactory manner to the liver therapy may be classified in three main groups."[103] In the first group were patients who had been given too little liver. Second were those with "definite and marked progression in the neurological signs" (three of twenty-five patients). Third were those with acute infections that apparently affected the potency of the liver. In all, the Simpson Institute study stated that about 20 percent of the patients with pernicious anemia did not benefit from Liver Extract No. 343. "With the advent of liver therapy, and its remarkable effects on the blood picture," wrote one British researcher, "it was thought by some and hoped by many that a panacea for all the evils of pernicious anemia had arrived. As far as the spinal cord symptoms are concerned this has not proved to be the case."[104] But were these nonrecoverers "truly" pernicious anemics, some physicians wondered? Or were these exceptional cases?

Already in 1928, there had emerged a pragmatic tendency among many physicians to use liver as a de facto diagnostic technology for pernicious anemia.[105] There were several reasons for this style of practice. Liver extract was more effective than any existing treatment for pernicious anemia; it was also less invasive, and it was an easily consumed product. So dramatic were the effects of liver extract that researchers were inclined to reclassify all unimproved patients as "anomalous," "atypical," or subject to "complications."[106] More than a few physicians objected to the way in which liver was becoming a kind of diagnostic technique—structuring not only medical practice and research, but also medical thinking about the identity of the disease. To some commentators, this shift in medical thinking was nothing more than crass commercialism.

Physicians and researchers who objected to this commercial pragmatism found themselves, however, on the horns of an ethical dilemma: with the prevalence of liver extract on the market, how could anyone *not* use it as a diagnostic test for pernicious anemia? William Middleton of Wisconsin argued that the "indiscriminate use of liver in all types of anemia should be discouraged as confusing the picture of undiagnosed blood diseases, [and] creating an empirical practice."[107] Yet "empirical practice" was financially and morally rewarding and efficient. In one study from the Simpson Memorial Institute, two researchers fell in step with the diagnostic trend, noting that they had studied "a series of 150 patients . . . in whom the diagnosis has been established by every known clinical procedure of value, *including the therapeutic response to liver extract*" (emphasis added).[108] Minot himself would later regret that "there has been a tendency in recent years . . . to decide at once that liver is indicated . . . Often [it] has been prescribed before a diagnosis and the actual needs of the patient have been firmly established or intelligently considered."[109] When faced with a patient suspected as a pernicious anemic, most physicians found liver extract a more satisfying diagnostic procedure than "intelligent consideration." By 1928, Liver Extract No. 343 was widely available, easy to use, and likely to provoke some kind of hematological and clinical response in anemic patients. The popularity of prescribing liver extract was a compelling force, altering the identity of pernicious anemia.

The consumer drug market and the availability of liver extract also limited alternative research views on pernicious anemia. In 1930, William Needles of the Neurological Division of New York's Montefiore Hospital observed that, although there was "profound skepticism in certain quarters as regards both its prophylactic and its remedial properties . . . at the present time, no one will be rash enough to deprive patients of treatment with liver to prove the point one way or the other."[110] Needles confirmed that, despite his own "profound skepticism" about the value of liver extract, most physicians believed they were morally obligated to deploy the drug in cases of anemia. For researchers with alternative views of pernicious anemia, he noted, the search for the truth was reduced to collecting "observations that were made by clinicians before liver was given."[111]

Faced with such constraints, many researchers chose a middle ground between praise and skepticism about the liver cure.[112] This ambivalence was well expressed by two Albany, New York, physicians (Thomas Ordway and L. W. Gorham) at the 1928 annual convention of the American Medical Association (AMA). They reviewed some 578 cases culled from the growing medical literature and reported on an additional 25 new cases. They excluded many cases that, ten years earlier, would have been labeled "pernicious anemia." "Cases above [red blood cell count of] 2,800,000 were excluded, together with borderline cases in which the diagnosis was uncertain" because they did not conform to new diagnostic criteria.[113] They employed Eli Lilly's Liver Extract No. 343 "furnished to us through the courtesy of the Pernicious Anemia Commission." Their results were largely positive, with exceptions being (1) cases with infection and other complications, (2) patients given insufficient liver, (3) cases where the management had been complicated with blood transfusion, and (4) a small number of "unexplainable failures."[114]

Was liver extract a cure for pernicious anemia? Ordway and Gorham concluded that, on one hand, liver "has no effect on the underlying pathological process and hence cannot be called a cure."[115] Nonetheless, they called the discovery "epoch-making, . . . [offering] a brilliant example of the successful application of scientific methods to the solution of clinical problems." Even if liver treatment was not a cure, it provided a strong endorsement of the clinical investigator and his by-products. A few hematological specialists like J. P. Schneider, who had worked with "blood diseases" for fifteen years, objected to this habit of "taking a narrow view of the disease." Others like E. B. Krumbhaar tried to remain consistent with their preliver commitments. Krumbhaar believed that pernicious anemia was not one, but *many* diseases: "To those who would look at the diagnosis of pernicious anemia [before 1926] as covering a group of diseases, we should say that due to our imperfections perhaps it still is today."[116] For a growing number of practitioners in late 1920s consumer-oriented culture, however, therapeutic empiricism had its distinct appeal. For them, there would be only one pernicious anemia, and its identity would be linked to liver extract. For at least one blood specialist in 1929, "a craving for liver" became part of the essence of the disease.[117]

At the core of medical ambivalence about the pharmaceutical definition of pernicious anemia, one finds deep-seated concerns about commercialism in medicine. Was medicine to be a economic trade or an intellectual pursuit? Was this new identity for pernicious anemia a kind of medical thinking that was (to paraphrase Roger Lee) designed to please the heads of pharmaceutical houses? As historian Roland Marchand has argued, the flowering of advertising, mass production, and mass consumption in the 1920s was a complex phenomenon, involving the mediation of taste by professional advertisers. Medical professionals also played a role in the mediation of taste. Historian T. J. Jackson Lears has noted that health, therapeutic, and physiological motifs were central to the advertising of the day.[118] One advertisement for Lucky Strike cigarettes stated that they were designed "to make the red blood leap and tingle!" Another spot for Home Billiards declared that the product "puts new blood into folks who work all day!"[119] The concept of a liver pill that cured by transforming the blood fit neatly into these motifs. Commercial appeals of this kind reinforced the new hematological identity of pernicious anemia.

Those who were skeptical about the therapeutic claims for Eli Lilly's Liver Extract No. 343 were voicing deep suspicions about these corporate developments and the various business interests that benefited from these claims. When a Seattle-based newspaper man gave his opinion of the medical profession in the pages of a 1929 issue of *Northwest Medicine*, he portrayed the "cure" of pernicious anemia as nothing more than a public relations ploy, a story promoted by the alliance of Eastern medical elites and the meat industry. "Within the last two years," the newspaperman wrote, "the medical profession has probably made a million or so dollars for the butchers and meat packers by turning what used to be considered almost a by-product of the slaughterhouse into a food of the highest class and reputation. I refer to liver and the new fad of eating it to offset anemia and other ailments."[120] A disease that twenty years earlier had been known only to a handful of specialists had become prevalent and had become the basis for legitimating all kinds of culinary taste and commercial enterprise.

The irony of this "new discovery," according to this writer, was that it ignored the true achievers in favor of the enrichment of Harvard doctors and the meat industry. He claimed to know two or three Portland doctors who had used liver for anemia years before the 1926 discovery was announced. "It was not a year after that until these eastern doctors translated this liver theory into language for popular comprehension and they rose to some degree of fame and the meat industry cashed in on it."[121] In this skeptical account, not only were local nonspecialists denied rightful credit for their simple observations, but a public relations coup—orchestrated by academics and industrialists—had captured the beliefs of a hapless public. In 1931, when *Popular Science Monthly* awarded Minot and Murphy for the conquest of pernicious anemia, no such skepticism appeared.

By the late 1920s, the identity of pernicious anemia had been recast. But what would be done with cases of pernicious anemia where liver extract was ineffective? Any ambivalence between previous definitions of the disease and a therapeutic-hematological definition would be resolved through reclassification. One approach was to identify these cases as "complications." Another solution, used by Minot's colleague William Castle, grouped unrelieved neurological cases under the rubric of "combined system disease."[122] Later, in 1929, Castle would discover that, in some cases where liver feeding had failed, improvement resulted from feeding patients *predigested* liver or beef muscle. Thus could some anomalous cases be reassimilated into the pernicious anemia category, since these patients could be said to lack an "intrinsic factor" necessary to digest the liver.[123] Such redistributions of "anomalous" cases were powerful examples of how academic medicine continued to manage the identity of patients and disease.[124]

Minot promoted this new identity of pernicious anemia, suggesting that response to liver extract was the crucial diagnostic marker:

> There are patients with conditions which may resemble pernicious anemia, and others with various simple sorts of anemia, who are not benefitted by this therapy. Thus, errors concerning the value of a diet rich in liver or an effective fraction may be made if the diagnosis of pernicious anemia is not correctly established. This is emphasized because, if the treatment is properly carried out and a distinct improvement in the health of the patient is not apparent in four weeks, it is probable that the diagnosis of pernicious anemia is incorrect.[125]

In 1934, the Nobel Committee announced that George Minot, William Murphy, and George Whipple had been awarded the Nobel Prize in Medicine or Physiology for this path-breaking work on pernicious anemia. In his acceptance speech Minot walked the same fine diagnostic line.[126]

By 1934, the *disease* had been *reconstructed around the antidote*. Pernicious anemia was a disease curable by liver therapy.[127] The key research question in the post–liver extract era was not "Why did liver extract not help many pernicious anemics?" Rather, physicians and researchers asked, "What disease did these patients 'really have'?" In their effort to resolve this question, the disease would become even more fragmented in subsequent years—pernicious anemia, researchers would gradually rediscover, came in many varieties. Some suggested that pernicious anemia was a folic acid deficiency, others argued that it was a vitamin B_{12} deficiency, others that it was an autoimmune disease. Years later hematologist William Dameshek would recoil at the implied association of liver extract and pernicious anemia, noting that "liver extract is of value in one condition only—liver extract deficiency."[128] (This growing complexity in the disease's identity after the 1930s is discussed briefly in ch. 6.) In 1934, however, medical researchers had achieved near consensus on the singular pharmaceutical identity of pernicious anemia.

Hematology, Consumer Culture, and Corporate Validation

The biography of pernicious anemia traces out three phases in the rise of academic medicine and its social relations. In all three phases, disease identity and medical identity were mutually constitutive. In all three phases, hematological tools and their interpretation played a crucial role in the validation of these identities.

In the 1890s academic scientists had focused on defining a natural history of this separate entity—a goal consistent with their scientific interests, their commercial skepticism, and their moralistic commitment to patient care. For them, pernicious anemia was an enigmatic blood disease closely intertwined with the lifestyle of patients. Putting one's faith in a drug or a tonic to cure pernicious anemia, they believed, was nothing short of commercial folly. It was also profoundly unscientific. For researchers like William Osler and George Dock, medical science could only be corrupted by commercial interests. The identity of pernicious anemia reflected their own identity as independent-minded medical scientists and moralistic practitioners.

In the disease's bureaucratic phase, pernicious anemia encountered the modern hospital, where competing specialists vied to define key organic aspects of the disease. By focusing on its organic aspects, these hospital-based specialists sought to remove the disease from all moral, dietary, and nutritional associations, exploring only those aspects that could be subject to organ-centered management. The hospital was rapidly becoming the specialists' workshop. How they perceived this disease reflected their own shifting alliances and institutional arrangements. Some saw pernicious anemia as a blood disease, others saw it as a neurological disorder, others viewed it as a gastrointestinal disorder, and yet others perceived it as a splenic malady. These identities of pernicious anemia revealed the faces of medical specialists themselves, their deployment of preferred technologies, and their struggles to adjust to a newly cooperative workplace.

The hematological-dietary image of pernicious anemia—in some ways a rather traditional view of disease—would be rediscovered by Minot and Murphy in 1926, but in a context set apart from nineteenth-century dietary moralism and from the bureaucratic hospital.[129] By the early 1910s, such university-based researchers were allowed to oversee novel approaches to knowledge production. But it was in forging alliances with the Eli Lilly Company that Minot and Murphy inspired an enthusiastic therapeutic redefinition of pernicious anemia. In this phase, Eli Lilly's Liver Extract No. 343 became a crucial technology, its mass production and use redefining established medical thought. By the late 1920s, American academic physicians had rationalized the disease's identity around the commodity—liver extract. They took liver as a kind of reductionist deus ex machina—at once diagnosis, cure, and their legitimation.

One patient's story highlights the difference between my story of the changing clinical construct called pernicious anemia and the neatness of the conquest narrative. In 1927, the aged mother of Eli Lilly (the founder of the pharmaceutical giant) had been diagnosed with pernicious anemia, and the family consulted George Minot. Minot suggested a calf's liver extract, which resulted in an apparently miraculous recovery.[130] The incident may have intensified the company's interest in collaborating with Harvard in the production of a liver extract, which the firm began selling in 1928. Taken to its conclusion, however, this story of dramatic rejuvenation ends ambiguously. George Minot's liver extract brought Mrs. Lilly only "temporary relief." By late 1929, Mrs. Lilly was bedridden. And in the same year that George Minot traveled to Sweden to receive his Nobel Prize, she died of pernicious anemia.[131]

As the ironic case of Mrs. Lilly makes clear, the "conquest" of pernicious anemia was a popular success, a marked advance in the technology of therapy, but it also involved a questionable act of academic reclassification. In 1938, any physician could state with assurance that "if an anemia does not respond to liver therapy, we may, it is true, rest assured that it is not pernicious anemia."[132] Osler and his contemporaries would have balked at such a claim. To a minority in the 1930s, it was clear that liver extract had not cured the disease, but merely altered its presumed identity—privileging and validating an academic-pharmaceutical construction.

As if to explain the plight of the Mrs. Lilly's of the world, in 1936 Wyndam Lloyd—author of A Hundred Years of Medicine—celebrated the discovery of liver treatment, but noted the ironic rise of "the progressively paralyzing complaint known by the cumbrous name 'subacute combined degeneration of the spinal cord' . . . Since 1927, after which liver extract was widely used, the number of deaths from subacute combined spinal degeneration have nearly doubled. Presumably this means that the patients who would formerly have died very rapidly have now been kept alive long enough for them to develop the late nervous sequel."[133] These deaths were never identified as deaths from pernicious anemia per se. They were attributed to some other disease that had appeared as a sequela of successful liver treatment. Such patients, who Osler would have described as pernicious anemics, were now classed as "anomalous" cases, complications, or sufferers of a new malady. Even with their death, the image of conquest could be preserved. Indeed, a signal achievement of modern academic medicine's system of knowledge production was its ability to redefine such therapeutic failures as new research problems.

This dialectic of mutual construction between technology and disease continued beyond the era of conquest. A certain kind of progress in the fight against pernicious anemia came with the deployment of liver extract, its extensive use, and the subsequent construction of new disease categories. In later years, other technologies—more precise hematological analysis like the Schilling test, folic acid, vitamin B_{12}—would also lead to shifts in classification. Some of these developments would lead to the reintegration of some "anomalous" cases into the class of "true" pernicious anemics; others would not.[134] The work of William Castle provides a case in point. Studying a group of patients with combined spinal degeneration in the early 1930s, Castle discovered that, while their illness could *not* be alleviated by liver extract alone, they gained some relief from partially digested liver.[135] With such diagnostic and therapeutic innovations, some of these anomalous patients could once again be considered pernicious anemics.

Disease identification continued to be a negotiated process, heavily informed in the 1920s and in later decades by clinical research and by collaborations between researchers and pharmaceutical firms. (In an era before the Food and Drug Administration became active in overseeing these corporate relationships, the validation of cures occurred within such business settings.) For physicians, drug manufacturers, and the medical profession at large, hematological analysis became a tool in the commercial validation of drugs. Commercial validation was the core issue, for example, in a 1935 discussion within the AMA's Council on Pharmacy and Chemistry, which sought to determine the efficacy of various liver extracts.

Manufacturers made it clear to the council that they favored definitions of disease and cure that reflected favorably on their own commodities. In accepting or rejecting liver preparations, the council wanted to use "as criteria of potency, the reticulocyte response in uncomplicated cases."[136] These standards, however, were not acceptable to liver extract manufacturers. "Some firms believed the reticulocyte response [in humans], if called for as a standard, is too high."[137] They argued that blood studies in animals were more reliable. They knew that hematology held a central place in identifying both disease and cure and therefore in endorsing their product. Whether patients like Mrs. Lilly actually improved, they argued, was not a reliable criterion for judging their product. As one physician noted, "There was practically universal objection to the use of humans in standardizing products . . . The firms now claim that human material is altogether too limited and it is impossible to get cases that come within the limitations of the specifications."[138] In keeping with company demands, the council advocated a narrow hematological determination of "cure."

At the same time, manufacturers and council physicians agreed that "all references be omitted to the relationship between raw liver and this standard [of hematological cure]," thus avoiding any evaluation of unprocessed commodities and maintaining an expert ownership of the disease. A cure could *not* be purchased at the corner butcher shop. Several independent physicians, by contrast, acknowledged that "dried hog's stomach worked just as well as liver extract . . . Furthermore," one writer stated, "it was shown that certain commercial vegetable products, notably marmite (a substance prepared from yeast), were equally effective."[139] Yet most academic physicians and manufacturers, in their public pronouncements, denied any relationship between these more widely available food products and pernicious anemia. It was this kind of collaboration between academics and the manufacturers that led Roger Lee later to decry how the "articles of medical men in the medical press often take on the flavor of advertisements for commercial nostrums."[140]

The therapeutic definition of pernicious anemia reflected a "corporate conquest" of pernicious anemia, a popular consumer-oriented style of disease definition. The disease's new identity depended upon the manufacturing, packaging, advertising, and promotion of the cure both within medicine and to the general public. It also depended upon the collaboration of academic researchers and empirical medical practitioners. The identity of the disease was thus a by-product of social relationships—particularly the evolving relationship of medical researchers, pharmaceutical companies like Eli Lilly, general practitioners, and consumption-oriented patients. As historian Owsei Temkin has noted, increasingly in the twentieth century "health began to take on the nature of a purchasable good . . . [and following from this,] the disease picture since the middle of the twentieth century differs from that of around 1900."[141]

Once liver extract appeared on the medical market, physicians worked hard to convince the public that the true cure for pernicious anemia could not be purchased from a butcher shop. It could be found only in a doctor's office. In a 1931 Massachusetts radio broadcast, for example, one physician warned his listeners against the "use and abuse of liver diet," suggesting that many people were becoming sick after unsupervised consumption of liver. "I dare say, many of you are taking liver, believing it will perform some miracle, when it is, in fact, only providing you with good food."[142] At the same time popular books on "liver diet" appeared.[143] Academic medicine, which had once eschewed the market, now sought to regulate consumer perceptions of the marketplace. Clearly, many patients believed that liver and blood were linked in many different ways. To the extent that they accepted the specific link between pernicious anemia and liver extract, they also expressed faith in the new corporate research relationships and the commercial forces that brought them such products in the 1920s.

5

Detecting "Negro Blood"
*Black and White Identities and the Reconstruction
of Sickle Cell Anemia*

The standard story of sickle cell anemia begins with James B. Herrick, who in 1910 discovered "peculiar, elongated and sickle-shaped red blood corpuscles" in a Negro patient with severe anemia.[1] His report has long been regarded as a landmark in clinical and hematological observation. After Herrick's observations, a second milestone came when Verne Mason and John Huck, using a new blood analysis technique, hypothesized that this was a hereditary disorder occurring only in Negroes.[2] Huck argued that the disease passed from one generation to the next according to the Mendelian laws regulating a dominant trait. That is, it could be transmitted from one parent to his or her offspring, independent of the other parent's genetic endowment. For those concerned with racial relations in the United States during the 1920s, the Mendelian dominant thesis meant that interracial marriages would probably spread the blood disease outward from the Negro population into negligent whites.

From 1910 through the 1940s, physicians developed and promoted this view of sickle cell anemia. As one Detroit physician wrote in 1926, "If . . . sicklemia [the tendency to develop sickle cells] is a dominant Mendelian characteristic, and if it is now as common as it seems to be in Detroit, shall we not in a few generations have a Negro population, the majority of whom show this peculiarity, and will not 'sickle cell anemia' then become a common condition?"[3] It was a disease of "Negro blood," whose very nature carried vital implications for black Americans and for others in American society. The concept of *blood* was a convenient catchall, collapsing within it ideas about heredity, kin, clan, and community in the same way that the term *genes* does today.

This chapter sheds light on the social forces and beliefs that acted in concert with the technology of blood analysis between 1910 and 1950 to shape the identity of this disease of Negro blood. In the late 1940s geneticist J. V. Neel and physical chemist Linus Pauling, using new techniques of blood analysis, put forth a new thesis. Viewed from the perspective of the molecular biologist, this was not a Mendelian dominant disorder, but a disorder that depended on the inheritance of recessive traits from *both* parents. This is the currently accepted view of the heritability of sickle cell anemia; the disease could not be spread outward by one member of an affected population.[4] Earlier generations of physicians had used blood analysis to detect the "tendency of blood cells to sickle," and according to molecular biologists they had confused this trait with the disease. These earlier physicians had gone on to make specious claims about the potential spread of this dangerous disorder.

Twentieth-century medical science has thus created two very different identities for sickle cell anemia. The social implications of the new post–World War II thesis were dramatically different from those stemming from the older Mendelian thesis.[5] According to the new construction, marrying "outward" would not spread the disease and might even reduce its incidence. This new thesis represented the beginning of a new chapter in the relationship of molecular biology and genetics with medicine.[6] With the advent of these disciplines, post–World War II physicians and historians could comfortably argue that earlier writers were simply mistaken and that former ideas about the hereditary and social implications of sickle cell anemia should be ignored. Lacking modern diagnostic tools and using inappropriate genetic theories, early twentieth-century authors had focused on what later became erroneous, unscientific beliefs like "Negro blood" to explain disease.[7]

These potent associations between blood, identity, and social relations—central to the growing authority of early twentieth-century hematology—were now seen as misguided. Scientists like Linus Pauling, J. V. Neel, and their hematologist peers represented a new order and new conceptions. They used new methods of electrophoretic analysis and focused on the hemoglobin molecule within red blood cells. The red blood cells were sickled not because they embodied Negro blood, but because the aggregation of abnormal hemoglobin molecules inside these cells caused the cells to take a sickled form. This led to clinical problems including thrombosis, infections, painful crises, and death.[8] In a now classic paper, Pauling and his colleagues labeled sickle cell anemia a "molecular disease," and within a few years this model had become a conceptual cornerstone in the construction of molecular biology.

The new identity of sickle cell anemia as a molecular disease demonstrated the clear applicability of the emerging discipline in medicine and in society.[9] Abnormal hemoglobins could now be detected through electrophoretic diagnosis, and scientists envisioned the day when the disease might be cured on the molecular level. In a 1951 article in *Scientific American*, researcher George Gray speculated that "it is conceivable, for example, that chemists may be able to devise a small, innocuous molecule which will lock permanently on to the defective hemoglobin and prevent the abnormal molecule from misbehaving, without interfering with the transport of oxygen."[10] A true medical scientist did not ponder "Negro blood," "white blood," or "Aryan blood." The disease was a "hemoglobinopathy," defined by molecular features and interactions. Pauling's work exemplified a significant step in the modern understanding of sickle cell anemia. It endorsed a new set of tools for studying disease and a new identity for medical scientists.

The transformation of sickle cell anemia reveals another aspect of the problem of technology and disease identity in America. In one sense, this seems to be a simple story of how a novel technological understanding of disease supplanted an older one; a new culture of disease thought took form. Yet historians have failed to confront this as a cultural process and to scrutinize the diverse ways in which technologies constructed both "Negro blood" and "hemoglobinopathy." For many physicians in the early twentieth century, *Negro blood* was a term with clear technological origins and with biological, social, and public health meanings. These physicians based their view on what was at that time hematological evidence and scientific understanding of the genetics of the disorder.[11] Just as electrophoresis has been a preferred diagnostic tool since the 1950s, before 1950 another technique (Emmel's blood test) was central to the definition of sickle cell anemia. In many ways, Emmel's technique played an even more central role in the definition of sickle cell anemia than has electrophoresis since 1950. Examining the cultural history of this technique explains much about why physicians thought that sickle cell anemia was passed on as a Mendelian dominant character and provides a rich understanding of technology's severe implications for the conceptualization of disease and public health in America.

But more than technology and genetics was at work. The early history of sickle cell anemia tells a story about hematological technique, "race," and social order. Prevailing social assumptions about black-white relations structured the use and interpretation of Emmel's diagnostic tool. Beginning in 1920 and extending into the 1940s, a small number of case reports on "sickle cell anemia in whites" appeared in the medical press.[12] These cases confirmed what most physicians believed—that the capacity for developing sickle cell anemia could be spread through miscegenation. In 1943, one Louisiana physician bluntly proclaimed that "sickle cell anemia is a national health problem, especially in the United States." He argued that "intermarriages between Negroes and white persons directly endanger the white race by transmission of the sickling trait . . . Such intermarriages, therefore, should be prohibited by federal law."[13] In less strident language, a 1947 editorial in the *Journal of the American Medical Association (JAMA)* confirmed that "its occurrence depends entirely on the presence of Negro blood[;] even in extremely small amounts it appears that the *sine qua non* for the occurrence of sickle cell anemia is the presence of a strain, even remote, of Negro blood . . . The disease . . . is regularly found in countries where there is frank interbreeding with African people . . . Race is thus a strong etiological factor."[14] Throughout this period, miscegenation was characterized as the key reason for the appearance of sickled cells in "whites" and as the primary vehicle of transmission of Negro blood and this disease.

How did this discourse evolve from 1920 to the 1940s? Why was this view revised in the years after World War II? It is not enough merely to attribute such beliefs to "biological racism" or to the purposeful use of hereditary theory to oppress African Americans.[15] In understanding such discourses, historians have emphasized that it is also important to understand the integral but changing role of medical sciences in constructing "race."[16] In her 1966 book *Purity and Danger,* anthropologist Mary Douglas observed that all cultures have rules and rituals for drawing lines between the pure and the polluted.[17] The expert use of diagnostic technology and genetic theory to analyze the blood in sickle cell anemia constructed these lines and demonstrates the subtle, ritualized ways in which some hematologists endorsed social order and lines of racial segregation in America, while others undermined these norms.[18]

Negro Disease and Negro Blood

Studies of the biological peculiarities of "the Negro" and of racial immunity or susceptibility to disease have a long pedigree in American medicine.[19] In the late nineteenth and early twentieth centuries, the new mobility of African Americans—the so-called Great Migration from the rural South into urban centers in the North and South—stirred discussions about Negro health in all regions and among many medical professionals. Dire predictions of the gradual decline and extinction of emancipated blacks had begun to subside in the face of demographic growth and mobility.[20] Through the imposition of Jim Crow restrictions, the rise in lynching, and other efforts, anxious whites sought to delimit black mobility.[21] Public discussions of the race problem abounded, and overt hostility toward black Americans and European immigrants peaked in what John Higham has labeled "the tribal twenties."[22]

Medical commentaries on so-called Negro diseases provided a powerful idiom for the expression of fear about this fluid social order. In 1910, one could hear a Southern physician evoke the "syphilitic Negro" as a comment upon political relations. "If the healthy Negro is a political menace, then the diseased one is doubly a social menace," he wrote, "and the invasion of the South by the North forty years ago has brought about an invasion of the North, and that by the man they freed."[23] Medical authors pondered the high incidence of tuberculosis, syphilis, and other venereal diseases among blacks, and their ideas established a framework for social policy.

Many of these commentators linked health differences to various aspects of Negro blood. Discussing mortality differences in "Negroes" and "whites," the authors of one 1903 textbook of legal medicine explained that "it is a generally known fact that . . . the mortality rate of mulattoes is greater than that of persons of pure Negro blood . . . On these accounts, it is essential for the medical examiner to investigate the question of ancestry carefully when there is suspicion of mixed blood." Exactness in blood findings (meaning family pedigree) could differentiate the acceptable insurance risk from the high-risk applicant. Such authors insisted that science, not prejudice, supported such findings, since "[insurance] companies do not discriminate against Negroes, but depend upon the warranty for correct information in regard to the race of which the applicant belongs."[24] Such questions of Negro blood had clear importance in the realm of social policy, for the possibility always existed that blood analysis might reveal authentic and valuable interrelations between identity and disease.

The close social proximity and economic relationships of blacks and whites was one factor that fed anxiety about the problem of Negro diseases. For some physicians, the very proximity of black workers in the homes of the white race and the large numbers of blacks in their region demanded attention to disease. According to one Alabama physician in 1923, "The Negro fills a most useful place in the economic welfare of the South, and there is every reason for so improving his condition that he will wish to remain . . . The medical professional and public health agencies in the South have never been called upon to render a greater service to their section than in this emergency of Negro labor exodus."[25] Another Dallas physician did not think it a digression, in discussing rectal pathology in the Negro, to note that "the obligation to concern himself with the question of disease in the more or less indolent, often dependent race, which makes up one tenth of our population and crowds our dispensaries, is mandatory—humanity impels and safety of the adjacent Caucasian race demands."[26] Negroes were the cooks, the maids, and the laborers in Southern households, and proximity posed clear, often hidden, hygienic concerns and responsibilities.[27]

Some authors argued that poverty and lack of access to medical information and care explained these differences in disease incidence between Negroes and whites. For others, disease indicated the inferior physical and moral constitution of the Negro race. Most frequently, physicians insisted that Negro disease resulted from a complex of factors. One Southern physician in 1932 suggested that "the safeguarding of the health of the Negro . . . [was] anything but an easy task, for the fight is not against disease, but against physical, mental, and moral inferiority, against ignorance and superstition, against poverty and filth."[28] Thus, writers on Negro diseases might focus on a wide range of issues: on moral character, on inborn features, on environmental conditions, or on economic deprivations. A significant sector of the American medical profession believed that health disparities stemmed from a natural inferiority.[29]

The questions of blood and blood degeneration touched these concerns particularly well, even as they highlighted the problem of black labor. In the 1910s, hookworm (known as the "germ of laziness" because of the anemia and lethargy that afflicted its sufferers) became a prominent Southern public health concern.[30] Enabled by the campaigns of the Rockefeller Sanitary Commission, many reformers saw the hookworm parasite as a symbol, if not as the cause of "backwardness, inefficiency, and laziness" among poor whites and blacks.[31] For some, disease explained identity. Anemia sapped energy and vitality, drew workers out of factories, and accounted for regional backwardness.[32] Public health enthusiasts like Charles Wardell Stiles proclaimed that the absence of outhouses and shoes in the rural south fed cycles of parasitic infection and anemia, but he believed that the Negro played a particular role in this cycle of regional laziness and disease.[33]

According to Stiles, "The Negro [is] a much more frequent soil polluter [and thus] a greater factor in the spread of the disease to others and its general dissemination throughout the community." He speculated that "this infection is more severe on the white race than on the Negro race . . . This thought must be very disquieting to the white race."[34] The Negro may even have brought the disease "with him from Africa and because of his soil pollution has spread it broadcast throughout the South, thereby killing thousands and causing serious disease among tens of thousands of others."[35] Thus, even in diseases with accepted origins in poverty, racial identity was a key to the proliferation of the pathology. The discussion of hookworm and anemia placed "the Negro"—soil polluter and disease vector—at the center of transmission.

In the early 1920s, similar concerns informed medical discussions of a new disease called "sickle cell anemia." When Virgil Sydenstricker of the University of Georgia presented one of the earliest talks on this new disease to a Southern medical audience in 1923, one of his colleagues rose to explain that this hereditary anemia was "of industrial, as well as medical importance. Efficiency is lowered in the adult and total disability is the result of recurrent attacks." "As we have plentiful supply of Negroes with us in the South," a fellow doctor offered, "it is important that we acquaint ourselves with this disease. I am quite convinced there is more [of it] in the South than is at present realized. It is therefore a Southern problem for us to work out."[36] It was not this regional theme, however, but the concern that sickle cell anemia was a latent, hidden disorder that physicians would repeat throughout the following decades. A potentially widespread, endemic, concealed, and hereditary anemia suggested trouble for Negro and non-Negro alike.

The individual Negro's inability to work featured prominently in clinical descriptions of the disorder. As one New Orleans physician noted in 1926, "The patient says that he has been 'sickly' and weak all his life and has never been able to 'pick up any strength.' Has never been able to do heavy work, or any kind of work when hurried. When attempting moderately heavy work, or on being hurried, he starts to 'tremble all over,' and has to lie down until it passes off."[37] Such a disease called for vigilance and careful study of the growing Negro population. One Pennsylvania physician suggested that "these cases should stimulate a more extensive search and study of similar cases in an increasing northern Negro population as well as among Southern Negroes."[38] By 1926, the new disease had confirmed and highlighted existing racial concerns—about black mobility, Negro disease, and the economic implications of disease in the Negro workforce.

Emmel's Blood Test and the Detection of Negro Blood

Concerns about the multiple dangers implicit in "Negro blood" informed the use and interpretation of Victor Emmel's diagnostic test, a tool that became the central method for identifying and detecting sickled cells.[39] To understand how sickle cell anemia became synonymous with "Negro blood," it is necessary to examine this technique closely. Its interpretation by physicians and hematologists sheds light on the central place of technologies in determining the meaning of sickled cells and thereby shaping disease identity and racial identity.

In 1916, Victor Emmel—an anatomist at the University of Washington—set out to investigate James Herrick's 1910 observations of sickle cell anemia. Since Herrick, only two other instances of the disorder had been reported.[40] In a 1917 paper, Emmel described a patient he saw in St. Louis' Barnes Hospital who had presented with the same symptoms described by Herrick. On a second visit by this patient, however, Emmel found none of the peculiar, sickle-shaped red blood cells in the blood he drew from her and observed under the microscope. Emmel then created what he called an "experimental technique" to observe these cells. He described how a ring of petroleum jelly could be drawn on a sterile glass slide, a fresh drop of the patient's blood was brought to rest in the center of the ring, and then the first slide was covered with a second. The technique confined the blood specimen in an "air-tight chamber" and held it at room temperature. After a few hours, Emmel found a "great abundance of these [sickled] structures" which made "a striking picture when viewed microscopically."[41] The test had induced the patient's cells to sickle.

A central feature of the disease's early history stems from how this technology was used to isolate so-called Negro blood. From 1917 onward, sickle cell anemia became less a *clinical* entity than a *technological* one. After his examination of the woman's blood, Emmel examined her father, who had (significantly) no symptoms of anemia or any other disease and in whose blood no sickled cells could be seen using the microscope. Using the experimental technique, however, his blood cells revealed a tendency to sickle. "Within one hour a large number of erythrocytes had assumed beautiful crescentic and sickle-shaped forms," Emmel wrote. Clearly, even though the man's circulating blood "had temporarily returned to an apparently more normal structure, they still retained the potentiality for transformation into the sickle-shaped forms."[42] Emmel cautiously suggested that his technique had diagnosed a "potential disease." As such, it was a hematological test for a latent disorder in a person who appeared to be healthy. Regardless of the patient's complaints, symptoms, or illness experiences, the technology could locate a disease. Truly, sickle cells were hidden, concealed and waiting to be found.[43]

As we have seen in previous chapters, practitioners during this era gave hematological analysis an expanded importance in clinical management and in arenas outside the hospital. Most physicians who studied sickle cell anemia in the 1920s and 1930s eagerly adopted Emmel's technique and his assumptions, and they turned to questions of comparative racial pathology and racial relations.[44] Many saw the sickle cell condition as a "latent condition," a potential disease.[45] In the early 1920s, for example, Virgil Sydenstricker used the technique to sample for the relative incidence of sickled cells in whites and blacks. "The blood of more than 300 white patients has been examined by us with special reference to 'latent sickling,'" he wrote, "and in no case has anything resembling it been seen. In a similar number of Negroes, it was found thirteen times." Sydenstricker had set out to test a statement put forth by Verne Mason in 1922 and believed that his finding "adds weight to Mason's hypothesis that sickle cell anemia is a condition peculiar to the Negro race."[46] Using Emmel's technique like most of his peers, Sydenstricker saw "latent" sickling as "the disease" itself.[47]

In the same year (1923), a young physician at Johns Hopkins Hospital, John Huck, and his colleague used Emmel's technique to study a black family. One family member had been diagnosed with sickle cell anemia. Huck, too, focused on the technological finding ("latent sickling" or what he called "sicklemia") rather than on patient complaints or clinical phenomena, seeking to determine the inheritance pattern of this potential disease. Most physicians agreed that this induced feature was *the* significant biological feature of the disease. Huck, for one, insisted that the "peculiar feature of the disease is the occurrence of crescentic or sickle-shaped erythrocytes when the blood is observed *in vitro* [that is, in Emmel's technique]."[48] On the basis of an incomplete study of the family's sickling potential, Huck created an inheritance chart of the disease which demonstrated that "sickle cell anemia behaves as a single Mendelian character which is dominant over the normal condition and . . . is not sex-linked."[49] Any parent could pass it on to his or her offspring, independent of the other parent's genetic endowment. This simple statement about a supposed hereditary mechanism had enormous biological and social implications.

The translation of hematological knowledge into social policy was, of course, a recognized area of expertise in the 1920s—as evident in the careers of George Minot, Alice Hamilton, and others.[50] Literature on sickle cell anemia also reflected another strain of social thought. As historian Peter Bowler has noted, the advent of Mendelism in 1900 represented "a shift in the way in which biology was used to provide a model for social policies."[51] Discourse on sickle cell anemia reflected both of these trends: the expanding use of both hereditary and hematological knowledge.

Yet, while other physicians and conservative social reformers used these sciences to limit the proliferation of the "unfit" and to restrict immigration, medical writers on sickle cell anemia pondered questions that were only implicitly eugenic.[52] As Detroit's Thomas Cooley and his assistant Pearl Lee observed in 1926, "If . . . sicklemia is a dominant Mendelian characteristic, and it is now as common as it seems to be in Detroit, shall we not in a few generations have a Negro population, the majority of whom show this peculiarity, and will not 'sickle cell anemia' then become a common condition?"[53] Few claimed to know what circumstances caused "sicklemia" to become a full-fledged anemia, and no one formulated specific social policies from these findings. But when physicians took up Emmel's diagnostic technology, most used it to sketch a threatening portrait of disease and American social relations.[54]

The potential disease posed a threat to Negroes and a hidden threat to industry. In 1930, G. M. Brandau of Houston, Texas, attempted to determine the "incidence of the sickle cell trait in industrial workers." This trait, he believed, was "a predisposing factor in the development of the anemia." Since "some authors even regard the trait as a very mild form of the disease," Brandau claimed that his investigation "was undertaken primarily to ascertain whether or not the sickle-cell trait is to be regarded as a definite industrial hazard."[55] He found that 6.67 percent (10 of 150) of the applicants for work at one factory showed the trait. Unlike other hematological analysts of his time, he avoided any specific recommendations about the proper management of this "industrial hazard."[56] Other industrial physicians might have seized upon such traits in the "scientific" management of the industrial workforce. Brandau may have believed that this hidden anemia dictated careful hematological screening of Negro workers. If so, these implications remained unstated.

By the late 1920s and into the 1930s, this tendency to sickle—even in the absence of any illness—was defined as a latent disease, a quality present in "Negro blood."[57] Modern clinicians have viewed these early twentieth-century beliefs as "mistaken," rooted in "confusions" between a technologically defined trait ("sicklemia," or what might be labeled "sickle cell trait" today) and a clinical disease ("sickle cell anemia").[58] But such confusions are part of the ongoing twentieth-century dialectic of technology and disease. Even today, we assume that technologically located genes are "diseases waiting to happen." Physicians have enthusiastically embraced genetic tools and moved aggressively along the path toward finding genes for latent diseases without authenticating the relationship between a technological finding and disease. Physicians of the early twentieth century did the same. They held an expansive view of the technologies of blood analysis, they enthusiastically discussed the medical and social implications of their findings, and in the process they created new identities for themselves and for patients.

In doing blood tests, physicians sought to define "the Negro" as he stood in relation to a social landscape.[59] Just as they spoke of latency to describe how the tubercle bacillus might reside in an individual's body for years before it ever gave rise to a clinical case of tuberculosis, physicians believed that the same term described the relationship of sicklemia to sickle cell anemia. Hidden threats lay nascent in Negro blood. Against this backdrop, physicians were hardly confused about the relationship between the sickle cell trait and sickle cell anemia—the relationship was a latent one. They assumed that some undetermined forces brought about the transformation from potential disease to actual disease.[60] The power of hematological technology was the power to see disease before doctor, patient, or society could experience or observe it.

Racial Identity and Fears of Miscegenation

Interpretations of Emmel's technique both reflected and shaped beliefs about the fundamental biological separateness of the "races"—black and white. The hematological view of racial identity became evident when physicians confronted cases of sickle cells in "white patients" and "white families." Beginning in the mid-1920s, a few such cases appeared in medical clinics and in the mainstream medical literature.[61] (We might be inclined today—from a modern medical standpoint—to label these as cases of "thalassemia," "thalassemia minor," "sickle cell/thalassemia," or "sickle cell anemia.") In their time, these patients were a volatile classificatory concern, stirring controversy that became more heated with the decades.[62] Physicians believed that the Mendelian dominant theory of inheritance merely confirmed that sicklemia (and thus the disease) had filtered into white populations through ancestral admixtures with Negro blood. Hematological technology, hereditary theory, and racial ideology created a self-reinforcing tautology.

A small number of physicians, however, believed that these cases of sickled cells in whites demonstrated that race was not the key to understanding the disease. Thomas Cooley suggested that these peculiar cells were also found in the "Mediterranean races." "Unquestionably," he concluded in 1929, "the general acceptance of the dictum that sickle cell anemia is peculiar to the Negro race has been too precipitate." By 1930 about ten such cases had been reported. One author suggested that "the demonstration that it is not peculiar to the Negro race emphasizes further its resemblance to congenital hemolytic icterus, to which we have referred in previous articles."[63] In 1927, a young hematological specialist named John Lawrence reported finding "elliptical and sickle-shaped" cells in "the circulating blood of white persons," and he questioned the supposed causal influence of "Negro blood" in this disease. Observing such cells in healthy black and white people, he estimated that "three percent of the normal white adults and five percent of 100 Negroes . . . showed some deformity of the red blood cells, some of which seemed to be similar to those described in sickle cell anemia."[64] Lawrence and a handful of others sought to set aside the notion that "deeply rooted racial characteristics" were responsible for the condition. "It would seem to me," he wrote, "that there may be an unknown factor at work even in the white race . . . Are we to assume that these apparently normal white

adults have quiescent sickle cell anemia?"[65] Perhaps all blood deforma-
tions of this type were related by some commonality.[66]

Most hematologically oriented physicians continued, however, to
see Negro blood as essential to the disease. Their descriptions of the disease constructed, idealized, and reified black-white identities and racial
relations. They insisted that, in so-called white patients with sickle cell
anemia, admixture with Negro blood could not be ruled out. This suspicion of admixture with Negro blood proved to be especially compelling
in patients of so-called Mediterranean stock—Greeks and Italians—because of their ancestral proximity to Africa. In one instance, the physicians noted that "in the case reported here there is no positive assurance
that the patient is 'pure white,' although his appearance is not Negroid,
and he [the patient] stated, 'If there is any Negro blood in my family, I
don't know about it.' Unfortunately, no other members of the family were
available for observation and study."[67] Through the 1930s, most physicians believed that, in these reports of sickle cell anemia in whites, "the
weight of evidence at the present time seems to point to the Negro origin
of sickling."[68]

Confronting white patients with a technological finding of sickled
cells, physicians repeatedly insisted that Negro intermarriage must have
occurred at some point in the family's history and that race mixing would
continue to spread the disease. As two New York physicians noted,
"Since interbreeding between the colored and the white races is more or
less constantly taking place in many regions, including this country, we
may in future generations expect the presence of this peculiar blood trait
in an increasing number of *apparently white descendants*" (emphasis
added).[69] By the middle and late 1930s, Emmel's test was enlisted in the
search for Negro ancestry and the detection of Negro blood.[70] Most
physicians were "inclined to explain the occurrence of this disease in the
white race on the basis of admixture of Negro blood in the family at some
time in the distant past," and many pointed to Hannibal's invasion of
Spain and Italy, the Moorish occupation of southern Spain, and the slave
trade as the processes that brought the races into closer proximity, spread
Negro blood, and transmitted disease.[71]

Emmel's blood test was thus part of a ritualized diagnostic interaction, pervaded with mistrust and suspicion about racial origins. Just as
they had used hematology to construct chlorosis in the 1890s, the same
processes of identity management constructed sickle cell anemia during
this later era. So convinced were some physicians of the ability of the di-

agnostic technique to detect Negro blood that, when faced with disagreement between the test and a patient's testimony about his or her
own family history, physicians suggested that *shame* would understand-
ably prompt patients to deny "Negro blood" in their pedigree. As one
physician noted in 1943, in the case of an apparently white child, "For a
long time Johnny's mother attempted to conceal her Negro ancestry by
making confusing statements concerning the Italian and Scotch ancestry,
which apparently constitutes only minor branches in her family tree . . .
[upon further questioning] she finally admitted Negro ancestry."[72] Disagreements between the hematological data and the patient's testimony
were easily resolved.[73] Technology, in the hands of a suspicious and
racially minded physician, pierced through duplicity and false pride, uncovering the truths of illicit relations, blood pedigree, health status, and
racial identity.

For these physicians, Emmel's technique and Mendelian law created appealing racial identities and endorsed their own role as society's
"race police." These diagnostic tools supported the belief that "the Negro" was the primary vector of the disease (analogous to the mosquito in
malaria and yellow fever, the bacillus in tuberculosis, and the uncinaria-
sis worm in hookworm). Blacks posed insidious threats to themselves
and to the non-Negro population.[74] Geographic proximity alone facilitated interbreeding, which had already accounted for the disease's
spread.[75] By the early 1940s, this interpretation of sickle cell anemia was
a common one in medicine. At the same time, the disease became part of
a wider public discussion, taking on new meaning when juxtaposed with
other controversies about racial blood and segregation in America.[76]

In the early 1940s, the disease provided rich biological material for
defenses of segregation and for restrictions on intermarriage and integration. A recent émigré to the United States, Julius Bauer cast sicklemia
as a distinct potential danger to society. He insisted that, because 7.5 percent of Negroes exhibited this constitutional sickle cell trait, "even if this
estimate is somewhat exaggerated, as we are inclined to believe, it is evident that the potential danger involved is by no means negligible, particularly as far as our armed forces are concerned." Bauer believed that,
on this basis, black Americans should not be admitted into the military,
and strident, racist generalizations followed.[77] "Persons with sickle cell
disease represent biological liabilities," he declared.[78] "Having sickle cell
trait, whether or not resulting in sickle cell disease with or without anemia, he [the patient] may become the victim of his constitutional biolog-

ic inferiority and succumb under circumstances which are innocuous to average normal people." These individuals were not normal and should be classified as "status degenerativus"—as weak, useless, and possessing an unusual number of degenerative stigmata.[79]

Many other physicians also defended the association between sicklemia and Negro blood, while avoiding Bauer's expansive claims. Even black pathologist Julian Herman Lewis, in his 1942 book *The Biology of the Negro,* agreed that "white" cases could not be perceived as authentic sickle cell anemia because miscegenation was highly probable. "It would seem," Lewis concluded after a review of the existing literature, "that there remain only three cases that have occurred in pure Caucasians—that of Sights and Simon in a white native American of Scotch-Irish descent and that of two children whose father is of a family that has lived for several generations in Illinois, Ohio and Missouri and whose mother has forebears from Virginia and Kentucky." But even these cases might be ruled out because of suspicions of race mixing. Indeed, Lewis agreed with his peers that "it appears that the burden of proof in presenting cases of sickle cell anemia or sicklemia in white people is to show, first, that they are true instances of the conditions and not other types of red cell deformity and, second, that the progenitors of the patient are entirely free of Negro blood, a task that may be difficult, owing to disappearance of obvious Negro features on dilution with white blood and to the tendency under such circumstances to deny Negro forebears."[80] Holding Emmel's test in high regard, Lewis voiced strong support for the hematological search for Negro blood. This was a form of hegemony via technological tradition, an endorsement and legitimation of cherished racial categories through blood analysis.

Other practitioners in positions of medical authority echoed Lewis's claims. In a 1943 study, M. A. Ogden argued that "the presence of the sickling trait in a white person is definite proof of admixture of Negro blood in the immediate or remote ancestry."[81] In the pages of the *Journal of the National Medical Association* (the national journal of black physicians), one editorialist called on black physicians to claim the disease as their own.[82] In 1947, *JAMA* offered its own editorial opinion on the disease, a defense of pure racial identities. "Sickle cell anemia . . . is independent of either geography or custom and habits. Its occurrence depends entirely on the presence of Negro blood, even in extremely small amounts . . . It appears that the *sine qua non* for the occurrence of sickle cell anemia is the presence of a strain, even remote, of Negro blood." Race mixing, according to *JAMA*, posed the greatest threat of the spread of sickle cell anemia. "The disease has never been found in countries such as Britain where the opportunity for miscegenation with Negroes has been small, and is regularly found in countries such as Latin America where there has been frank interbreeding with African people."[83] "Race," the editorial proclaimed, "is thus a strong etiological factor; the role of other factors is not clear."[84]

Varieties of Disease Identity

Even as mainstream medical journals endorsed Emmel's test and its severe implications, criticisms appeared from within and outside of organized medicine. Some analysts brought new tools, novel methods of genetics analysis, and different social and political assumptions about race to bear on the problem of "Negro blood." Howard University's Montague Cobb, a black pathologist and an astute student of racial pathology, questioned Lewis's reliance on Emmel's technique. Cobb believed that the concept of a "race test" was a "*reductio ad absurdum* which the Negro himself denounces . . . Lewis' argument might be said to imply that a bona fide diagnosis of sicklemia in a white man is tantamount to evidence of some Negro blood," Cobb stated, "but in reality no known fact precludes the possibility of occurrence of authentic sicklemia in the white."[85] Other authors found "several [authentic, white] cases in which there is little or no possibility of Negro blood."[86] Others turned away from Mendelian law (as much of the human genetics community was doing the same) and took up an interest in the new population genetics, a field concerned with natural mutations, gene pools, and evolutionary theory.[87] For these authors, factors other than racial crossing explained the disease's transmission and incidence.

Tensions over the identity of sickle cell anemia reflected newly exposed anxieties in science and society during the World War II era. Blood banking during the war made blood a national resource and blood donation a source of civic pride and military necessity. Nazi Germany's pride in Aryan blood further highlighted the relationship between blood, race, and national identity. On the American home front, the meaning of blood became an issue of wide public discussion. Blood donation and blood plasma transfusion created new technologies, informing the public explication of blood beliefs. A March 1942 *New York Times* article scoffed that "'senseless' insistence on 'Aryan' blood in transfusions for wounded soldiers had complicated German surgical care on the Russian front."[88] But later that year, America's blood policies laid bare the racist assumptions that prevailed at home. The American Red Cross segregated the blood of Negro donors from that of others, and this policy came under fire from African-American civic leaders, religious groups, and reform-minded anthropologists.

That "Negro blood" had a largely symbolic meaning became evident to many of these observers. Another *New York Times* editorial of June 1942, entitled "Blood and Prejudice," reported that, "because the American Red Cross for no scientific reason segregates the blood donated by whites and blacks, the Committee on Race Relations of the American Association of Physical Anthropology comes forth with a protest." Belief in Negro blood seemed to be nothing more than superstition and prejudice masquerading as science. "We ask ourselves in vain why there should be this prejudice against Negro blood and why no one shudders at the origin of many a substance that is now injected to save human life . . . We cannot explain the prejudice that the Red Cross is keeping alive[; it] is a survival of the superstitions and mysticism associated with the blood."[89] A variety of organizations, scholarly disciplines, and individual scholars undertook a reexamination of race and blood, focusing on their mutual construction and their uses in medicine and social policy.[90]

In *An American Dilemma,* the influential study published in 1942, Swedish sociologist Gunnar Myrdal could have easily been writing about the early history of sickle cell anemia when he came to the section on "Racial Beliefs of the Unsophisticated." "Without any doubt there is also in the white man's concept of the Negro 'race' an irrational element," he wrote. "It is like the concept of 'unclean' in primitive religion. It is invoked by the metaphor of 'blood' when describing ancestry. The ordinary man means something particular but beyond secular and rational understanding when he refers to 'blood.' The one who has got the smallest drop of 'Negro blood' is as one who is smitten by a hideous disease." American blood beliefs, Myrdal argued, were among the cornerstones of segregation. "It does not help if he [the Negro] is good and honest, educated and intelligent, a good worker, an excellent citizen and an agreeable fellow. Inside him are hidden some unknown and dangerous potentialities, something which will sooner or later crop up."[91]

Myrdal's language was strikingly evocative of the medical thinking about the "potentialities" of Negro blood in sicklemia. For Myrdal, these views were not only unsophisticated, but also "a manifestation of the most primitive form of religion." "The Negro," he concluded, "is seg-regated, and one deep idea behind segregation is that of quarantine what is evil, shameful, and feared in society."[92] Myrdal's assertion that mysti-cism and primitivism lay behind beliefs about Negro blood sheds some light on the early history of sickle cell anemia, on the interpretation of Emmel's test, and on the symbolic importance of hematology. Mysticism and primitivism took many ritual forms. In the construction of hemato-logical beliefs about sickle cell anemia, the disease's meaning emerged from a ritualistic use of diagnostic technology and from the sophisticat-ed invocation of Mendelian theory.

Such implicit critiques of the science of hematology in the 1940s led some hematologists to reexamine their use of terms like *blood,* to seek new tools of scientific analysis, to embrace new theories of heredity, and there-by to distance themselves from their predecessors. However, for most physicians in the 1940s, Emmel's diagnostic technique continued to be used as a de facto diagnosis of Negro blood and as validation of the hid-den dangers of racial proximity and admixture. Within twenty years, however, a new dogma had been established. One hematologist would later recall with disgust how people of this earlier generation had be-lieved that, "through some mystical property, blood presumably carried the essence of the individual, the family, the clan, the nation, and the race. People speak of white blood and Negro blood . . . In our day, these beliefs reached their most vicious climax with the absurd myth of Aryan blood."[93]

In the 1940s, several more narrowly clinical identities for sickle cell anemia began to appear in medical writing. When faced with a black child showing signs of anemia, joint pains, abdominal pains, lethargy, enlarged spleen, leg ulcers, infections, or other symptoms, specialists in-terpreted what they saw in terms of what they already believed.[94] A con-stellation of symptoms led physicians to different diagnoses.[95] Abdom-inal pains often suggested appendicitis or other abdominal diseases to the surgeon.[96] Surgeons also perceived the enlarged spleen as an inde-pendent affection or as a cause of the disease and hastily removed it.[97] Others attributed splenic enlargement to malaria. Joint pains were fre-quently diagnosed as rheumatism. Cardiac symptoms were commonly diagnosed as mitral insufficiency.[98] Specialists thus saw different facets of the disease through their specialized lenses—focusing on blood and anemia, on abdominal pain, on splenic enlargement, or on cardiac symp-toms and fitting these symptoms into existing professional assumptions.

In 1943, two authors labeled the disease "a great masquerader" (a term traditionally applied to syphilis), since "the disease is often not diagnosed, and patients are operated on unnecessarily because an erroneous diagnosis of appendicitis, gallbladder disease, or some type of acute abdominal disease has been made." They sought instead to create one coherent story from this clinical complexity during those same years when the concept of a diagnostic race test came under assault.[99]

In many respects, the history of sickle cell anemia as a clinical entity is the mirror image of the history of splenic anemia. Where splenic anemia became obsolete precisely because its various symptoms were reclaimed by various specialists (leaving the surgeon with nothing to work with), sickle cell anemia *began* as an obscure and fragmented assortment of symptoms. Different specialists fit these symptoms into discrete, readily available diagnostic categories. A few physicians tried to convince their colleagues, however, that cases of so-called appendicitis, mitral insufficiency, and tuberculosis were actually sickle cell anemia.[100] As public and professional awareness of the disease intensified in the early 1940s, a growing number of physicians urged surgical restraint, breadth of vision, and sensitivity to the complexities of the disease.[101] Physicians writing in the 1940s suggested that the malady's rareness was an artifact of professional structure. Sickle cell anemia, they would suggest, was fragmented and obscured by specialism and by assumptions about the central place of appendicitis, joint pain, splenectomy, cardiac disease, infection, and race (as discrete problems) in the medical mind.[102]

As pediatricians and hematologists described the "rare" disease in journals and meetings, they created an increasingly complex portrait focusing not merely on blood or any single symptom but on the ensemble of clinical signs. As early as 1927, two authors noted that the "prognosis in sickle cell anemia is poor in the active cases, simply because of the likelihood of intercurrent infections; the patient does not die from the severity of the anemia, per se."[103] Infections killed patients, and the blood picture played a minor role in mortality. Another reviewer noted that "in this disease it is not the anemia but thrombosis [the clotting of blood in veins and organs] which constitutes the most important pathologic process . . . It is [also] well known that cardiac enlargement is a usual finding in patients with sickle cell anemia."[104] Multiple phenomena defined the disease.[105] By focusing on why patients died, rather than on the meaning of particular hematological symptoms, some physicians expressed a primary concern for patients, families, and the problem of mortality.

Pediatricians saw sickle cell anemia as "a disease of childhood," a label evoking particular moral and social meaning in the 1930s and 1940s. Writing in 1932, Thomas Cooley insisted that the "earliest reports led one to think that it was about as frequent and as important in adults as in children. Obviously, from further study, this is not the case."[106] Responsibility thus fell on pediatricians to take this disease as their own problem, to define their concerns by it, and to care for its sufferers. As historian Sydney Halpern has argued, in the 1920s and 1930s pediatrics "brought health supervision into the mainstream of the specialty, leaders articulated a new professional ideology . . . [with] a focus on children's growth and development . . . The child specialist was advisor to the family, educating parents on child management . . . stressing 'the importance of guiding parents in the proper training of children.'"[107] Cooley (later to become president of the American Pediatrics Association) suggested that special vigilance and a variety of tools were needed in detecting, managing, and alleviating this disease. "None of the patients I have lost have died of actual effects of sickle cell anemia," he wrote. "One died of tuberculosis, another of endocarditis and a third of surgical accident."[108] By the mid-1930s, some pediatricians identified sickle cell anemia as one among their special clinical (and social) concerns.[109] Their writings placed the Negro child (rather than Negro blood) at the center of disease identity.

Individual signs and symptoms derived their meaning from the structure of medical specialties and from the professional agendas and social values of practitioners. Hematological meaning depended upon social context. One Tennessee pathologist suggested that, in his region, physicians might overdiagnose sickle cell anemia because of the prevalence of malnutrition and anemia in the mid-South. He warned that "the presence of sickled cells in the moist preparations [Emmel's test] does not alone make the diagnosis of sickle cell anemia."[110] "The presence of sickle cell trait in association with secondary anemia, which often occurs in hospital patients as a result of infection, faulty nutrition or cachectic disease, likewise does not make the case one of sickle cell anemia, but merely secondary anemia superimposed on the sickle cell trait."[111] Poverty, malnutrition, and anemia in the region made disease identity a complex affair.

For some clinicians and many patients, one particular symptom of the disease emerged as symbolically crucial—the "sickle cell crisis." Recurrent episodes of joint and abdominal pain often brought patients into the clinic.[112] This feature has its own cultural history, its status rising as the voice of patients gained greater import in twentieth-century medicine. By the 1950s and 1960s, "the crisis" came to represent the failures of medicine to address suffering, particularly in the black community. Civic groups lent support for the "fight against sickle cell anemia." Their appeals highlighted the pain of the disorder. By the early 1960s, one newspaper writer noted that, "while much of this nation fiddles in unawareness, a mysterious and crippling chronic blood disease of considerable prevalence burns unchecked, causing much pain and suffering."[113] In time, as the medical focus on Negro blood faded, the crisis would become a key feature of the clinical and social portrait of sickle cell anemia, capturing for many black Americans the true identity of this disease.[114]

Medical images of sickle cell anemia were wedded to various medical identities, social commitments, and professional concerns. Thus, in the 1940s, some hematologists upheld the validity of Emmel's test for Negro blood, while pediatricians labeled sickle cell anemia a childhood disease. For some clinicians, the crisis was slowly taking center stage while more traditional characterizations endured. In 1948, for example, one hematology handbook noted that "if the incidence of active sickle cell anemia is taken as 15 per cent . . . according to Ogden, 135,088 Negroes in this country have the disease and consequently are doomed to complete extermination either in the first or second decade of life."[115] At the same time, a novel technology—electrophoresis—appeared, promising a new basis for defining sickle cell anemia and fostering a revision of traditional views of the heritability of the disorder. The history of electrophoresis exemplifies a new movement in American medical science; it encouraged a new kind of medical scientist, and it endorsed a new identity for this disease, one that would raise as many new questions as it resolved.

Molecular Hematology and Ideals of Human Engineering

Into this controversy over racial origins and complex symptomatology entered a new molecular-based technology—electrophoresis—that seemed to resolve all disputes. Electrophoresis was a tool of physical chemistry, used by chemists since the early 1930s to determine the structure of complex molecules by analyzing their behavior in varying electrical currents. As physical chemists like Francis Crick turned to human biology, the medical value of these tools seemed great. Historian Pe-

ter Bowler has suggested that "the discovery of the structure and function of DNA is often presented as the key that has unlocked the most fundamental secrets of life itself."[116] In the late 1940s and 1950s, molecular
biologists used such tools to affirm a new medical science, to promote a
"molecular vision of life," and to highlight the role of such tools in the
treatment of disease. Electrophoresis exerted a powerful force on medical thinking about sickle cell anemia and about disease in general. For
hematologists, seeking a new basis for how we think about disease, molecular tools also offered a new identity for themselves.[117]

Linus Pauling is a key figure in postwar molecular biology and in
the story of sickle cell anemia. He later wrote that "the discovery of the
abnormal human hemoglobin was the result of having been appointed
to a committee . . . called the Medical Advisory Committee [to advise
President Roosevelt on the future funding of science] . . . in 1944."[118] The
committee's work, which eventually led to the report *Science, the Endless
Frontier,* helped to chart the federal government's increasing role in medical and scientific research. (Ch. 6 focuses on this expansion of federally
funded science and its influence on blood investigation, technology, and
the politics of disease.) During one of the committee's conferences, Pauling first learned of sickle cell anemia and guessed that it might have a
molecular genesis. "Dr. William B. Castle . . . began talking about the disease sickle-cell anemia, with which he had some experience . . . When Dr.
Castle said that the red cells in the blood of a patient are sickled in the ve-
nous blood but not in the arterial blood, the idea occurred to me that sickle-cell anemia might be a disease of the hemoglobin molecule."[119] Based
upon his experience analyzing protein structures, Pauling speculated
that a molecular abnormality might cause the disease.

> I thought at once of this possibility: that the hemoglobin molecules of these
> patients might have, as a result of a gene mutation, a structure formed so
> that one portion of the surface of the molecule would be sufficiently com-
> plementary to another portion to permit the molecule to aggregate into
> long chains. Further, these long chains would then line up side by side to
> form a needle-shaped crystal, which . . . would twist the red cell out of
> shape. These deformed cells would have properties sufficiently different
> from normal cells to give rise to manifestations of the disease.[120]

Electrophoretic studies of sickle cell hemoglobin confirmed Pauling's hypothesis. In Pauling's telling of the story, it was the chance conversation
between Castle (the clinical hematologist) and himself (the physical

chemist) that created a new identity for sickle cell anemia.

This radically new portrait of disease also suggested a new medical and scientific agenda. Throughout the early twentieth century, Emmel's technique had constructed a blood disease, and it provided a biological understanding of racial differences in health and society.[121] This tool had helped to sustain an image of "the Negro" as a public health threat and highlighted the dangers of racial proximity, intermarriage, and miscegenation.[122] Molecular biology, however, promised a new optimism in its portrait of the disease—highlighting the role of race mixing in its eradication and envisioning the possibilities of an engineering solution to the "molecular problem." The molecular disease thesis must be understood as part of identity politics in postwar medicine—as a product of historically specific biomedical interests and also as a contribution to the discourse of race relations in America. The use of electrophoresis in the 1940s and increasingly in the 1950s transformed the identity of sickle cell anemia, shifting medical thought from "blood" cells to "hemoglobin" molecules.[123] Pauling and his colleagues, using the technique, found structural anomalies in the hemoglobin of patients with sickle cell anemia and on this basis labeled it a "molecular disease" defined by the abnormal "hemoglobin S."

At the same time, geneticist J. V. Neel reexamined the Mendelian dominant thesis.[124] As such investigators shifted their sights away from the blood per se, Emmel's test could be said to locate a *trait*, not a *disease*. "Sickle cell trait," as one geneticist now defined it, "is a heterozygous condition . . . It is detectable by the fact that, when a few drops of blood of an affected subject are examined under the microscope . . . the red cells sometimes . . . appear like crescents or sickles."[125] Hemoglobin studies, on the other hand, located the disease. And hemoglobin studies in families suggested that inheritance did *not* follow Mendelian dominance principles. Although the trait could be spread by an individual parent, the disease could not. It required a "double dose" of the trait—that is, it required inheritance of the sickling trait from *both* parents. Family studies made in Kenya and by Neel in the United States suggested "that the double dose of this gene, which occurs in homozygous individuals, causes a very severe anaemia which usually prevents them from surviving infancy."[126]

Electrophoresis opened a path for new studies in human biology, as had Emmel's test in earlier decades.[127] In the early 1960s, one biologist stated that "the study of sickle cell hemoglobin has not only provided much information about normal and abnormal hemoglobins but has opened an era of biochemical genetics."[128] With the use of electrophoresis in many clinical settings, in genetics research, and in medical anthropology, scholars realized that various "hemoglobinopathies" were widely distributed. A global cataloging of abnormal hemoglobins followed. Reports discussed their transmission in terms of population mobility, intermarriage, and historical evolution, but avoided their association with "races."[129]

Indeed, hemoglobin variations (without evidence of clinical disorder) and abnormalities turned up everywhere. In 1955, one of Pauling's co-workers (Harvey Itano) could write that "five more abnormal hemoglobins have been found, two in clinical states resembling Cooley's anemia [i.e., thalassemia] and two in asymptomatic cases."[130] Enamored of the new diagnostic tool, two clinicians reminded their peers in 1954 that "it is no longer satisfactory to use the term *sickle cell anemia* without attempting to establish . . . the forms of hemoglobin responsible for the disease." The new era of molecular diagnostics (and growing federal funding for research in molecular biology) meant new patterns of hematological practice and growth of the enterprise of producing knowledge about hemoglobin variations.[131]

By focusing precisely on hemoglobin, molecular hematologists believed that they had found the root, cause, and essence of the disease. They had also avoided the unfortunate metaphorical associations that had plagued blood studies in the past. In his 1958 book *The Story of Blood*, physician Kenneth Walker insisted that modern hematologists had abandoned the linkage of "blood" and "race" in favor of a more global, biomolecular view. Hemoglobin signified a common inheritance, a molecular and chemical bond shared by all humans. "We talk of pure blood, of mixed blood, of bad blood and of Jewish, Negro and Chinese blood," wrote Walker, "but from the standpoint of the scientist the blood of one race is quite indistinguishable from the blood of another race."[132] Hemoglobin studies suggested that hemoglobin abnormalities (hemoglobinopathies) were not confined to any race. If particular abnormalities like hemoglobin S appeared in higher frequencies in one population, it was because of evolutionary and historical reasons. (This construction is discussed further in ch. 6.) Molecular biology provided an ostensibly objective, nonracial language for thinking about blood.

Even as molecular biologists explored the meaning of hemoglobin abnormalities, a few acknowledged the ambiguous relationship among technological finding, clinical symptomatology, and patient experience. The same hemoglobinopathies did not always result in the same symptoms and, even when they did, those symptoms might vary dramatically from one patient to another. In 1963, historian Owsei Temkin noted the limitations of this scientific approach to disease: "Since about twenty kinds of abnormal human haemoglobin are said to exist, the number of combinations and possible 'specific diseases' in this one province seems very large . . . Danger arises lest specific diseases be postulated which have no clinical reality."[133]

For some observers, the technological notion of a hemoglobinopathy was estranged from clinical concerns and also from the crises and illness experiences of patients.[134] Displeasure with the "science" of sickle cell anemia resonated from one clinician who protested that "sickle cell patients have been paraded before beginning graduate students as evidence that biochemistry is relevant, that genetics can be fun. Yet for all this 'understanding,' no treatment or effective palliation exists for the disease, and no real effort has been made to increase public awareness of its nature."[135] Electrophoretic diagnosis solved many problems, yet it highlighted the gap between biomolecular and other conceptions of disease. In replacing one technological identity with another, medical science had revised the former, harsh symbolism of the disease and yet played down the centrality of pain, infection, and infant death.[136]

The reconstruction of sickle cell anemia in the 1950s and 1960s suggested that the physician of the future would be a kind of engineer—tinkering with molecular mechanisms to cure disease.[137] As Pauling stated in a 1948 talk entitled "Molecular Architecture and the Processes of Life," "we [scientists] do know what the nature of life is (aside from consciousness), in terms of molecular architecture." For Pauling, the molecular disease thesis stood as an archetype of modern biomedicine's mechanistic ideals. "The problem of attacking . . . diseases is made most difficult because of the lack of complete understanding of their nature . . . in terms of molecular structure," Pauling continued.[138] Future struggles against disease would involve the detection and manipulation of underlying molecular mechanisms.[139] Chemist George Gray forecasted in 1951 (as noted above) that in sickle cell anemia we "may be able to devise a small, innocuous molecule which will lock permanently on to the defective hemoglobin and prevent the abnormal molecule from misbehaving."[140] Molecular biologists and molecular hematologists ardently believed that intransigent biological and hereditary problems might be eradicated by technological fixes. Victory over heredity seemed to be at hand.[141] The concept of molecular disease endorsed these values and aspirations, reflecting a cultural enthusiasm for engineering solutions that was only to be expected after America's wartime experience.[142]

Scientists, physicians, and patients wondered, however, where such enthusiasm would lead. Columbia University's L. C. Dunn asked, "What should happen if a cure for sickle-cell anemia is found and the homozygotes which now die should be enabled to contribute their quota of children and genes to succeeding generations?" What burden would growing numbers of sickle cell patients place on the shoulders of America? Such concerns, Dunn believed, highlighted that we should use technologies not to cure patients, but to engineer society. With technological cures, Dunn forecasted, "the fall in the gene frequency would be arrested . . . and we should have to be prepared to continue to cure the disease as a permanent obligation of the social system." The success of future technology would only increase social obligations. Technology might also lead in another direction if policymakers promoted gene detection, since "we could dissuade or prevent all persons known to harbor the gene from having children. We could order them sterilized, a measure which . . . encounters difficulties in societies in which individual freedom is prized." Dunn neither advocated nor condemned these measures. He merely outlined the consequences of hemoglobin manipulation. For Dunn and other geneticists, sickle cell anemia provided an archetypal example of the modern technological dilemma. It posed the paradox of technology and disease cure and highlighted many of the other "questions which have to be considered when we think about evolutionary processes in human populations."[143] If Emmel's technique symbolized the racial politics of pre–World War II America, then electrophoresis symbolized a new set of technological ideals and eugenic possibilities for dealing with race in America.

Blood, Technology, and "Race"

Technologies are critical elements in the construction of diseases and in their reconstruction. The use of two technologies—Emmel's test and electrophoresis—framed two very different portraits of sickle cell anemia in twentieth-century America. Each offered, for example, contrasting identities for the disease, the physician, and the patient. Emmel's test showed the physician as "race detective"; electrophoresis revealed an optimistic "molecular engineer." Emmel's test portrayed the Negro as "disease vector"; electrophoresis revealed the black people as part of the biochemical diversity of humankind.

Each tool also provoked different speculations on American race relations. Emmel's test had been used to endorse racial segregation. But in the early 1950s, A. C. Allison suggested that the sickle cell trait (or what the previous generation had labeled "sicklemia") "apparently protects young children against the malaria parasite during the dangerous years until they acquire an immunity."[144] An inferior trait was redefined as a beneficial adaptation. Allison's work suggested that "mixed mating with Indian and white people and movement from a malarious region to one free of this disease" would tend toward the disease's disappearance. This was "a cheering thought on the genetic future of civilized man."[145] Those very factors—migration and miscegenation—that had been labeled "insidious" in earlier years were now presented as "cheering." Others continued to see the trait as a profound threat, speculating that *trait* might become *disease* at high altitudes when the blood became deprived of oxygen. "Since such a large segment of the population is involved," wrote physician William Levin of Galveston in 1958, "awareness of the problem should be encouraged among members of the medical profession, the air transportation industry, the medical services of the Armed Forces and among Negroes themselves."[146] The new technology engendered a new disease discourse and legitimated new forms of disease surveillance and social policy. "The simplicity of performance of hemoglobin electrophoresis makes it practical to recommend that all Negroes entering military service be screened for this hemoglobin," wrote Levin. "Further, the demonstration of sickle cell trait should be the basis for exclusion of affected personnel from flight status. Similar principles may be applied in civilian practice."[147] (These controversial policies and the politics of electrophoresis are discussed in greater detail in ch. 6.)

Molecular biologists were well funded, rising in medical and social status, and well situated to define disease, inform social policy, and promise technological fixes for this disease. It was not until the early 1970s, however, after increased political pressure from black Americans, that biochemists sought to make good on their therapeutic promises. When a urea-based "desickling" treatment for hemoglobin was announced in 1972, Pauling prematurely proclaimed that the promise of molecular biology had been fulfilled. The disease had "a known molecular basis for pathogenesis, a molecular basis for diagnosis, and a molecular basis for treatment."[148] The treatment, however, proved to be toxic and therefore clinically useless. Indeed, treating the symptoms has been far more effective than any molecular therapy in extending the lives of patients with sickle cell anemia.[149]

The story of sickle cell anemia highlights a crucial irony about the relationship between technology and the discourse of "race." While both Emmel's technique and electrophoresis supposedly disclosed biological data about disease, both tools required interpretation if they were to have clinical or social meaning. This constructed meaning depended heavily both on previous medical assumptions about the location of disease (blood or hemoglobin) and on reigning genetic theory. Both tools provided a substrate for building compelling but myopic narratives about race relations.[150] As expressions of modern technological medicine and modern hematology, Emmel's technique and electrophoresis mirror one another and, at the same time, they stand side by side. They reveal the diverse ways in which hematology produced ideas about disease, and they highlight the ways in which objective and subjective notions about racial identity, medical identity, and disease identity related inextricably.

6

"The Forces That Are Molding Us"

The National Politics of Blood and Disease
after World War II

"In 1961," as one hematologist later recalled, "there was a flurry of activity in the cellular and molecular biology. The war . . . had given a boon and a boom to biomedical sciences. Sputnik had enhanced this profusion of research. The scientific climate was exuberant."[1] As this young researcher saw it, "much of what was going on was related (so it seemed to me at least) to hematology: the structure of hemoglobin, the story of sickle cell disease, the reticulocyte as a model for protein synthesis, leukemia as a model for cancer, etc." The possibilities of biomolecular blood analysis in this new era suggested insights into diverse diseases and into crucial questions of human identity. Looking back, this researcher "was under the naive impression that blood cells were less complicated and more accessible than other cells."[2] Blood seemed accessible and at the same time remarkably malleable.

In contrast to the era before World War II, postwar blood researchers embraced a comprehensive engineering approach to health and disease. Wartime developments in blood transfusion had demonstrated that blood could be divided in many ways and that the plasma component had enormous value as a life-giving tool. A 1957 NBC television health program on "Blood" proclaimed that "blood is yielding more and more of its secrets to the tireless and ingenious research workers in laboratories and hospitals."[3] Blood analysis and manipulation, wrote another author in 1961, set the stage for other technical innovations. To the aspiring organ transplant surgeon, for example, "the protective action of the blood is sometimes considered one of nature's enormous blunders."[4] Altering hematological immunity now seemed necessary, since blood impeded "one of the greatest potential advances in the preservation of life and health."[5] Lingering postwar anxieties about nuclear weapons prompted the U.S. government to support studies of chemotherapy and radiation and of their positive and negative effects in diseases like the leukemias. Blood was a fluid to be divided, studied, and manipulated in the name of higher technical achievement and national security. Specialists and general physicians in the 1940s, 1950s, and 1960s embraced this engineering ideal, redefining yet again their relationship to the vital fluid.

One of this book's key concerns has been the ways in which changing social relationships shaped the use of technology and the meaning of blood. From the heyday of chlorosis and the family doctor through the conquest of pernicious anemia, I have explored the ways in which relations between families and their doctors, researchers and the pharmaceutical industry, and other client-practitioner pairs have influenced medical pronouncements about blood and disease. After World War II, a new medical patron—the federal government—would enter this negotiation. This chapter explores the many ways in which government involvement in science, technology, and medicine transformed the meaning of blood by making it a national concern. Blood specialists began the postwar era expecting that their new technologies would transform disease, medicine, and society. By the late 1960s, many hematologists found that political forces beyond their control had actually transformed the hematologists themselves in dramatic ways. They also found that a new problem had emerged: who would control technology in this modern medical era?

The variety, power, and proliferation of new technologies of blood manipulation created new problems for hematologists and increasingly for the government agencies that fostered and regulated these tools. The U.S. government acted as a powerful broker in the development of blood manipulation technologies. After the war, the federal government increased the funding of the medical sciences, regulated new drugs, and encouraged particular research programs. Many of the disciplines that form the core of medicine today gained recognition in that era—among them, molecular biology. New, expensive, and powerful technologies of blood manipulation seemed to resolve previously unsolvable clinical problems and to reduce mortality and morbidity. In the same way that the discovery and use of insulin in the 1920s and 1930s had created a new category of diabetic, as historian Christopher Feudtner has shown, interactions between new technologies and blood created new disease identities in the postwar context.[6] In bringing new clarity and complexity to our understanding of disease, these technologies—powerful, expensive, and widely deployed—raised new problems for the government, for patients, and for hematology.

Federally funded chemotherapy and radiation studies created, in many senses, modern oncology and the modern leukemia patient. The rising status of the discipline and of these patients became a professional problem for hematology. New drugs also created problems in hematology. The discovery and use of a new antibiotic—chloramphenicol—dramatically reduced mortality for many infectious disorders and at the same time caused cases of aplastic anemia, raising the problem of "iatrogenic disease" (diseases caused by medicine). This, in turn, led to calls for increased drug regulation. Electrophoresis (as we've seen in ch. 5) created new classifications of patients with sickle cell anemia, focusing medical and public health attention on hemoglobin S—and eventually on "the heterozygote" as the "carrier" of the disease. Here, too, national politics would inform the deployment and interpretation of this diagnostic technology. This chapter examines these encounters between technology and disease. Each encounter suggests the complex problems raised by medical tools during the postwar years and the ways in which national politics affected the control of technology and the meaning of blood.

Earlier technologies—such as the hemacytometer, hemoglobinometer, arsenic therapy, splenectomy, bone marrow puncture, liver extract, and Emmel's blood test—had their own politics and implications for patient identity. Whether they were used in family practice, academic research, routine hospital care, industrial management, or public health debates, these hematological tools had stood at the center of the medical and popular imagination, suggesting clear and compelling identities for disease, patient, and physician. In the 1950s and 1960s, however, their legitimacy would be undermined by the promise of new tools, by tensions with other specialists, by a changing politics, and by an increasingly vocal and skeptical public. Such factors explain what became of "the anemias." With new tools in hand for hematological study in 1953, one leading hematologist suggested that "anemia is no longer a disease," illustrating how new ideas in hematology supplanted such traditional concepts.

Just as microscopy had brought the anemias into focus in the late nineteenth century, innovations in medical technology after World War II produced new ideas about the blood and ensured that "the anemias" would become outmoded diseases. Molecular-level analysis of blood provided compelling new visions of disease and of the physician as biomolecular scientist. The new biomolecular sciences of blood suggested that patients were little more than complex, malfunctioning, biomolecular processes. "Man," one geneticist could claim in 1959, "can be described as an extremely complicated and successful demonstration of chemical engineering."[7]

Developments in molecular biology suggested that hematological thought should be organized not around blood cells per se, but around the molecular mechanisms within (and around) the blood cells.[8] "The anemias" (various depletions in the numbers of blood cells) seemed to be altogether vague as diseases. In his 1961 book, *The River of Life: The Story of Man's Blood from Magic to Science,* Bernard Seeman pictured the anemias as mere clinical phenomena, end points of complicated biomolecular processes.[9] These processes were, themselves, "the diseases." This view of disease placed the biochemical scientist atop medicine's cultural hierarchy. For Seeman, the blood took its true identity from its unique biochemistry, not from specious associations of blood with family, nation, or race or even from blood's clinical significance. "The identity between blood and the sea is no mere figure of speech but a biochemical fact," Seeman proclaimed. "Sea water today is almost identical with blood serum except that it has a higher concentration of inorganic salts" (12). All living things took their identity from biomolecular forces precisely because "some distant portion of the original sea still flows . . . in ourselves" (30). In the 1950s and 1960s, physicians followed these developments closely, adopting the tools of molecular analysis and embracing these insights into the human body and disease identity.[10]

The era posed national challenges for hematologists and their diseases. The American Society of Hematology and the journal *Blood* appeared in these years. Even as hematologists consolidated as this national society and journal, they were no longer the only specialists studying blood. New disciplines emerged, funded by federal largesse, claiming expertise in blood analysis and manipulation. Agencies like the Food and Drug Administration gained new powers to oversee medicine's expanding therapeutic capacity. Gradually, various patient groups built national constituencies, voicing their own concerns and speaking through their legislators and through social movements of the 1960s. In 1968, hematologist William Dameshek sketched out for his colleagues "the complex state of the present-day world . . . We must," he proclaimed, "have an intelligent appraisal of the forces that are molding us, modifying our position."[11] For hematologists, the political forces that had led to their consolidation now gradually led to their fragmentation. The flurry of activity surrounding blood studies had also brought scientific competition and a crisis in the specialty. Hematology's control—over the use of blood manipulation technologies and the meaning of blood—was put to severe tests by national political forces in post–World War II America.

Leukemia and the Formation of Hematology-Oncology

As Maxwell Wintrobe noted to his colleagues in the early 1980s, "The emergence of hematology as an identifiable discipline in the delivery of health care poses a major challenge for us . . . With increasing involvement of Government in the delivery of health services, decisions may be made which would have a significant influence on the practice of hematology as we understand it."[12] Government legislation—Medicare, Medicaid, the Food and Drug Administration (FDA), as well as disease-related legislation—reflected an intensified public interest in medicine and research, and this heightened federal activism led to stiff competition for research funds.

In this context the rise of oncology (cancer research) as a field had gradually eroded hematology's status. Ownership of leukemia had become, since the 1950s, a key point of contention. Wintrobe reflected that "hematology has suffered a degree of fragmentation" partly because of "the continued growth of the field of oncology in the United States."[13] Federal support of research in leukemia had helped to develop oncology as a discipline, fostering tensions over disease identity and professional identity. Was leukemia a "blood disease," a "cancer," or both? As Wintrobe saw it, "the initiative in these areas has been seized by groups and organizations with oncology as their primary interest . . . [because such groups] have recognized the need to speak to both the public and to government, and to develop a constituency within the public which knows of and supports their views." Hematologists had simply not spoken forcefully enough on the cancer problem, and "our inability to speak to the larger issues which face our society and our health care system has been a striking defect."[14]

This professional crisis and Wintrobe's lament about it were part of a larger drama involving careers, disciplines, diseases, and technologies of blood manipulation. Radiation and chemotherapy were central players in this professional transformation. In a letter to Max Wintrobe, Leon Jacobsen recalled that his interest in hematology had begun in the early 1940s, but wartime nuclear research, radiation studies, and national security matters had quickly altered his hematological interests. Military officials at the University of Chicago recruited Jacobsen to work in secret research related to the atomic bomb project. Concerned about the role of radiation in causing leukemia (an uncontrolled proliferation of white blood cells), they asked Jacobsen to oversee studies of "exposure to penetrating radiations and radioisotopes . . . a project that eventually resulted in the first controlled atomic reactor with all the consequences, good and bad." Jacobsen found himself manipulating blood and pondering hematological problems "that were heretofore beyond anyone's imagination."[15]

Through the early 1940s, his interests in hematology coalesced around leukemia, radiation, and chemotherapy. He recalled that "we conducted hundreds of experiments on fission products, including lethal ranges, general metabolism in the body, localization of fission products in the body, methods of reducing the body burden of these radioactive atoms, and treatment of any overexposure, whether it be from external sources or from ingested, inhaled, or injected fission products."[16] Such studies produced insights into the effects of these external agents on blood and blood-forming tissue—both as causes of blood dyscrasias and as treatments. The first human chemotherapy trials of nitrogen mustard "on patients with cancer of the blood" took place at this time.[17] At war's end, Jacobsen and many other hematologists like him had experienced a dramatic transformation. They had amassed experience with a specific disease and with new tools of blood manipulation. This experience informed their postwar work, validating a perception of themselves as radiation and chemotherapy specialists within the field of hematology and cancer, rather than as hematologists or blood experts. After the war, Jacobsen noted, "we . . . turned our attention to the exploitation of interesting and provocative findings that could not be pursued in depth during the war."[18]

United States radiation laboratories became major suppliers of technologies for leukemia researchers in the 1950s. With public enthusiasm for science at its peak, these government-research relationships expanded. Alvin Mauer, later to be director of St. Jude's Children's Hospital, recalled that "in 1959 the investigators at Brookhaven Laboratories provided us with tritium labeled thymidine."[19] The radioactive substance could be introduced into cells and used to monitor chemical processes of cellular growth. "With this tool and those techniques," noted Mauer, "we were ready to try to make some basic observations concerning the nature of the leukemic cell population . . . With our newly found tools it seemed that information concerning the leukemia cell population and its proliferative characteristics was like ripe fruit waiting for plucking."[20] Even as hematologists organized their own national and international societies and created new journals in record numbers, radiation and chemotherapy had begun to change their research field dramatically.

Cases of leukemia seemed to be on the rise, attracting intense public and professional interest. Was this increase a by-product of medicine's and society's newfound interest in the disease, or was the increase "real"? In a 1949 article on "The Leukemic Terror," a *Newsweek* writer noted that, during the last thirty years, "the case rate has doubled in the United States from 2 to 4 per 100,000 population . . . [accounting for] between 3,000 and 5,000 deaths per year."[21] Some speculated that the increase was due to the proliferation of specialists and their increased diagnostic abilities. One 1947 editorial in *Blood* noted that "the advent of the technician into the community hospital laboratory and the large numbers of routine blood counts consequently being made undoubtedly uncover many a case which was formerly called anemia or purpura."[22] Most blamed exposure to x-rays, other radiation, waste materials, gasoline fumes, sulfa drugs, cosmetics, and mineral oils for the increase.[23] Gardeners, radiologists, photographers, automobile owners, wearers of cosmetics, and many others came into regular contact with suspicious chemicals every day. Many physicians suggested, as did one in a 1958 *Saturday Review*, that this increase was "a by-product of more and more powerful therapeutic procedures and the production of chemical substances outside the biological experience."[24] "In this chemical age," wrote William Dameshek in the pages of *Blood*, "how do we know which chemical is someday going to start off a leukocytic 'spree' in a susceptible individual?"[25] Whatever the reason for the rising incidence of leukemia, blood analysis promised clues and answers.[26] But many of the novel interpretations of blood and its role in disease were being generated outside the boundaries of conventional hematology. Many researchers saw leukemia as a new and lucrative field of "cancer" investigation.

Access to chemotherapy and radioactive materials through federal agencies transformed entire research institutes, like the Thomas Henry Simpson Institute for Medical Research. Previously dedicated to research on blood diseases, the institute had been created in memory of a Detroit industrialist who had died of pernicious anemia in 1923. In one year in the 1920s, "a total of 81 patients with pernicious anemia were studied and treated at the Institute."[27] Beginning in the 1930s, however, "leukemia took up more and more the Institute's research program, while pernicious anemia took up less and less."[28] Before the war, x-rays and radioisotopes had been minor parts of the institute's therapeutic armamentarium. But in 1946–47, according to Simpson Institute annual reports, "an improvement in the availability of radioisotopes to the Institute took place through the formation of the University Radioactive Materials Research Group, which was able to obtain P 32 from the United States Atomic Energy Commission at Oak Ridge." By the mid-1950s, such tools contributed to their expansion of leukemia research and their decision to study other cancers.[29] "The mission of the Simpson Institute was extended to encompass 'oncology.'"[30]

With their expanding "mission," leukemia specialists suggested that leukemias were not merely blood diseases but forms of cancer. Their primary contributions were toward the general understanding of "cancer."[31] Studies of the effects of chemotherapy and radiation in various leukemias suggested, in fact, that these diseases might be subdivided and reclassified based on their different responses to chemical and radiation treatments. The public understood that, if such principles "can be shown to work in leukemia, it may be possible to extend it to other forms of widespread cancer."[32] As an indication of their rising status in medical culture, radiation and chemotherapy were rapidly rewriting the identity of diseases, becoming new tools for reclassifying diseases operationally—much as splenectomy and liver extract had in earlier eras.

The image of a "cancer of the blood" proved compelling to many specialists, though not always to traditional hematologists. Some speculated that leukemia was not a cancer.[33] One Simpson Institute author noted that, while most "thought that leukemia is a species of cancer . . . [characterized by a process of] atypical, persistent, and purposeless multiplication entirely unrelated to the requirements of the organism," there were good reasons to think otherwise. "One reason for hesitating to call leukemia a cancer," he noted, "is that typical cancers originate as a localized disturbance and develop as solid tumors before they spread, whereas the disturbance in leukemia is general throughout the blood-forming tissue."[34] The "true" identity of leukemia was no trivial abstraction. Its identity determined who would control research and treatment for this growing market of patients. Existing hematological tools had become well established by the 1940s and 1950s. But these were no longer perceived as leading-edge technologies, and few believed that these tools were up to the task of cancer study and treatment. In the area of leukemia research, hematologists slowly ceded this valuable turf to their competitors.

At the same time, hematologists saw their ranks fragmenting as academic hematologists lost touch with the majority of front-line practitioners. In the 1960s, it became clear that, outside the academic setting, pathologists "pretty much control all the hematology in hospitals . . . They say that bone marrow punctures and biopsies are their province . . . [and, moreover] the radiologist controls all the radioactive isotope procedures."[35] Another practitioner, Joe Ross, later noted that this inability to establish a solid institutional turf for hematology had crippled the specialty. "The performance of bone marrow aspirations and biopsies, and the recognition and interpretation of cytological and morphological abnormalities . . . that were the 'turf' of the hematologists," he wrote, "now increasingly are performed by hematopathologists."[36] Having generously shared its research tools with pathologists and others, hematology "to a major extent has worked itself out of a monopoly by educating the general internist to competently manage most disorders of the blood and hematopoietic system. This has left to the hematologist . . . the neoplastic diseases of the hematopoietic and lymphatic system."[37] But even this category of disease (the leukemias and lymphomas) were being encroached upon by oncology. The "War on Cancer" Program initiated in 1971 under the Nixon administration, shifted massive federal research priorities in cancer research, thus further emphasizing the importance of leukemia as a cancer concern.

Such political turf battles over technologies and disease ownership were often abstract and hidden from public view. But they pervaded post–World War II medicine. The public marvelled that these new tools were saving lives and giving hope to the desperate.[38] Practicing hematologists knew that these technological and intellectual struggles meant loss of clients, loss of status within the culture of medicine, and bespoke a need to control one's own tools. These struggles meant a crisis of professional identity. "Until now," wrote Dameshek in 1968, "the American

Society of Hematology has been reluctant to step into this 'political' arena, but with the problems as outlined here and the need for a definition
of a hematologist as a specialist . . . the Society may have to alter its
stand."[39] (Dameshek believed that "the Medicare and Medicaid people"
had also contributed to the problem by failing to acknowledge hematologists as legitimate and reimbursable "specialists.")

This decades-long struggle to define and control leukemia resulted
in the formation of a new discipline in the 1970s—hematology-oncology.
Writing in 1976, one hematologist noted that the major change in his field,
particularly since 1971, was "the advent of medical oncology as a recognized medical specialty." Because of "overlapping disease areas," a heated "boundary dispute" seemed inevitable, with hematologists suffering
the worse losses. The front-line hematologists saw that 27 percent of the
patients normally seen by them would eventually fall "under the confines of the medical oncologists," and this would be economically disastrous for hematological practice.[40] Without the integration of hematology and oncology, the extinction of the hematologist was inevitable.

For trainees who sought professional respect and status during this
period, moving into oncology seemed the best option. Although the
number of hematologists had almost tripled from 1960 to 1971, more and
more of them identified with the field of oncology. According to one 1971
survey, nearly 30 percent of all academic hematologists worked in cancer or white blood cell research.[41] "Increasingly," Joe Ross observed,
"hematologists are becoming oncologists, and are extending their concern to the management of neoplastic diseases of organs and tissues other than those of the hematopoietic system."[42] In the end, the embrace of
radiation and chemotherapy had reshaped the identity of many hematologists over several decades. As Wintrobe noted, "the initiative in these
areas has been seized by groups and organizations with oncology as their
primary interest."[43]

The new subspecialty of hematology-oncology took its bifurcated
identity not from any intellectual connection between diseases of the
blood and the cancers, but from the national politics of leukemia in
post–World War II America. With the founding of new journals, certifying examinations, and societies, a subfield like pediatric hematology-oncology could "achieve its own identity."[44] As blood studies reached new
heights of popular and medical appeal in the immediate post–World War
II years, such appeal paradoxically led to the fragmentation of blood
studies. The contested identity of leukemia did not exactly bring two

fields together; instead it drove hematologists toward cancer, where many remain today. These identity concerns among specialties and about diseases were products of a new federal patronage system, one which responded to political constituencies and dictated more than ever the trajectory of medical research. Institutions and practitioners created agendas in accordance with this new politics. But, as we will see in the following section, pharmaceutical companies and the medical profession at large continued to exercise considerable influence in this political arena and in the deployment of technologies.

Chloramphenicol: The Politics of Blood Effects

The modern story of chloramphenicol and aplastic anemia offers another tale about hematology's ambivalent relations with powerful new technologies and about the role of federal oversight in this unfolding drama. The industrial use of benzol during World War I had caused numerous cases of aplastic anemia (discussed in ch. 3), but public health concerns had faded with the shift away from benzol. The industrial use of benzol again during World War II had resulted in a similar pattern. With the synthesis and production of a new antibiotic in the late 1940s (chloramphenicol), few hematologists or drug manufacturers could have forecasted the disturbing resurgence of aplastic anemia that would follow in the drug's wake. Discovered in 1948, the drug was hailed as a wide-spectrum antibiotic, and it proved to be more powerful than even penicillin. Physicians prescribed it liberally. By the early 1950s, a few hematologists noted that chloramphenicol had been linked to a few "blood dyscrasias" and cases of fatal aplastic anemia.[45]

Did chloramphenicol cause these blood diseases? Could it (like benzol) shut down the body's production of blood cells? From 1952 through the early 1960s, the drug and the disease became closely linked in an evolving politics of hematological analysis and drug regulation. In the 1920s, aplastic anemia had been tied to factory life, but these findings were more disturbing to hematologists because they suggested that modern medicine itself was to blame for these human tragedies.

Cooperation among government, industry, and the military during World War II had produced many technological triumphs, such as modern blood transfusion, penicillin, and the atomic bomb. In the late 1940s, private industry had extended these accomplishments with the artificial synthesis of several new antibiotics. Chloramphenicol (marketed as

Chlormycetin by Parke, Davis, and Company) had become the most popular of these new antibacterial agents. Because of its value in the treatment of rickettsial infections, typhoid fever, and a wide range of infectious organisms, chloramphenicol was enormously popular with American physicians.[46] In 1951, sales of the drug by Parke-Davis hit $51 million, making it the best-selling drug of the year.[47] From 1949 to 1951, sales of chloramphenicol to federal agencies alone (such as the Veteran's Administration and military hospitals) had skyrocketed from 58,900 chloramphenicol capsules to nearly 22 million.[48] One hematologist later recalled that "chloramphenicol was being used . . . to treat all kind of infections, and even was used, I know, in treating things like the common cold, which was bad judgement."[49] The availability of such therapeutic tools sustained high public faith and elevated expectations in the drug industry and in medicine.

Hematologists began to note the disturbing side effects of this wonder drug at the same time that they began to ponder the effects of radiation and chemotherapy on the blood. They noted that a tiny percentage of patients treated with the drug developed severe blood dyscrasias, low blood counts, and fatal aplastic anemia with stunning suddenness. The first reports in 1951 and 1952 prompted a meeting between FDA officials, U.S. Public Health Service administrators, National Research Council (NRC) physicians, and representatives from Parke-Davis.[50] With an increasing number of powerful drugs on the market, the FDA was now under "legal obligation to certify certain drugs . . . limited to five antibiotics, insulin, and coal tar dyes used in foods, drugs, and cosmetics."[51] The 1952 meeting was convened by the NRC at the request of the FDA.

Those attending expressed unanimous concern about the rising incidence of aplastic anemia, but disagreed about the role of chloramphenicol in these tragedies. Federal officials, in their roles as regulators of such technologies, wondered whether this was a matter of causation or mere coincidence? Should the drug be banned? Should there be limits on its use? The meeting continued what had become a twentieth-century pattern, in which the identity of this disease and its relation to chemical influences would be determined through negotiation—now among pharmaceutical concerns, expert hematological advisors to government agencies, and federal regulators.

Dr. E. A. Sharp, Parke-Davis's Director of Clinical Investigation, denied that aplastic anemia was caused in any direct way by chloramphenicol. Its mere association with these terrible side effects did not demonstrate causation or culpability. "The Company had observed no blood dyscrasias in [their own] studies now under way in humans." Sharp emphasized that "the reported cases have been sporadic and isolated instances." Blame could be widely distributed. He believed that doctors frequently misused the drug and "that many patients had taken the drug continuously for fancied illness or to prevent tonsillar infection." Sharp concluded that "one can accept only on a presumptive basis the association of aplastic anemia with the administration of chloramphenicol."[52]

Speaking for the FDA, however, Medical Director Irving Kerlan insisted that "the Administration is equally concerned not only with chloramphenicol but also with other drugs such as Mesantoin, the thiouracil group, the sulfonamides, the nitrogen mustards and radioactive substances." Most of the conferees agreed that "everything pointed to an allergic susceptibility [of some patients] to chloramphenicol" and that this "allergy" frequently manifested itself as blood dyscrasia and aplastic anemia.[53] But what was the next regulatory step? Should chloramphenicol be pulled from the market?

The problem, as many saw it, was medical ignorance—that most physicians knew nothing of aplastic anemia and its relationship to chloramphenicol. The return of aplastic anemia reexposed problems in disease identification (enduring problems of blood- versus marrow-based diagnosis, discussed in ch. 3) that had never been resolved. Conferees admitted that aplastic anemia was not easy to identify. Some eight million people had been administered chloramphenicol since 1949, and "the United States count of deaths credited to aplastic anemia was 638."[54] These numbers, however, were not entirely reliable because of the many diagnostic terms used for naming blood dyscrasias and aplastic anemia. The FDA's Kerlan noted that, in one grouping of cases, "half of the 300 deaths from aplastic anemia were diagnosed as idiopathic [that is, of unknown origin]."[55] Physicians used various confusing terms to describe what might be called aplastic anemia.

Hematology, William Dameshek pointed out, was itself partly responsible for this confusion since "many physicians make a diagnosis of aplastic anemia when there is pancytopenia . . . Some cases of aleukemic leukemia or of benzol (benzene) toxicity may show pancytopenia in the peripheral blood stream." Some physicians continued to feel, as he did, that "examination of the bone marrow is necessary for a correct diagnosis." He concluded that "it is difficult to get physicians to define the term,

aplastic anemia." Carl Moore agreed with Dameshek that "the term 'refractory anemia' is used as a synonym for aplastic anemia."[56] If hematologists could not agree on the identity of the disease, then how were
generalists to agree, and how were they to confirm and document its incidence, much less establish its actual relationship to chloramphenicol?

After Parke-Davis's representatives left the 1952 meeting, hematologists and government administrators decided to leave regulation to
the average doctor. They voted to keep the drug on the market and to
place the decision of how to use this new and dangerous tool into the
hands of the average physician. They rejected the most drastic regulatory options since, as Dr. Joseph Smadel insisted, "chloramphenicol is a
valuable drug in several specific circumstances and . . . its dangers must
be considered in the light of its benefits . . . The basic problem," Smadel
decided, "was to find means by which to assist the average physician to
practice medicine sensibly."[57] A warning label, they decided, would educate physicians about chloramphenicol's side effects.

Despite acknowledging that the onset of aplastic anemia was both
rapid and irreversible, hematologists and administrators agreed that
blood testing of patients could guide the average doctor through this
dangerous terrain. They placed their faith in the "periodic blood test" as
the protector of patients who were being administered the drug. Could
peripheral blood studies indeed detect the onset of aplastic anemia? Most
evidence suggested not. Dameshek believed that it would "require alert-
ness on the part of the clinician to detect a beginning depression of the
marrow in time to stop the drug before the onset of irreversible changes."
Yet, the conferees placed their own trust and faith in the managerial skills
of average doctors. As Chester Keefer wrote, "it was the responsibility of
each practicing physician to familiarize himself with the possible toxic
effects of the drug." The administrators and hematologists eschewed
federal micromanagement of medical practice. "It would be impractica-
ble," wrote Keefer, "to specify in the labeling that the drug should be used
only for typhoid and resistant infections . . . Each physician would use it
as he saw fit."[58] Hematologist Carl Moore believed that "daily blood and
platelet counts would be required in order to give any real protection to
the patient," but this monitoring should not be mandated.[59] The 1952
conference concluded that the protection of consumers from the fatal effects of chloramphenicol was appropriately, if precariously, placed in the
hands of the average American doctor and his or her use of blood testing.[60]

This wishful hematological thinking turned out to be misguided. The adverse publicity on chloramphenicol and aplastic anemia temporarily affected the use of the drug and the incidence of the disease. By the late 1950s, however, aplastic anemia again became a federal regulatory concern.[61] In the intervening years, physicians and readers of most medical journals may have assumed that the FDA's approach had worked. But, as one 1959 article noted, "this was only because American hematologists . . . hardly consider it worthwhile to report another case or two. Actually, there has been a steady increase during the past few years . . . an increase presumably resulting from the freer use of the drug."[62] A 1960 report in the *Journal of the American Medical Association* attracted the attention of the FDA's William Kessenich, who called another conference on chloramphenicol. "As a result of the 1952 publicity," Kessenich wrote to the NRC, "use of the drug by physicians dropped sharply for a time." The brief decline was followed by "a significant reversal in recent years as shown by the following quantities [in grams] certified for sale":

1952	34,043,183	1956	27,320,359
1953	5,806,087	1957	28,872,529
1954	10,091,051	1958	40,593,884
1955	18,638,518	1959	50,070,646

Physician education had failed to protect the consumer. Kessenich concluded that "aplastic anemia deaths attributed to the use of Chlormycetin [chloramphenicol] continue to occur and in some instances, it appears that the drug was prescribed without a clear-cut indication for its use and apparently without a full appreciation on the part of the physician of the hazard involved."[63] With a new sense of urgency nurtured by growing public sensitivity over chemicals, radiation, and their effects, Kessenich asked the NRC to convene another meeting of physicians and hematologists.

The voices of consumers and parents who had lost children to the drug were more evident to Kessenich than they had been to FDA administrators a decade earlier. As Kessenich noted, "letters received from some parents of children who died of aplastic anemia following Chlormycetin therapy, assert that the drug was used improperly . . . These parents express severe criticism of the medical profession and the Food and Drug Administration."[64]

The suggestion to perform blood studies had done little to reduce physicians' use of chloramphenicol. Even to physicians who were aware of the side-effects controversy, the drug's benefits in treating infectious disease clearly outweighed the possibility of blood dyscrasias or aplastic anemia. A January 1961 article noted that, "despite warnings of the need for greater caution and more rigid limitation in the use of the drug, the past few years have seen a marked increase both in the use of the drug and in the number of cases of aplastic anemia associated with its use."[65]

NRC physicians had not lost faith in the blood tests or in the individual doctor as the regulator of dangerous technology in the medical domain. Kessenich suggested that blood studies were still valuable, but "such studies cannot be relied upon to detect bone marrow depression prior to development of aplastic anemia." The NRC conferees hastily endorsed a new warning label, but they continued to believe that if individual physicians were given the correct tools they would do a better job. "A serious need exists for a simple, easily applicable method of detecting early changes in the blood elements," they believed. The problem was time. "The study of the bone marrow, as well as changes in the plasma iron content, are valuable tests, but they are not readily performed on a day to day basis." The conferees agreed that "more effective education of physicians in the proper use of drugs must be a continuing consideration." There was little room for government regulation; instead, they called on pharmaceutical companies and leaders in medicine to "face this situation boldly and realistically." Building a better blood test, they believed, would protect and reassure consumers.[66]

In 1960, the politics of consumer protection from side effects was already becoming heated. In the next three years, the American public would hear of the birth of deformed babies whose mothers had been given thalidomide. Rachel Carson's *Silent Spring* would further sensitize Americans to the insidious dangers lurking in the so-called miracle chemicals of the 1940s and 1950s, most notably DDT. Historian Alan Marcus has documented the debate that began in this period over the use of the growth-producing hormone DES in the cattle industry and its links to human cancer.[67] By 1963, Senator Estes Kefauver of Tennessee would hold hearings on the drug industry, the medical profession, and the problem of side effects.

What emerged from these hearings was an indictment of the average doctors and of the pharmaceutical industry's manipulation of them. It seemed to Kefauver and others that the medical system was unable to manage itself or disease. Testimony portrayed the system as the very origin of disease.[68] One insurance official suggested that "five percent of all the patients in hospital wards were being treated for ailments resulting from doctor's treatment, particularly from side effects of drugs—a situation he declared, that made the problem equivalent to a major disease."[69] Public hearings of this kind highlighted the declining consumer confidence in miracle drugs and other technologies and declining faith in the ability of doctors to regulate themselves and protect their patients.

The expanding role of the federal government in regulating drug consumption and the health effects of drugs did not, however, have any dramatic effect on chloramphenicol. Warning labels were expanded to further highlight the limitations of blood studies. The American Medical Association had responded by creating a Council on Drugs, which educated physicians and the public. As the controversies over drugs subsided, however, the council was abolished.[70] It was left for clinical audits and reviews, academic exposés, and malpractice cases to arbitrate the correct uses of chloramphenicol and to determine the wisdom of using such dangerous tools.[71] Hematologists served as witnesses in this arena, and their experiences with aplastic anemia would serve as expert testimony in these tragic cases, although they often admitted having only a limited understanding of the full range of chemicals that could induce the disease.[72]

Aplastic anemia has had many identities during this century. Environmental disease, iatrogenic disease, disease of susceptible workers and patients, disease of civilization, blood disease, and bone marrow disease. These labels link disease to vastly different social processes, distributing blame and responsibility in different directions. Hematologists play a dominant, if still ambivalent, role in this social allocation of responsibility. Their constructions of aplastic anemia have defended or implicated particular interests—drug companies, patients, or physicians. Other constructions (like the term *idiopathic*) are meant, whether because of sincere lack of information or because of deceit, to avoid such direct blame.

In the early 1990s, some medical authors wondered whether chloramphenicol was "saint or sinner."[73] As developing nations gain access to such drugs and as the veterinary uses of chloramphenicol have increased, related cases of aplastic anemia have appeared. Taking a long historical view, one pathologist wrote in 1979 that, "since [Ehrlich's time] . . . the reports [of aplastic anemia] reflect, to some degree, the changing patterns of exposure to drugs and chemicals." Benzene, arsenic, Salvarsan, gold, and chloramphenicol followed one after the other. "Since the chemotherapeutic and antibiotic era," this author concluded, "chloramphenicol has been the drug most commonly implicated."[74] Hematologists continue to sit as judges, uncertain of how to label this disease and still arbitrating questions of blood testing, disease identity, and moral culpability.[75]

In one sense, the story of chloramphenicol and aplastic anemia is a story of medicine's ongoing attempt to come to terms with its own technical innovations by deploying ever more sophisticated technologies. In the 1920s, aplastic anemia captured the dilemma of industrial workers caught in an economic and social system not of their own making. The use of benzol by industry created the doctor's dilemma. Toxicologists like Alice Hamilton were seen as experts in reading the blood and in determining blame and responsibility. Today aplastic anemia illustrates the dilemma of patients who are caught in a burgeoning consumer-pharmaceutical-medical system. In this context, as one recent author has stated, "marrow damage [has become] one of the most feared of all drug reactions since it is, so frequently, irreversible."[76]

The dissemination of chloramphenicol into the hands of the average practitioner has clarified numerous disease problems. For patients, it has transformed many life-threatening infections into somewhat trivial events. Physicians, with a minimum of oversight, have deployed this technology. Yet the new drug and the pattern of its deployment created many new dilemmas about the control of technology. Despite the rareness of side effects like aplastic anemia, the technology has engendered public fear, periods of strict and lax federal oversight, and a lingering skepticism within the profession. Without being too deterministic, one might say it has also changed the mentality of practitioners—making many of them cautious, defensive, and fearful in their practice. It has made others into critics of the medical system. To many professionals, the story of chloramphenicol confirms that "miracle drugs" are inextricably linked to "iatrogenic disease."[77] Throughout its twentieth-century history, aplastic anemia has raised concerns not only about exposure to chemicals and about the management of side effects, but also about the technological system that produces such diseases. It has helped to produce many new systems of regulation—legal, bureaucratic, and medical—as well as ongoing debates about which of these constitutes the best method of controlling what is, in effect, a social and technological disease.[78]

Civil Rights, Electrophoresis, and the Hemoglobinopathies

Sickle cell anemia exemplifies another aspect of the transformation in hematological thought in the United States after World War II—the rise of patients' advocacy groups, their increasing role in the federal politics of disease, and the ways in which the modern technology of electrophoresis created a troubling new category of patient and further highlighted issues of control. As I emphasized in the previous chapter, with their ability to detect abnormal hemoglobin molecules using electrophoresis, molecular biologists opened a new investigative pathway.[79] The hypothesis of the molecular origins of sickle cell disease suggested that the human animal might be an elaborate protein-based machine and that disease might be a fixable molecular malfunction. Like Victor Emmel's blood test in an earlier era, electrophoresis became the basis for a new discourse on disease, technology, and social relations.

In the 1950s and 1960s, biochemists began documenting hemoglobin variations in many different populations in the United States and worldwide.[80] From these studies inside and outside clinical settings, they built a comprehensive understanding of "hemoglobinopathies" and their many consequences.[81] In an era of increasing patient advocacy and social activism, however, many patients' groups and eventually legislators seized upon electrophoretic findings for very different reasons. In the decades after Pauling's work, electrophoresis spread as a diagnostic tool. It became clear to many physicians that electrophoresis detected both heterozygotes—people with abnormal hemoglobins but without disease—and homozygotes—those suffering from clinical disorders. Embracing electrophoresis, different groups constructed very different narratives of disease and identity.

As a direct consequence of the hemoglobin studies in Africa, a new portrait of the evolutionary history of sickle cell anemia emerged (now called *hemoglobin S disorder* because of the particular form of hemoglobin present). This image moved beyond the level of the blood cell into geographic and ecological explanation and even claimed to offer compelling insight into African history. According to A. C. Allison, a British biomedical scientist working in Kenya in the early 1950s, people with sickle cell trait (the heterozygotes) actually had an acquired resistance against the malarial parasite.[82] Sickle cell trait was therefore proclaimed a "helpful defect" in malarial regions.[83] In passing the trait to their children, African heterozygotes granted their offspring a competitive advantage for survival in these regions.[84] If both parents passed this help-ful trait to one child, however, the disease became a grave clinical prob-lem. The heterozygote continued to exist as a social type because he or she had clear survival advantages in malarial surroundings, while oth-ers without this protection died off. This was a portrait of disease that highlighted the fundamental relationship between genes and environ-ment, nature and nurture, for it demonstrated how environmental forces determined whether this trait was a "good" gene or a "bad" gene. Sickle cell anemia was thus described as a "helpful defect" or (as J. V. Neel la-beled it in 1953) a "balanced polymorphism."[85]

This particular example of a balanced polymorphism gave cre-dence to an evolutionary theory that had long sought legitimacy. It also suggested that the difference between life and death, disease and health, strength and weakness was determined by a subtle ecological balance.[86] As one observer wrote, "the gene causing sickle cell trait . . . helps to de-fend against malaria, but when there is no malaria, it has no use and is only disadvantageous."[87] In the view of population geneticists, the sur-vival of heterozygotes could not be considered a social disaster. Sickle cell anemia told both a tragic and a triumphal story of human populations and delicate natural balances. The subtle hemoglobin abnormality of het-erozygotes indicated their great adaptedness to various kinds of adver-sity.[88]

In the mid-1960s, anthropologists like F. A. Livingstone suggested that African cultural evolution itself played the crucial role in this disease narrative—the story of the heterozygote. Livingstone asked, If these peo-ple continued to exist because of their adaptation to malaria, then what caused the malarial environment? These regions of malaria were not ac-cidents of evolution, Livingstone argued. These were the by-products of the evolution in African agriculture.[89] The stagnant bodies of water where the mosquito vector of malaria prospered emerged only after land had been cleared for agriculture; that is, malaria appeared as a conse-quence of the emergence of a stable agricultural tradition among former hunter-gatherer societies. Other anthropologists like Steven Weisenfeld agreed that this "new agricultural system allows expansion and involu-tion of the population and, at the same time, is the ultimate cause of an increase in malarial parasitism."[90] In this view, cultural change created the context in which the mosquito, malaria, the heterozygote, and thus sickle cell anemia would thrive. The disease and the "carrier" thus be-came deeply embedded in African history, linked particularly to tradition and to the emergence of distinct ways of life. It was *culture*, Livingstone and other anthropologists declared, that ultimately molded, shaped, and determined genetic evolution, nature, identity, and disease.[91]

Such portraits historicized "racial identity," embedding genes in culture, context, and social history.[92] Genes themselves were by-products of complex social, cultural, and historical processes. Electrophoresis merely detected the abnormality, but for anthropologists there was more to this disease or the heterozygote than nucleic acids, hemoglobin variants, and clinical problems. Hemoglobin studies using electrophoresis provided a window on evolution, culture, and the complexities of human identity. As one scholar has written, "the sickled cell, with its varied distribution among the varied peoples of tropical Africa, is a particularly powerful grain of sand that leads naturally into broader considerations of evolution and culture."[93] From the study of hemoglobin molecules, anthropologists, biomedical scientists, and historians in the 1950s and 1960s constructed a rich, proud, and textured historical narrative of African identity. Such tales offered existential reassurance to heterozygotes, disease sufferers, and their communities rather than specific medical interventions or preventive advice.

It was intense national black activism during the 1960s that effectively highlighted another aspect of the disease experience—the sickle cell crisis—and created another context for the evaluation of technology. Through the first six decades of the twentieth century, blood transfusion, splenectomy, bed rest through the crises, and a few drugs made up the standard medical armamentarium against sickle cell anemia. Physicians focused on an expanding and confusing set of symptoms. For patients in the 1960s, however, *pain* became one of the key signifiers of the disease—refocusing its identity not around the hemoglobin, but around an experiential concern. Whereas geneticists tried to understand the evolutionary status of the heterozygote, community activists highlighted the pain and suffering of "the sickler" as a long-ignored individual with a unique illness experience.[94] They called attention not to the heterozygote, but to vital patients' experiences which demanded prompt medical attention and research.[95]

As federal agencies assumed increasing powers in the funding of basic science and medical research, in consumer protection, and in the war on poverty, American citizens turned to government for answers about this and other maladies. Political forces altered the social meaning of this disease and brought "the heterozygote" and "the sickler" onto a national stage. A November 1965 information pamphlet on sickle cell anemia from the Department of Health, Education, and Welfare spoke to health care practitioners, asking "What is it?" "What causes it?" "Who gets it?" and "How is it recognized?"[96] Three years later, an updated pamphlet addressed patients directly: "How it makes you sick." "How you get it." "Can it be cured?" "How the patient can help."[97] The shift came in the midst of mounting public pressure during the era of Civil Rights, turning physicians and bureaucrats from scientific concerns about "the disease" to questions about patients and consumers of medical services.[98]

These were eventful years for patients' advocacy and consumer groups as their concerns gained national legislative attention. This was particularly true in specific disease areas.[99] Between 1970 and 1973, for example, cancer research, renal disease, sickle cell anemia, thalassemia, and cardiovascular disease would all become important national disease concerns. Disease foundations and advocacy groups highlighted the experience of disease. One representative of the Black Athlete's Foundation for Research in Sickle Cell Disease noted that "the problems of the trait carrier [the heterozygote] are mild in comparison to the agonizing pain and the terror that the sickle cell anemia victim endures."[100] Pursuing a health initiative supported by Republican President Nixon, Memphis' Congressman Dan Kuykendall announced his own support for legislation on this "excruciatingly painful" disease. "A terrorizing collection of symptoms attend the disease," he acknowledged. "But there is more to it than pain and suffering."[101]

Legislators like Kuykendall shifted attention back to the heterozygote, noting that this individual (detectable by electrophoretic testing) had become highly stigmatized in public and medical discussions. An extensive public relations effort was necessary. Kuykendall believed that "the trait is not a disease . . . The word 'carrier' brings to all of us the image of 'Typhoid Mary.'" He urged "that the words 'disease' and 'carrier' be stricken from our vocabularies when we are talking about the trait."[102] "The best way to explain this disease," he continued, "is to give the true historical background. Being a carrier of the sickle cell trait is not a weakness. It is not a stigma. Actually, it is a historical strength. The sickle cell trait is historically a protection from malaria" (46). Electrophoresis, having sharpened medical understanding of the heterozygote, had also helped to create a stigmatized category of pseudopatient, individuals of problematic social status. From the standpoint of family planners, genetic counselors, genetic screeners, and social policymakers, the heterozygote was a compelling problem—not only in sickle cell anemia, but also in cystic fibrosis and other genetic diseases.[103] Kuykendall suggested that some identity work was necessary to allow mass screening to succeed. "An individual who has the sickle cell trait," he believed, "is stronger [in Africa] than other people are, and I wonder why we do not use some of the strengths and the positive aspects of the trait instead of emphasizing the 'disease'? . . . When we talk about selling the sickle cell anemia screening programs, we must emphasize the positive aspects of the sickle cell trait."[104] The heterozygote should be a symbol of black pride.

The 1971 congressional hearings resulted in passage of Public Law 92-194, the National Sickle Cell Anemia Control Act of 1972.[105] This controversial legislation promised to increase research on new molecular-level therapies and to fund treatment and counseling at new community-based centers.[106] Many states initiated their own mandatory screening programs, deploying electrophoresis in classrooms, hospitals, and clinics, sending hematologists and their tools out to detect heterozygotes.[107] Emphasis on screening and "control" of the disease raised many concerns in the black community, particularly with regard to the stigma, insurance risks, and other consequences of being labeled a "carrier."[108] "In some areas," wrote Doris Wilkinson in 1974, "mandatory testing of infants has been proposed or enacted . . . In a most dehumanizing fashion, increasing numbers of state and local governments have begun to re-intervene in the marital decisions of black people."[109] For many such observers, federal and state responses to sickle cell anemia aggravated the problem.[110] "Certainly," concluded Wilkinson, "the growing negative by-products are not in the best interest of the black community." For other observers, even counseling and treatment centers were simply a "new ghetto hustle"—a cynical attempt by medical professionals to cash in on the black disease.[111]

Electrophoresis proved difficult to interpret, master, and control in this volatile political context. One representative of the Sickle Cell Foundation had testified before Congress that, "because electrophoresis is clearly the best method for carrying sickle cell testing on the massive scale contemplated by the bill, it is our strong belief that the legislation should specify that this method of testing be used."[112] Physicians and legislators agreed that electrophoresis was the most dependable of numerous diagnostic devices.[113] Although expensive, electrophoresis could accurately distinguish between sickle cell trait and sickle cell anemia. However, patients, medical practitioners, and genetic counselors were often confused about the difference between trait and disease. Writing in 1978 on the "genetic diversity in hemoglobins," two medical authors noted that "one can readily appreciate the difficulty involved in trying to explain these genetic concepts without making the person believe that he has a disease."[114]

Identifying the heterozygote remained a problem, even among the experts. "The specter of stigmatization of persons who carry some potentially deleterious recessive trait has been felt in the hemoglobin screening in recent years."[115] One survey found that physicians also confused the heterozygote with the diseased.[116] One researcher wrote in 1972 that "the ignorance even among experts as to what constitutes sickle cell disease and what does not is appalling . . . Some athletes who have represented their country at the Olympic Games in Mexico (at a height of more than 7,000 feet where sicklers are supposed to flake out) and beat the world, went back to their country to be found to be sicklers on mass screening campaigns and were promptly labeled sick."[117] Charged racial attitudes and social policies (such as the U.S. Air Force's ban on allowing heterozygotes to become pilots) shaped even the expert's interpretation and thus highlighted the social control function of electrophoretic testing.

Managing the disease not only became a task *for* technology but also involved the alleviation of social and racial stigmata *associated with* technology. Writing in the pages of *Blood*, hematologist Helen Ranney noted that "a child who is found to have sickle cell trait is hardly benefited if he is then treated as 'different,' or if this information is utilized to deny him employment or life insurance in the future."[118] Much of the hematological literature, government hearings, and counseling reports focused upon the stigma associated with the electrophoretic finding of the trait—even though the sickling trait was not, in itself, seen as a clinical problem.[119] By the late 1970s, then, broader social dilemmas implicit in electrophoretic screening had become explicit parts of the disease picture. Technology's psychological, social, and political effects had become central aspects of "the disease" to physicians, patients, and public policymakers alike.[120]

The original message of molecular biology had proclaimed to physicians, patients, and policymakers that electrophoresis located the core of the disease process, the hemoglobinopathy. These disorders were scattered throughout human populations. In subsequent years, however, national politics, race relations, competing disciplinary portraits of the evolution of hemoglobins, and hematology's relationship to federal and state social policy–makers all created more complex environments for technology and disease. Electrophoretic interpretation in the late 1960s and early 1970s entangled medical technology in a changing politics of race relations and racial identity. In 1973, one year after the Sickle Cell Anemia Control Act had been signed into law, another "hemoglobinopathy" associated with Greek and Italian Americans (thalassemia) gained its own legislative recognition.[121] Advocates and legislators asked, "Were its sufferers not also entitled to their hearings, and the benefits of federally-funded research?" The existence and political identity of self-conscious racial and ethnic groups in America demanded that these diseases be treated separately yet equally. Although they are closely related according to the terms of diagnostic technology and often are clinically indistinguishable, these two hemoglobinopathies remain quite distinct in name, in politics, and in identity.

Blood and National Politics

The federal government and the technologies it supported—radiation, antibiotics, electrophoresis, and many others—played a key role in medicine's postwar triumphs and transformations. Increased federal funding for the study of blood helped to build new approaches to disease, new disciplines, and new social possibilities for doctors and patients. As one enthusiast noted in the late 1950s, "a pathway has been opened, in man himself, for exploring the mechanisms by which the machinery on which life depends (the proteins) is put together."[122] But where would this pathway lead? In this chapter, I have traced three narrow threads in the history of radiation research, antibiotic therapy, and electrophoretic diagnosis, which were three among technologies' victories after World War II, evoking faith, drawing praise, and attracting federal dollars. In time, however, a national enthusiasm for technology would evolve into a politically complex effort to control these new tools. This national politics posed new challenges for hematologists, their tools, and their subject—blood disease.

The proliferation of radiation, chemotherapy, and blood testing had completely altered the practice of hematology, changed the identity of the hematologist, and altered hematological diseases. In the immediate postwar decades, hematology had been at the center of almost every medical advance. The link between chloramphenicol and aplastic anemia revealed that medicine's new tools had unintended hematological consequences, and this suggested (at first) that regulation was in some sense the hematologist's concern. Hematologists advised the FDA to leave the regulation of these tools to the average doctor; they hoped to educate these lesser experts in the proper use of blood testing. But, at the same time, other methods of blood testing and blood manipulation were also migrating out of their expert province. By the mid-1970s, a practicing hematologist would suggest that he was in danger of becoming "about as rare as . . . the coelacanth" and that his survival could only be assured "by hematology and medical oncology fellowships offering dual training programs."[123]

Because the new technologies were perceived as powerful and because their proliferation was so great, they also stimulated anxieties within the profession, in public discussion, in state and national legislatures, and in many other settings. Scandals over the harmful side effects of modern chemicals undermined public faith, beginning in the 1950s and increasing through the 1960s. Patients' advocates, consumer groups, environmentalists, and citizens opposed to the nuclear arms race all encouraged Americans to revise their earlier assessments of technological triumphs. Legislative oversight became an all too familiar mode of technology regulation. New technologies led medicine to discover new disease mechanisms and new therapies, but they also led medicine into new political and epistemological terrain. National political forces shaped the distribution of technologies and thereby changed the very meaning of disease, altering the status of specialties like hematology and gradually legitimizing the disease experiences and beliefs of patients themselves. Gradually throughout the postwar decades, the question of who should control technology gained prominence in national politics, for patients and consumers, and for specialists, like hematologists, who realized that their discipline, careers, and very identity depended on the answer.

Conclusion

*Disease Identity in the Age
of Technological Medicine*

In this century, medical technologies have frequently been celebrated for their value in combatting disease and, just as frequently, been scorned as frivolous gadgetry. Looking into the future from 1961, one thoughtful hematologist envisioned only the promise of technology. He saw the day when blood tests would reveal all of the body's ills and mysteries. "Blood tests should be able to detect the presence of many serious ailments in their incipient stages," wrote Bernard Seeman. "Should further experiments bear this out, medicine may reach one of its greatest goals—*a universal diagnostic test of the blood to detect the presence of disease in its earliest and, often, most curable stage.*" Blood testing would reveal the destiny and identity of both individual and disease. "In a sense," Seeman concluded, "these characteristic blood changes might be considered 'biological fingerprints' of disease."[1] Seeman's futuristic pronouncements highlighted a particularly intense post–World War II enthusiasm. Decades later, however, technologies of genetic analysis (often using blood) make the same promise—to uncover hidden information, to illuminate disturbing problems of individuality and disease. How are we to understand and assess such promises (so frequently voiced throughout this century)?

In this book I have argued that we must situate such medical pronouncements in a broader cultural context; the promise of technology cannot be fully assessed apart from a careful consideration of the diseases it purports to fight, the cultural ideals it embodies, and the professional tensions that give rise to technological innovation and interpretation. The preceding chapters—on the evolution of blood analysis and hematological beliefs—provide a basis for evaluating technology's claims. In each chapter, I investigated how the technologies of blood analysis have been deployed, what promises they inspired, whether those promises were fulfilled, and the social and professional issues their histories reflected. Many of these technologies—diagnostic blood tests, iron and liver pills, surgical procedures, electrophoretic analysis of hemoglobin, radiation, and chemotherapy—can be judged successes, in the sense that they succeeded in guiding physicians' theories and practices, assigning coherent meaning to patients' complaints and symptoms, and even informing social policy. They could liberate or oppress patients, they could resolve anxieties or create new ones, they could bring both clarity and complexity to doctors' encounters with disease. My assessment of these technologies has depended not only on whether they were successful in this sense, but also on particular contextual factors—on the institutional relations they engendered, on the economic interests they served, on the web of interacting cultural expectations and ideologies they embodied, and on the diseases they sought to construct and combat. To assess technologies fully, I have also taken a particularly close look at the physicians who derived so much of their identities from the tools they used.

In the late nineteenth century, independent practitioners—family doctors, surgeons, pathologists, and others—were faced with the relatively new phenomenon of blood analysis. All embraced tools of hematology, attempting to become practitioners of a more "scientific" medicine and thereby to raise their professional status. For some family doctors in the 1880s and 1890s, blood work endorsed an explicitly social and moral view of chlorosis (a disease of women, originating in the stresses of higher education and activity outside the home). Blood analysis confirmed what many physicians of the time believed, that these unconventional activities had demonstrably negative health consequences for American women. In time, this interpretation of blood would disappear. For abdominal surgeons at the turn of the century, hematology became one of several tools supporting their new zeal for splenectomy and their use of abdominal operations to combat disease. After only a few decades, the tools of hematology were turned against surgeons themselves, to reveal the excesses of this surgical vision. In the 1910s, hospital workers and a new breed of "blood specialists" embraced hematology as a basis for constituting an independent professional identity, for rationalizing clinical management, and also for disciplining surgical excess.

By the 1920s, blood work was thus well established in medicine. The proliferation of blood analysis meant that diseases like pernicious anemia, sickle cell anemia, aplastic anemia, and splenic anemia became well known, attracting increasing scrutiny in medical practice, public health, industrial medicine, and the public press. In part, this prominence reflected the supposed relevance of blood work to what many Americans perceived as pressing social concerns—the proper role of women, the health consequences of modern industrial work, professional work relations in the hospital, the rise of the pharmaceutical industry and changing patterns of drug consumption, and the problem of "Negro blood" and American race relations. By the late 1920s, hematologists could claim to speak authoritatively on all of these vital problems. In a society where the state and federal governments, insurance companies, hospitals, and large corporate interests assumed increasing responsibilities in health management, experts in blood disease could claim an expanding regulatory role. Blood analysis—in hospitals and factories, in workers' compensation hearings and court cases—became part of the arbitration of many medical, social, and cultural disputes. By the late 1930s, hematologists could also point to their own Nobel laureate (Harvard's George Minot), and they could begin to think of building a specialty organization to protect their professional interests.

What does the development of hematology in the first half of the twentieth century tell us about the changing role of technology in twentieth-century medicine? Blood analysis technologies produced biological findings that stood in ambiguous relation to disease. Most technologies—like liver extract and even splenectomy—succeeded in becoming central to patient management for only a limited period. Although much of our general understanding of technology in medicine is based on analyses of technologies that have endured, much can be learned from these technologies that informed medical practice for only brief periods. Looking closely at them, we see that success or failure occurred in particular institutional and cultural environments. George Whipple recalled, for example, that clinicians in a nonacademic, therapy-oriented hospital in the late 1910s had scorned the suggestion that liver had "cured" pernicious anemia. Their scorn reflected a set of assumptions about the disease that were prevalent in clinical culture. A few years later, university researchers from Harvard made similar pronouncements, and most physicians rallied around their findings, embracing the new gospel. To understand the history of liver extract (which in time became a diagnostic technology in its own right), I explored not only the evolution of the cultures of hospitals and academic research, but also the collaborative relations between university researchers and pharmaceutical enterprises and the dramatically new consumer and commodity orientation of medicine during the 1920s. Ultimately, it is these factors that explain the "conquest" of pernicious anemia and the temporary success of liver extract as a prominent diagnostic technology.

What did technology tell physicians about the identity of patients—particularly, of women, black people, and industrial workers? Technology was frequently used to reinforce and extend existing biases, suggesting, for example, that disease could be explained by the "natural" biological limitations of women, by Mendelian dominant blood traits inherent in "Negro blood," and by the biological susceptibilities of industrial workers. In so writing about chlorosis, sickle cell anemia, and aplastic anemia, blood experts often created disease identities that legitimated conventional social values and social roles. Other physicians and observers of medicine could look skeptically upon these technology-based claims, as did pathologist Montague Cobb in the 1940s, when he analyzed Emmel's blood test, and as did Mary Dunham Hankinson-Jones in 1904, when she wrote on the tragedy of splenectomy. Other observers described vividly, as did sociologist Gunnar Myrdal in the early 1940s and Simone de Beauvoir in the early 1950s, the ways in which beliefs about blood and disease provided a powerful basis for the reinforcement of threatened social relations. In assessing technology, I have emphasized that one must be aware of how its message is constructed and is made to speak to questions of social order.

But technologies have also been used to challenge such orthodoxies—both within medicine and in society. When Frederick Henry used hemacytometers to diagnose anemia and chlorosis in the 1880s, he was using technology not merely to identify a disease, but to construct a new kind of sick patient. By revising the belief that women were "naturally delicate," Henry sought to revise outmoded medical thinking and to promote an ideal of moral management that spoke more directly to contemporary concerns about women during his era. The embrace of a new technology has often thus involved practitioners in a politics of diagnosis and treatment and raised tricky epistemological problems of disease identity. When pathologists in the early twentieth century (wedded to the autopsy as the "supreme court of diagnosis") evaluated the new diagnostic claims of laboratory scientists, they understood that these new methods subtly undermined their own established status and knowledge. New technologies of blood analysis reflected the emergence of a new medical sensibility, focusing the pathologist's lens upon patients rather than corpses as the preferred subjects of analysis. Similarly, the use of electrophoresis in the 1950s and 1960s promoted a new trend in hemoglobin studies in medicine and challenged the orthodox view of sickle cell anemia as a disease of Negro blood. A central goal in this book has been to demonstrate how such new technologies supplanted older beliefs and came to endorse new orthodoxies in diagnosis and perception.

Whether challenging orthodox belief or reinforcing social and professional ideas, technological controversies always point to broader problems of professional identity and status. Physicians themselves often perceived these dimensions of the technological challenge. Their debates about the proper role of technology indicated an awareness of historically specific professional tensions. Debate over the true identity of pernicious anemia in the 1910s, 1920s, and 1930s cannot be separated, for example, from the intense competition among the specialties of hematology, surgery, neurology, and gastroenterology or from the changing relationship of researchers and general practitioners, to say nothing of researchers and the pharmaceutical industry. Likewise, the evolution of splenic anemia provides a particularly clear example of how professional identity and disease identity informed one another. The post–World War II history of leukemia highlights the enduring role of technology in professional struggles for disease ownership. Throughout this century, such debates took the form of almost ritualized struggles over specialty boundaries and professional status in a changing medical marketplace. In assessing technology, then, one must always consider the relationship of innovative or routine technologies to such questions of professional legitimation.

These debates point to an enduring problem of technology and "disease." The correlations between technological findings and disease (as clinically perceived, personally experienced, or culturally constructed) have always been problematic. Did splenectomy cure splenic anemia? The answer, of course, depends on how one defined splenic anemia in the first place—or whether one believed this was ever a legitimate disease construct (and many did not). Did the blood of women with chlorosis improve with moral management? Did liver extract cure patients with pernicious anemia? Again, such questions point us toward closer scrutiny of the problem of disease identity. Certainly, these tools provided important modes of patient management. But an important part of the history of technology has been the ways in which such medical technologies—splenectomy, liver extract, and so forth—actually constructed diseases. The very definition of pernicious anemia in the 1920s and 1930s depended upon the availability and marketing of liver extract. The legitimacy of splenic anemia depended upon the freedom of surgeons to perform abdominal surgery. Emmel's blood test and electrophoresis helped physicians invent two versions of sickle cell anemia that stood in problematic relation to disease as clinically perceived and personally experienced. In assessing technology, it is necessary to analyze and make explicit this enduring disjunction.

The very power of technology in twentieth-century medicine has raised enduring problems of control. Who should control and regulate the use of technologies? What interests and groups should guide technological interpretation? Which practices of social control have technologies endorsed, and which should they continue to endorse? The story of the anemias highlights the ways in which such questions emerged early in the history of particular technologies as they related to splenic anemia, pernicious anemia, sickle cell anemia, aplastic anemia, and chlorosis. It also highlights the ways in which medicine, industry, consumers, and later the federal government took leading roles in arbitrating these questions. The story of the anemias chronicles the voice of technology's critics and particularly the powerful force of patients' advocacy groups in the 1960s in shaping the use, control, and cultural critique of technologies.

The history of the anemias in the early twentieth century traced, therefore, not only the expanding authority of hematology, but also the rise of technology as a significant force in defining disease and in arbitrating a range of medical, legal, political, and ideological disputes relating to disease and society. It might be tempting to argue that this story is unique to the anemias because they were particularly malleable; vague ailments, they might have been especially prone to such shaping by competing specialists. While the anemias *were*, in fact, unusually malleable diseases, their histories illuminate all the more clearly the power of technology to take vague and imprecisely defined ailments and give them clarity, definition, and identity. Technologies today are used in similar ways—to construct medical stories about disease, to guide clinical management, to define professional boundaries, to create novel categories of persons, to manage the identity of both the sick and the healthy individual, to validate medicine's economic and political relations, and to inform both medical practices and social policies. To what extent can such observations be turned toward the assessment of technologies in current use?

Controversies over the meaning of the blood are everywhere in contemporary American society; they are not merely artifacts of the historian's imagination. In what follows, I highlight three ways in which contemporary Americans "assess" technology and then turn to particular issues regarding technology and contemporary blood beliefs (in the case of bone marrow transplantation and prostate specific antigen). Even with the rising symbolic importance of genes, the blood continues to have an appeal for public and professional alike. Indeed, with the possibility of blood tests for genetic disease, modern specialists imply that the blood is indeed the "biological fingerprint," a key vehicle for uncovering insidious diseases waiting to manifest themselves—from Alzheimer's to alcoholism. Such analyses of the blood, we are told, can be used to identify diseases early, to treat them before they appear, and to shape the future of human health. Skeptics have already voiced concern about the potential abuse of such blood tests by employers seeking to weed out "sick" workers and by insurance companies in determining the "risk" of insuring such individuals and their families. No doubt, in decades to come, physicians, bureaucrats, patients, communities, and legislators will be called upon to arbitrate such disputes and controversies and to define the proper uses of such tests.

The emergence of such tests, however, reflects much about the current culture of disease construction. As new genes supposedly linked to disease are being discovered, tests for those genes are being produced by biotechnology companies; such activity is promoted by medical geneticists and endorsed by a federal research program, the Human Genome Project. To the extent that genetic tests can predict the "future identity" of individuals, they define a patient and a disease (such as the breast cancer victim) that may become manifest sometime in the distant future. Such tests also become the basis for early medical treatment under the rubric of disease prevention (mastectomy in the case of breast cancer, although interventions for Alzheimer's, alcoholism, and other "genetic diseases" have yet to be imagined). What distinguishes these tools from their predecessor technologies is their far-reaching futuristic appeal. The diseases at the center of medical and social debate are, indeed, diseases

that are predicted on the basis of genetic evidence (and sometimes legitimated by family history). They are primarily "future diseases." Such
technologies, as I have argued throughout this book, do not reflect disease per se but stand in relation to disease. This point has become accepted in the history and sociology of science, and philosophers of technology have revisited the problem of technology and knowledge and the
ways in which this relationship is mediated by ideology, politics, or ideas
of moral and social order.[2] But these aspects of technology warrant further attention in genetic medicine, public discourse, and public policy.[3]

An extensive actuarial calculus in government, insurance companies, and health maintenance organizations has become particularly
prominent in the deployment of these tools.[4] Such technologies promise
to prevent enormous suffering and reduce health care expenditure dramatically; the cost of screening and preventing disease today, it is said,
will reduce the cost of treatment later. Of course, all of the calculations
have yet to be worked out. Health administrators and health maintenance organizations are constantly weighing the cost of performing particular diagnostic tests against long-term savings from finding disease
early. The idea that business economies shape their decisions about deploying technology is not, of course, new. What is new is that increasingly
these economies are limiting the individual consumer's access to technology. Administrators weigh the monetary expenditure for performing,
say, a particular diagnostic test against the long-term savings that may
come through finding disease early. Why pour dollars into technology-
intensive neonatal services, some ask, when the fewer dollars devoted to
prenatal care might reduce the burden of premature births? These days,
mass screening for prostate cancer, the use of fetal heart monitors in
childbirth, and the use of experimental interventions are also often discussed in these actuarial terms.[5]

At the same time, some scholars have eschewed either actuarial or
futuristic thinking in favor of a psychosocial evaluation of technology's
meaning. For these observers of technology and medicine, hidden dangers lurk in many technologies—new drugs, x-rays, invasive cardiac diagnostics, HIV tests, and so on.[6] Concerned with the problem of social
stigma, these scholars highlight the ways in which diagnostic testing
may produce useful information for physician and public health worker
while engendering social discrimination for the person "tested." Individuals who test positive for some disease (whether genetic disease, HIV,
or prostate cancer) may lose insurance benefits, suffer social ostracism,

or be adversely affected in numerous other ways. Such issues highlight a very modern and complex image of medical technology—at the center of actuarial concerns, futuristically promising, and both psychologically and socially dangerous. Any assessment of technology in our time cannot avoid these pervasive cultural concerns that shape the meaning of technology.

Today, more than nine hundred tests can be performed on the blood—and thus the substance can be used to build many portraits of disease, human frailty, and social pathology. A recent best-selling author on the benefits of the antidepressant Prozac suggests, for example, that studies have correlated the level of serotonin in the blood with emotional life, feelings of dominance, and self-esteem.[7] The interpretation of blood and other body fluids from serum cholesterol to serotonin continues to serve physicians well as a moral guide to good living. Let us consider two blood-related technologies and their cultural complexities.

In the decades after World War II, bone marrow transplantation (BMT) became (along with chemotherapy and radiation therapy) another promising tool for the treatment of blood disease—particularly the leukemias. With successes in treating some forms of leukemia, this tool has been extended into the treatment of other congenital hematopoietic diseases (for patients with aplastic anemia and most recently with sickle cell anemia).[8] The expansion of BMT fits a familiar pattern—the movement of a successful technology into new disease terrain (a move enabled in this case by numerous supporting technologies and promoted by the growth of hematology-oncology). The technology has been a boon for hematology-oncology, and it has engendered both therapeutic promise and professional controversy.[9]

As BMT expanded in the late 1980s and early 1990s, it has created new dilemmas in the case of sickle cell disease.[10] The problem of finding HLA-matched bone marrow donors has been one of the factors limiting the use of this technology. The success of the tool depends, in part, on the construction and maintenance of a social network of faithful donors. At the same time, although many researchers see BMT as a life-saving procedure, they admit that it has risks—there is a small likelihood of producing unpredictable and fatal side effects (as in the use of chloramphenicol).[11] One of these technological side effects is the iatrogenic graft-versus-host disease (GVHD).[12] This is only one of the risks of BMT. According to one study, the transplant-related mortality in children with sickle cell anemia has been (without considering GVHD) between 10 and 20 percent.[13] Thus, the choice of BMT for children with sickle cell anemia is a high-stakes gamble: the procedure could result in a complete cure, in death, or in the development of chronic or fatal GVHD. (In a recent survey of forty-two BMT subjects, one died of GVHD and six experienced chronic GVHD.)[14]

This tradeoff vividly captures the story of the expansion of a modern technology. Yet this is also a story of professional expansion and the changing identity of disease. Committed to the expansion of these tools, how has the hematology-oncology community faced the ethical and epistemological problems posed by this expansion? In some instances, the treatment has compelled a rethinking of the very nature of sickle cell anemia. As in the case of splenectomy in splenic anemia and liver extract in pernicious anemia (where particular treatments became the basis for redefining the disease), a similar redefinition is at work with BMT and sickle cell anemia. The professional urge has been to reconstruct sickle cell anemia—a highly variable disease—by using this available and promising "cure." According to one observer, the next challenge is the "need for *a clinical severity index* that can prospectively identify patients who are at high risk for a turbulent clinical course and a poor prognosis [after BMT]."[15] BMT—a modern blood manipulation instrument—becomes the occasion for rethinking the nature of the disease, subdividing sickle cell anemia according to indices of severity. Mock symposia have been organized to discuss whether it is possible to separate sickle cell patients who are likely to benefit from those with a poor prognosis.[16] New tools have always had this collective fascination for twentieth-century specialists, individual patients have always sought to gamble on the promise, and diseases are reconstructed in the process. Moreover, the BMT enterprise promises to reconstruct the identity of disease in ways that promote the further development of hematology-oncology.

Nothing better exemplifies the relationship among blood testing, professional identity, and patient identity than the controversy over a new blood test for prostate cancer (PSA, or prostate specific antigen). In 1989, this new test was advocated and prompted by urologists. These specialists embraced it as a sensitive screening test for this often-ignored disease of men. Physicians hailed PSA as a vital tool in the early detection of a deadly cancer. It offered the possibility of saving lives by getting a jump on disease.[17] To some observers, the test became a vehicle for putting the spotlight on prostate cancer as a disease of men (equal and analogous to breast cancer, a high-profile cancer in women). According to *Newsweek* magazine, while "breast cancer has emerged as one of the most ubiquitous afflictions on the broadcast spectrum, spawning a steady barrage of talk shows, health specials and public-service announcements, and a nationwide network of support groups and health collectives . . . prostate cancer, which kills a comparable number of men . . . commands nowhere near the attention or resources."[18] In this view, male health and sexuality was finally getting equal time—comparable public awareness and research support to its female counterpart.

But since its initial appearance, a variety of specialists, general practitioners, and lay persons have wondered about the relationship of this blood test to the disease. One medical specialist noted that "prostate specific antigen (PSA) based screening nearly doubles the detection rate of early prostate cancer. However, it is unknown whether the additional tumors detected are medically important."[19] If there is an ambiguous connection between test and disease, then what consequences does testing have for the anxieties and concerns of patients, for the policy of mass screening, or for the treatment of the disease?[20] The test itself has altered both the perception and the prevalence of prostate cancer. "The screening craze has had dramatic effects already. Though there's no evidence that prostate cancer is actually on the rise, the rate of new diagnoses has increased by 85 percent since 1973 and is jumping by as much as 16 percent annually."[21] Was this leap real or an artifact of suspect technology?[22] Because of PSA's ability to detect minute, even inconsequential, levels of cancer, some researchers wondered whether (with the proliferation of the PSA) anyone could be said to be truly cancer free.[23] PSA expanded the pool of the sick. Moreover, both disease and test have become a vehicle for a medical subspecialty—oncological urology—to demonstrate its value to society, not only in screening for disease but by raising public awareness and highlighting the continuing war against cancer. Despite the problems associated with the test, PSA has helped these specialists prevent many cases of prostate cancer, while catering to desires among many men for open discussion of mortality, sexuality, and identity.

At the same time, however (and this too is characteristic of new technology), the PSA test has raised concerns within the medical profession at large—not only about the relationship of the blood test to clinical disease, but also about the professional relationship of urologists to general physicians and about the actual harm of early medical interventions. Challenged by these questions, specialists insisted that PSA is a useful diagnostic tool; the only problem, they stated, was proper use and interpretation of its findings.[24] Others believed that the test was perhaps *too* sensitive (especially compared to standard physical diagnosis using the digital rectal examination).[25] It detected evidence of prostate cancer at such an early stage and prostate cancer often developed so slowly (especially in older men) that they wondered what the blood test actually found. Moreover, surgical treatment often resulted in new complaints—impotence and incontinence.[26] For many (but certainly not all) men with PSA-defined "prostate cancer," death came from other causes rather than from the slow-developing disease. In late 1995, an independent panel sponsored by the U.S. Public Health Service recommended that the use of the PSA test be reduced because of these ambiguities; the American Urological Association, protecting its own diagnostic, therapeutic, and professional interests and speaking on behalf of many patients, immediately disagreed.[27] How, then, can we assess this new technology? One way is to explore further the broad range of identity issues—problems of patient identity, professional identity, and disease identity—shaping this contemporary discourse.

Seen against the background of the previous chapters, these debates should by now be familiar dramas characteristic of the age of technological medicine. In previous chapters I explored the ways in which new medical technologies, like the PSA test, constructed and perpetuated similar anxieties within the profession and among patients' groups and the technology's overseers. It behooves us to understand that these debates about "disease itself" are also political debates about the nature of diagnosis, the relative status of specialists and generalists in the marketplace of patients, and the implications of new technology for the economic well-being of the practitioner and the physical and emotional well-being of the patient. An intense commercialism informs this debate as well. In the case of PSA, two different marketed tests often reveal very different PSA results in the same patient—raising the question of which to rely upon.[28] In short, the current story of the PSA blood test and prostate cancer is, on one level, about a biopathological entity and the alleviation of suffering. But, on another level, it concerns the variety of interests that speak to, oversee, construct, and manipulate the problem of disease. The future of prostate cancer screening will depend in large part on how these interests and social forces interact.

The preface of this book began with an anecdote about my father, his various identities, and the various readings of his "abnormal EKG."

The book has offered a detailed historical analysis of the politics of medical technologies throughout this century and of their relationship to questions of medical, patient, and disease identity. It has concluded with discussion about the contemporary politics of PSA and the contested identity of prostate cancer. One critical idea runs throughout: disease thought is inextricably bound to social thought and social relations. It behooves us all—scholars, students of medicine, health care practitioners, advocates, and patients—to bear this relation in mind and to study it. It behooves us as well to find a language—apart from the cost-benefit calculus—with which to assess the meaning of technology in modern medicine. I have sought to explore some of those meanings, to make explicit the ways in which problems of identity have been, are now, and will continue to be bound up in the use of medical technology and in the discourse of disease.

Notes

Introduction: *Putting the Question to Technology*

1. See Robert C. Gallo et al., "Frequent Detection and Isolation of Cytopathic Retroviruses (HTLV-III) from Patients with AIDS and at Risk for AIDS," *Science* 224 (1984): 500–502; for observations on the subsequent construction of AIDS, see Simon Watney, *Practices of Freedom: Selected Writings on HIV/AIDS* (Durham: Duke University Press, 1994); see especially ch. 8, "'AIDS' or 'HIV Disease'?" See also Gerald Oppenheimer, "In the Eye of the Storm: The Epidemiological Construction of AIDS," in *AIDS: The Burdens of History*, ed. Elizabeth Fee and Daniel Fox (Berkeley: University of California Press, 1988).

2. For insight into the meaning of HIV seropositivity, see, for example, D. W. Lyter et al., "The HIV Antibody Test: Why Gay and Bisexual Men Want or Do Not Want to Know Their Results," *Public Health Reports* 10 (1987): 468–574; K. McCann and E. Wadworth, "The Experience of Having a Positive HIV Antibody Test," *AIDS Care* 3, no. 1 (1991): 43–53. For more on the implications of thinking of AIDS as a "gay disease," see P. L. Westerman and P. M. Davidson, "Homophobic Attitudes and AIDS Risk Behavior of Adolescents," *Journal of Adolescent Health* 14 (1993): 208–13.

3. B. F. Haynes, "Scientific and Social Issues of Human Immunodeficiency Virus Vaccine Development," *Science* 260 (1993): 1279–86; R. B. Belshe et al., "Interpreting HIV Serodiagnostic Test Results in the 1990s: Social Risks of HIV Vaccine Studies in Noninfected Volunteers," *Annals of Internal Medicine* 121 (1994): 584–89.

4. As philosopher Hubert Dreyfus has written recently, in a thoughtful essay on Heidegger's view of technology, "once one recognizes the technological understanding of *being* for what it is—a historical relation—one gains a free relation to it." Dreyfus, "Heidegger on Gaining a Free Relation to Technology," in *Technology and the Politics of Knowledge*, ed. Andrew Feenberg and Alastair Hannay (Bloomington: Indiana University Press, 1995), 97–107.

5. One genre of technology assessment is Dorothy Nelkin and Laurence Tancredi, *Dangerous Diagnostics: The Social Power of Biological Information* (New York: Basic Books, 1989). Others include Louise Russell, *Educated Guesses: Making Policy about Medical Screening Tests* (Berkeley: University of California Press, 1994); Jeffrey Fisher, *The Plague Makers: How We Are Creating Catastrophic New Epidemics—And What We Must Do to Avert Them* (New York: Simon and Schuster, 1994); and Joseph Bronzino et al., *Medical Technology and Society: An Interdisciplinary Perspective* (New York: McGraw-Hill, 1990). Other assessments of technology include M. Janet Barger-Lux and Robert Heaney, "For Better or Worse: The Technological Imperative in Health Care," *Social Science Medicine* 22 (1986): 1313–20, and Stanley Joel Reiser, *Medicine and the Reign of Technology* (New York: Cambridge University Press, 1978).

6. For a recent statement on the need for such perspectives on medical technology, see Henk A. M. J. ten Have, "Medical Technology Assessment and Ethics: Ambivalent Relations," *Hastings Center Reports* 25 (1995): 13–19.

7. Several works have examined the ways in which technologies give rise to particular clinical or laboratory constructions of facts. See, for example, Ludwig Fleck, *Genesis and Development of a Scientific Fact* (Chicago: University of Chicago Press, 1979), and Bruno Latour and Steve Woolgar, *Laboratory Life: The Construction of Scientific Facts* (Princeton: Princeton University Press, 1986).

8. Alexandra Oleson and John Voss, eds., *The Organization of Knowledge in Modern America, 1880–1920* (Baltimore: Johns Hopkins University Press, 1979). For a discussion of similar trends toward corporate control of science and technology, see David Noble, *America by Design: Science, Technology, and the Rise of Corporate Capitalism* (New York: Knopf, 1977).

9. A synthetic discussion of disease thought and its implications in these terms is Charles Rosenberg, "Disease and Social Order in America: Perceptions and Expectations," in Fee and Fox, eds., *AIDS: The Burdens of History*.

10. In a recent collection on the laboratory revolution in medicine, Andrew Cunningham and Perry Williams examined why the laboratory became so dominant in modern medicine. The essays in this collection contribute much to our understanding of the tools, intellectual products, and cultural context that created laboratory medicine. Cunningham and Williams, eds., *The Laboratory Revolution in Medicine* (Cambridge: Cambridge University Press, 1992).

11. A theoretically nuanced interpretation of the meaning of anemia in the context of tropical medicine is Annemarie Mol and John Law, "Regions, Networks, and Fluids: Anaemia and Social Topology," *Social Studies of Science* 24 (1994): 641–71.

12. Michel Foucault, *The History of Sexuality: An Introduction* (New York: Vintage Books, 1990), 147.

13. Richard Cabot, "The Blood Stream as a Public Highway," *Yale Medical Journal* 1903 (August): 1–5.

14. Writing in 1919, William Osler, a leading figure in Anglo-American medicine, noted that "those . . . whose professional careers coincide with its modern study will remember how important was the part played by . . . severe anaemia." Osler, "The Severe Anaemias of Pregnancy and the Post-Partum State," *British Medical Journal* 1 (4 January 1919): 7.

15. "To Your Health: Blood," 1957 NBC program (in conjunction with the New York County Medical Society), National Museum of Television and Radio (New York).

16. Maxwell Wintrobe to Owsei Temkin, 19 January 1978, Maxwell Wintrobe Papers, box 4, folder: "History of Hematology, correspondence, 1975–79," Marriot Library, University of Utah.

17. Here I paraphrase Foucault, who argued that "power spoke *through* blood" before the nineteenth century, but not in our society, where power "spoke *of* sexuality and *to* sexuality." Foucault, *The History of Sexuality*, 147.

18. For a discussion of the ways in which biological thought has sustained its integrity by drawing upon metaphors from the wider world and for insight on the relation of microcosm and macrocosm in biological thought, see Owsei Temkin, "Metaphors of Human Biology," in *The Double Face of Janus* (Baltimore: Johns Hopkins University Press, 1977), 271–83.

19. Alfred McCann, *The Science of Eating* (New York: George H. Doran, 1918), 75.

20. The International Society of Hematology was founded in 1946. The American Society of Hematology was founded in 1954. See Maxwell Wintrobe, *Hematology: The Blossoming of a Science* (Philadelphia: Lea and Febiger, 1985), 147. This is a standard reference in the history of hematology, combining autobiographical memoir with reflections on the history of the specialty.

21. Frederick Henry, *Anaemia* (Philadelphia: Blakiston, 1887), 16.

22. Throughout the twentieth century authors have linked chlorosis variously to corset wearing, to exploitative industrial work, and to the dietary habits of Victorian women. According to such theories, a general emancipation of women from the constraints of nineteenth-century life led to the decline of chlorosis. Others wondered whether chlorotic anemia ever really existed, arguing that the disease was merely a symbolic construct, created by bourgeois physicians in a capitalist society increasingly calling for the medical regulation of women laborers. Yet others insisted that the disease did exist, but that its integrity was undermined by the use of more technically precise diagnostic methods and language. Chapter 1 offers an extended discussion of the historical origins of these theories.

23. Recent medical authors continue to disagree about its reality. See, for example, W. H. Crosby, "Splenectomy: In and Out of Fashion," *Archives of Internal Medicine* 145 (1985): 225–27; W. H. Crosby, "The Spleen," in Max Wintrobe, ed., *Blood, Pure and Eloquent: A Story of Discovery, of People, and of Ideas* (New York: McGraw-Hill, 1980), 96–138; and A. H. T. Robb-Smith, "Osler's Influence on Hematology," *Blood Cells* 7 (1981): 513–33.

24. Roger Lee, *The Happy Life of a Doctor* (Boston: Little, Brown, 1952), 225.

25. Erving Goffman, *Stigma: Notes on the Management of Spoiled Identity* (New York: Prentice-Hall, 1963).

26. Among the works that have most influenced my historical view of medical thought, see Knud Faber, *Nosography: The Evolution of Clinical Medicine in Modern Times* (New York: Hoeber, 1930); Robert Hudson, *Disease and Its Control: The Shaping of Modern Thought* (Westport, Conn.: Greenwood, 1983); Owsei Temkin, *The Falling Sickness: A History of Epilepsy from the Greeks to the Beginnings of Modern Neurology* (Baltimore: Johns Hopkins University Press, 1995); and Charles Rosenberg, *The Cholera Years: The United States in 1832, 1849, and 1869* (Chicago: University of Chicago Press, 1962).

27. "Blood and Iron," *Time Magazine*, 2 November 1953, 105. Quote is from Maxwell Wintrobe. As the article noted, "only a generation ago, anemia was both a common and fashionable complaint."

28. Bernard Seeman, *The River of Life: The Story of Man's Blood, from Magic to Science* (New York: W.W. Norton, 1961), 12.

29. See R. Scott and R. Gilbert, "Genetic Diversity in Hemoglobins: Disease and Nondisease," *Journal of the American Medical Association* 239 (1978): 2681–84. For an earlier observation of the distinction between hemoglobinopathy and clinical disease, see Owsei Temkin, "The Scientific Approach to Disease: Specific Entity and Individual Sickness," in *The Double Face of Janus*, 444–45.

30. Paul Clough, *Diseases of the Blood* (New York: Harper, 1929), 1.

31. Quoted in "William Dameshek, 1900–1969" (obituary), *Blood* 35 (1970): 580.

32. One can think of twentieth-century specialties as being organized around one of four primary features—tools, patients, organs, or diseases. These have been key overlapping factors supporting the integrity of specialization in medical practice and knowledge production. Some specialties, like obstetrics and gynecology, geriatrics, and family medicine, have sought to maintain their integrity by appealing to the health concerns of specific patient clienteles. Their identity and status has depended, to a large extent, on the social and economic histories of these client groups. Specialties like cardiology, nephrology, and pulmonology have arisen primarily because of the perceived place of particular organs in the body economy. Their integrity depends on the degree to which specific diseases can be located in these organs. A third group of specialists—oncologists and diabetologists, for example—have come to tie their identity to specific disease concepts. Their identity is therefore inextricably linked to the perception of diseases, their prevalence, and their politics. A fourth kind of specialist organizes primarily around the mastery of particular tools. For radiologists and anesthetists, their integrity depends on their control of such technologies and on their ability to convince patients and physicians of the value of these tools. An excellent discussion of the dynamics of specialization in twentieth-centruy America is Rosemary

Stevens, *American Medicine and the Public Interest* (New Haven: Yale University Press, 1971).

33. For a recent example, see the rhetoric of Carl Pochedly, "From the Editor," *American Journal of Pediatric Hematology/Oncology* 1 (spring 1979): 1; Carl Pochedly, "From the Editor," *American Journal of Pediatric Hematology/Oncology* 2 (spring 1980): 3; and Carl Pochedly, "Emergence of Pediatric Hematology/Oncology as an Independent Specialty," *American Journal of Pediatric Hematology/Oncology* 7 (summer 1985): 183–89.

34. On the need for definitions of technology that go beyond instrumentation, see Steve Shapin and Simon Shaffer, *Leviathan and the Air Pump: Hobbes, Boyle, and the Experimental Life* (Princeton: Princeton University Press, 1985), 25. On technological systems, see the excellent collection of essays in *The Social Construction of Technological Systems: New Directions in the Sociology and History of Technology*, ed. Wiebe Bijker, Thomas Hughes, and Trevor Pinch (Cambridge: MIT Press, 1987).

35. Sir Humphry Davy Rolleston, *Aspects of Age, Life, and Disease* (London: Kegan Paul, Trench, 1928), 79.

36. A recent example of scholarship along these lines is Charles Rosenberg and Janet Golden, eds., *Framing Disease: Studies in Cultural History* (New Brunswick, N.J.: Rutgers University Press, 1992). The pioneer of such studies is Ludwig Fleck, *Genesis and Development of a Scientific Fact*, a study using the Wasserman test as the focus for exploring the early twentieth-century reconstruction of syphilis. Also see Ronald Bayer, *Homosexuality and American Psychiatry: The Politics of Diagnosis* (Princeton: Princeton University Press, 1987); Mark Micale, "On the 'Disappearance' of Hysteria: A Study in the Clinical Deconstruction of a Diagnosis," *ISIS* 84 (1993): 496–526; Carroll Smith-Rosenberg, "The Hysterical Woman: Sex Roles and Role Conflict in Nineteenth Century America," in Carroll Smith-Rosenberg, *Disorderly Conduct: Visions of Gender in Victorian America* (New York: Oxford University Press, 1985); Steven Peitzman, "From Bright's Disease to End Stage Renal Disease," in Rosenberg and Golden, eds., *Framing Disease*; and Peter Wright and Andrew Treacher, eds., *The Problem of Medical Knowledge: Examining the Construction of Medicine* (Edinburgh: University of Edinburgh Press, 1982). Useful works on disease epistemology include Lester King, *Medical Thinking: A Historical Preface* (Princeton: Princeton University Press, 1982), and Georges Canguilhem, *On the Normal and the Pathological* (New York: Zone Books, 1991).

Chapter 1   "Chlorosis" Remembered: *Disease and the Moral Management of American Women*

1. William Osler, "Chlorosis," in *Text-book of the Theory and Practice of Medicine by American Authors*, ed. William Pepper, vol. 2 (Philadelphia: W.B. Saunders, 1894), 197.

2. A classic chlorotic, according to some analysts, is Milly Theale in Henry James, *The Wings of the Dove* (New York: Scribner's, 1902); see also W. Somerset Maugham, *Of Human Bondage* (New York: Sun Dial Press, 1915). For two discussions of James's Milly Theale, see Caroline Mercer and Sarah E. Wangensteen, "'Consumption, Heart-Disease, or Whatever': Chlorosis, a Heroine's Illness in *The Wings of the Dove*," *Journal of the History of Medicine and Allied Sciences* 40 (July 1985): 259–85, and Sarah E. Wangensteen and Caroline Mercer, "Addenda: Henry James, Chlorosis, and Heart Disease," *Journal of the History of Medicine and Allied Sciences* 43 (April 1988): 183–90. See also Diane Price Herndl, *Invalid Women: Figuring Feminine Illness in American Fiction and Culture, 1840–1940* (Chapel Hill: University of North Carolina Press, 1993).

3. J. Lange, *Medicinalium Epistolarum Miscellanea* (Basel, 1554), trans. Ralph H. Major, in *Classic Descriptions of Disease* (Springfield, Ill.: Charles C Thomas, 1932). "I therefore say, I instruct, virgins afflicted with this disease, that as soon as possible they live with men and copulate . . . Wherefore, be of good courage, you shall give away your daughter: also I shall be present at the nuptial with pleasure" (pp. 446–47).

4. By 1830, *Gunn's Domestic Medicine* describes chlorosis, the green sickness, as merely a retention or stoppage of the menses. John Gunn, *Gunn's Domestic Medicine* (facsimile of 1st ed.), with introduction by C. E. Rosenberg (Knoxville: University of Tennessee Press, 1980). For some early twentieth-century lay authors, however, the linkage of marriage and chlorosis continued. See discussion of "Diseases of the Blood in Relation to Marriage," in H. Senator and S. Kaminer, *Marriage and Disease* (New York: Hoeber, 1909), 183, 188–90.

5. Frederick Porteus Henry, *Anaemia* (Philadelphia: Blakiston, 1887), 16.

6. New York's Francis Delafield, speaking of a case in 1889, noted that "I do not mean to say that the sufferings of these patients are imaginary; they are perfectly real. They are sick; they require treatment; and yet you can not ascribe the sickness to any of the ordinary categories. They are often somewhat anaemic; they have a diminution of the quantity of hemoglobin." Francis Delafield, "The Clinic—On Blood Diseases," *Journal of the American Medical Association* 13 (1889): 776.

7. Henry, *Anaemia*, 16.

8. The concern with productivity and efficiency in late nineteenth-century America has been examined by Daniel Rogers, *The Work Ethic in Industrial America, 1850–1920* (Chicago: University of Chicago Press, 1978), and also by Samuel Haber, *Efficiency and Uplift: Scientific Management in the Progressive Era, 1890–1920* (Chicago: University of Chicago Press, 1964).

9. Advertisements for the treatment of chlorosis, anemia, and other ailments appeared regularly in the pages of the *Boston Medical and Surgical Journal*. See, for example, "What is Hematherapy?" *Boston Medical and Surgical Journal* 139 (1898): 11. See also "A Flat Fact," *Boston Medical and Surgical Journal* 139 (1988): 4. For writ-

ings on illness due to social stress, see "Editorial: More 'Cruelty to Women',"
Boston Medical and Surgical Journal 103 (1880): 209–10; Robert Edes, "High Pres-
sure Education: Its Effects," *Boston Medical and Surgical Journal* 106 (1882): 220–23;
Jane K. Sabine, "The Effect of Public School on the Health of the College Girl,"
Boston Medical and Surgical Journal 146 (1902): 386–90.

10. See C. W. Townsend, "Chlorosis, with Especial Reference to Its Treatment
by Intestinal Antisepsis," *Boston Medical and Surgical Journal* 134 (1896): 529.

11. Franklin Martin, *Fifty Years of Medicine and Surgery: An Autobiographical
Sketch* (Chicago: Surgical Publishing, 1934), 108.

12. Recently, Mark Micale commented upon the contemporaneous decline of
"hysteria." Mark Micale, "On the 'Disappearance of Hysteria: A Study in the
Clinical Deconstruction of a Diagnosis," *ISIS* 84 (1993): 496–526. On the prolifer-
ation of hospitals during this period, see George Rosen, *The Structure of American
Medical Practice, 1875–1941,* ed. Charles Rosenberg (Philadelphia: University of
Pennsylvania Press, 1983).

13. Henry, *Anaemia,* 16.

14. Ibid., 38.

15. Female invalidism was a prominent theme in much late nineteenth-century American writing. One version of the female invalid appeared in Charlotte
Perkins Gilman, "The Yellow Wallpaper," reprinted in *The Charlotte Perkins
Gilman Reader,* ed. Ann J. Lane (New York: Pantheon, 1980), 1–19; see also *Women
and Economics: A Study of the Economic Relation between Men and Women as a Factor
in Social Evolution* (Boston: Small and Maynard, 1898). Gilman was also an astute
critic of the rest cure. The female invalid has attracted the attention of numerous
historians. See Lorna Duffin, "The Conspicuous Consumptive: Woman as an Invalid," in *The Nineteenth Century Woman,* ed. Sara Delamont and Lorna Duffin
(New York: Harper and Row, 1978).

On the way in which ideas about female biology were used to circumscribe
the lives of women, see Carroll Smith-Rosenberg, "The Hysterical Woman: Sex
Roles and Role Conflict in Nineteenth-Century America," in *Disorderly Conduct:
Visions of Gender in Victorian America* (New York: Knopf, 1985), 197–216; Ann
Douglas Wood, "The Fashionable Diseases: Women's Complaints and Their
Treatment in Nineteenth-Century America," *Journal of Interdisciplinary History* 4
(1973): 25–52; Sarah Stage, *Female Complaints: Lydia Pinkham and the Business of
Women's Medicine* (New York: W.W. Norton, 1979); Diane Price Herndl, *Invalid
Women: Figuring Feminine Illness in American Fiction and Culture, 1840–1940*
(Chapel Hill: University of North Carolina Press, 1993); and Marina Benjamin,
ed., *A Question of Identity: Women, Science, and Literature* (New Brunswick, N.J.:
Rutgers University Press, 1993). See also Mary Jacobus, Evelyn Fox Keller, and
Sally Shuttleworth, eds., *Body/Politics: Women and the Discourses of Science* (New
York: Routledge, 1990). Another overview of the relations between women and
physicians in the late nineteenth century is Nancy Theriot, "Women's Voices in

Nineteenth-Century Medical Discourse: A Step toward Deconstructing Science," *Signs* 19 (autumn 1993): 1–31.

A classic and cogent exploration of these themes is Charles Rosenberg and Carroll Smith-Rosenberg, "The Female Animal: Medical and Biological Views of Women," in Charles Rosenberg, *No Other Gods: On Science and American Social Thought* (Baltimore: Johns Hopkins University Press, 1976).

16. Barbara Ehrenreich, *For Her Own Good: 150 Years of Experts' Advice to Women* (Garden City, N.Y.: Anchor Press/Doubleday, 1978). For literature on the social, economic, and political transformation of womanhood in the late nineteenth century—and specifically on the "problem" of appropriate female activities, see Nancy Cott, *The Grounding of Modern Feminism* (New Haven: Yale University Press, 1987); Kathy Peiss, *Cheap Amusements: Working Women and Leisure in New York City, 1880 to 1920* (Philadelphia: Temple University Press, 1985); Smith-Rosenberg, *Disorderly Conduct*; and Leslie Woodcock Tentler, *Wage-earning Women: Industrial Work and Family Life in the United States, 1900–1930* (New York: Oxford University Press, 1979).

For an excellent discussion of women's health during this period, see Martha Verbrugge, *Able-bodied Womanhood: Personal Health and Social Change in Nineteenth-Century Boston* (New York: Oxford University Press, 1988).

17. Robert Edes, "High-Pressure Education: Its Effects," *Boston Medical and Surgical Journal* 106 (1882): 223. The hazards of both underwork and overwork were echoed by T. Clifford Allbutt, "Chlorosis," in *A System of Medicine*, ed. T. Clifford Allbutt (New York: Macmillan, 1898), 6:516–17.

18. T. Gaillard Thomas, "Clinical Lecture on Chlorosis" (delivered at the College of Physicians and Surgeons, New York), *Boston Medical and Surgical Journal* 103 (1880): 389–90.

19. Lionel S. Beale, *Our Morality and the Moral Question* (Philadelphia: Blakiston, 1887), 13.

20. Ibid., 25.

21. Thomas, "Clinical Lecture on Chlorosis." There are unmistakable parallels with S. Weir Mitchell's *Fat and Blood: An Essay on the Treatment of Certain Forms of Neurasthenia and Hysteria* (Philadelphia: Lippincott, 1885), and particularly with Mitchell's rest cure, which gained wide popularity in the late nineteenth century. A synthetic cultural analysis of the origins of this therapeutic worldview can be found in T. J. Jackson Lears, *No Place of Grace: Antimodernism and the Transformation of American Culture, 1880–1920* (New York: Pantheon Books, 1981).

22. According to Thomas, "small doses of Fowler's solution, I have found, will often do much more good than iron. In addition, a proper amount of exercise is imperatively demanded in most cases of chlorosis." Thomas, "Clinical Lecture on Chlorosis," 390.

23. In her study of working women's leisure and social life at the turn of the century, Kathy Peiss has argued that "the reformers' response to working girls'

style [often couched in terms of middle-class moralism] represents one facet of a larger cultural transformation occurring between 1880 and 1920." Peiss, *Cheap Amusements*, 185. For more on moral reform during this era, see Paul Boyer, *Urban Masses and Moral Order in America, 1820–1920* (Cambridge: Harvard University Press, 1978), and Samuel Haber, *Efficiency and Uplift: Scientific Management in the Progressive Era, 1890–1920* (Chicago: University of Chicago Press, 1964).

24. Ellen Richards, "Hospital Diet," *New England Kitchen Magazine*, April 1894, 22.

25. Henry, *Anaemia*, 43; see also Frederick Porteus Henry, "Remarks on Chlorosis and Its Treatment," *University [Pennsylvania] Medical Magazine* 7 (1895): 830–37, and J. Tyson, "A Clinical Lecture on Chlorosis," *University [Pennsylvania] Medical Magazine* 5 (1893): 420–26.

26. Delafield, "The Clinic—On Blood Diseases," 774–76.

27. One practitioner who depended heavily on blood monitoring was Charles Dowd. See Dowd, "The Condition of the Blood in Chlorosis," *American Journal of Medical Science* 99 (1890): 549–67.

28. Delafield, "The Clinic—On Blood Diseases," 774.

29. Ibid., 774.

30. C. E. Simon, "A Study of Thirty-one Cases of Chlorosis," *American Journal of Medical Science* 113 (1897): 399–423.

31. Ibid., 416. Masturbation was regarded as both a cause of disease and a disease in its own right. See H. Tristam Engelhardt, "The Disease of Masturbation: Values and the Concept of Disease," in *Sickness and Health in America*, ed. Judith Leavitt and Ronald Numbers (Madison: University of Wisconsin Press, 1985): 13–21.

32. Simon, "Thirty-one Cases of Chlorosis," 413.

33. Beale wrote: "As the object of our attention is to relieve and cure the patient, we are not regarded with suspicion, and more likely to be able to receive a true account of the actual facts than those who make enquiries from the purely moral or religious rather than medical side." Beale, *Morality and the Moral Question*, 162.

34. Eliza Bisbee Duffey, *What Women Should Know: A Woman's Book about Women Containing Practical Information for Wives and Mothers* (Philadelphia: J.M. Stoddard, 1898), 49.

35. Figures on labor participation are from Mary Ryan, *Womanhood in America: From Colonial Times to the Present* (New York: Watts, 1983), 119. A useful discussion of working women and morality in late nineteenth-century America is Lynn Werner, "From Working Girl to Working Mother: The Debate over Women and Morality in the U.S., 1820–1920" (Ph.D. diss., Boston University, 1981).

36. Ryan, *Womanhood in America*, 138.

37. Peiss, *Cheap Amusements*; Tentler, *Wage-earning Women*.

38. On the texture of nineteenth-century women's relations and collective

women's activities and concerns about them, see Carroll Smith-Rosenberg, "The Female World of Love and Ritual: Relations between Women in Nineteenth-Century America," *Signs* 1 (autumn 1975): 1–29.

39. Simon, "Thirty-one Cases of Chlorosis," 416.

40. David Rosner, *A Once Charitable Enterprise: Hospitals and Health Care in Brooklyn and New York, 1885–1915* (New York: Cambridge University Press, 1982), 9.

41. Several historians of hematology have chronicled and celebrated this development of hematological analysis and thought. The most thorough of these is Maxwell Wintrobe, *Hematology: The Blossoming of a Science, a Story of Inspiration and Effort* (Philadelphia: Lea and Febiger, 1985), and Maxwell Wintrobe, ed., *Blood, Pure and Eloquent* (New York: McGraw-Hill, 1980).

42. Hobart Hare, "A Brief Review of Some of the Recent Practical Advances in Medicine and Therapeutics," *Journal of the American Medical Association* 20 (1893): 651–56.

43. Frederick Henry, "Relations between Chlorosis, Simple Anaemia, and Pernicious Anaemia," *Transactions of the Association of American Physicians* 4 (1889): 163.

44. Simon, "Thirty-one Cases of Chlorosis," 412.

45. Ibid., 412. According to Frederick Henry, "the only constant anatomical characters of chlorosis are those of the blood itself . . . [but] even the blood changes are not uniform . . . It has since been established that this view of the blood-change in chlorosis is altogether too narrow . . . The essential point is that the percentage of hemoglobin is reduced in this affection, and this is common in many forms of anemia." Henry, *Anaemia*, 55.

46. F. W. Higgins, "Examination of the Blood for the General Practitioner," *Journal of the American Medical Association* 38 (1902): 235. Writing in William Pepper's widely read medical textbook from 1894, William Osler suggested that "the influences of unsatisfied sexual desire and of masturbation have, it seems to me, been over-estimated." William Osler, "Chlorosis," in *Text-book of the Theory and Practice of Medicine by American Authors,* ed. William Pepper (Philadelphia: W.B. Saunders, 1894), 2:197.

47. Allbutt also encouraged his colleagues "to test the blood not only for the number of red corpuscles and apparent hemoglobin value, but also to ascertain whether they are equal and of full size, is the only trustworthy way of gauging the rate and degree of cure." Allbutt, "Chlorosis," 6:516–17.

48. G. Stanley Hall, *Youth: Its Education, Regimen, and Hygiene* (New York: Arno Press, 1972), 313.

49. Winifred Richmond, *The Adolescent Girl: A Book for Parents and Teachers* (New York: Macmillan, 1926), 34.

50. Richard Cabot, *A Layman's Handbook of Medicine with Special Reference to Social Workers* (New York: Houghton Mifflin, 1920), 301.

51. One British physician who began his career in the 1920s recalled, "When I was a medical student immediately after the First World War my teachers used to speak of going into the outpatient departments in the old days, seeing benches crowded with greenish or pasty-faced girls and young women, and murmuring to themselves, 'Nothing but chlorosis.'" L. J. Witts, *Hypochromic Anemia* (Philadelphia: F.A. Davis, 1961), 33.

52. Originally written by William Osler, *Modern Medicine* went through many editions after his death, with contributions from many authors. Although not listed as such, Cabot is the author of the cited chapter. Richard Cabot, "Diseases of the Blood and the Blood-forming Organs," in *Modern Medicine*, ed. Henry Christian (New York: Appleton, 1938), 729. For attribution, see 1915 edition.

53. Richard Cabot, "Diseases of the Blood: Pernicious Anemia and Secondary Anemia, Chlorosis and Leukemia," in *Modern Medicine*, ed. William Osler (Philadelphia: Lea and Febiger, 1915), 647. See also 1908 edition, p. 641.

54. This way of thinking about disease as imbalance was common in the nineteenth century. See Charles Rosenberg "Prologue: The Shape of Traditional Medical Practice, 1800–1875," in George Rosen, *The Structure of American Medical Practice, 1875–1941* (Philadelphia: University of Pennsylvania Press, 1983).

55. Cabot, "Diseases of the Blood" (1915), 647.

56. Richard Cabot, "Diseases of the Blood-forming Organs," in *The Principles and Practice of Medicine*, 9th ed., ed. William Osler and Thomas McCrae (New York: Appleton, 1920), 725.

57. Thomas Oliver, *Occupations from the Social, Hygienic and Medical Points of View* (Cambridge: Cambridge University Press, 1916), 71. See chapter on "Female Labor—Female Employment and Motherhood."

58. "Anemia," in *The Principles and Practice of Modern Medicine*, 13th ed., ed. William Osler, Henry Christian, and Thomas McCrae (New York: Appleton, 1938), 912.

59. Physicians like Arthur Beifeld objected to the connection between chlorosis and work conditions. He argued that "hard work and long working hours played only accessory roles . . . That these are not the immediate causes is shown by the fact that chlorosis is seen by no means infrequently in girls of the better situated strata of society." Arthur Beifeld, "Chlorosis," *Medical Clinics of North America* 2 (1917): 981.

60. Reisman continued: "In some cases the disappearance is only apparent, having been brought about through a change in name. Others have disappeared because they were really not diseases at all but symptoms wrongly interpreted as clinical entities . . . Some were entirely fanciful and had to give way to increasing technical knowledge, and some have disappeared as the result of a general enlightenment of the people." David Reisman, "Deceased Diseases," *Annals of Medical History* 50 (1932): 160.

61. Ibid., 166.

62. In one article on chlorosis, two Boston physicians argued that "the environmental changes and the emancipation of women from a cloistered sedentary life . . . undoubtedly lead to a better appetite and a better diet." A. Patek and C. Heath, "Chlorosis," *Journal of the American Medical Association* 106 (1936): 1465.

63. In his examination of women in America, William Chafe suggested that in the 1920s *emancipation* possessed several meanings. Along with economic and political freedom, emancipation referred to freedom from older conventions of behavior. See William Chafe, *The American Woman: Her Changing Social, Economic, and Political Roles* (New York: Oxford University Press, 1972). For other discussions of this emancipation motif, see Ryan, *Womanhood in America*; Glenna Matthews, *The Rise of Public Woman: Woman's Power and Woman's Place in the United States, 1630–1970* (New York: Oxford University Press, 1992); and Cott, *The Grounding of Modern Feminism*.

64. In 1925, one British physician reflected that "it seems now almost certain that the main exciting cause of the disease was the wearing of corsets, and that the gradual abandonment of the tight-lacing has ultimately led to its almost complete disappearance." F. Parkes Weber, "Two Diseases Due to Fashion in Clothing: Chlorosis and Chronic Erythema of the Legs," *British Medical Journal* 1 (1925): 961. In his 1934 autobiography, one Chicago gynecological surgeon asked: "Was the prevailing mode of dress responsible for the invalidism of so many of our race of civilized women? . . . On the few occasions when I made bold to inquire . . . the patient replied . . . 'I would die without the support of my corsets.'" Martin, *Fifty Years of Medicine and Surgery*, 109.

65. William Elder, "Diseases Due to Fashion in Clothing," *British Medical Journal* 2 (1925): 88 (letter). See also Rupert Waterhouse, "Diseases Due to Fashion in Clothing," *British Medical Journal* 2 (1925): 232 (letter).

66. The best known is the 1892 book, Charlotte Perkins Gilman, *The Yellow Wallpaper* (New York: Feminist Press, 1973).

67. Joan Jacobs Brumberg, "Chlorotic Girls, 1870–1920: A Historical Perspective on Female Adolescence," *Child Development* 53 (1982): 1468–77. For another view, see Lorna Duffin, "The Conspicuous Consumptive: Woman as an Invalid," in Delamont and Duffin, *The Nineteenth Century Woman*, 38, 40. Where Duffin emphasized the doctor's agency in "labeling" patients, Brumberg emphasized the patient's agency in taking on "sick roles." Brumberg, "Chlorotic Girls," 1476. See also Joan Jacobs Brumberg, *Fasting Girls: The Emergence of Anorexia Nervosa as a Modern Disease* (Cambridge: Harvard University Press, 1988).

68. Nancy Theriot, another scholar who took up the issue of chlorosis, drew heavily on Barbara Welter's analysis of the "cult of true womanhood," as well as upon the social theory of Karl Mannheim, particularly his observations on intergenerational dynamics. Nancy Theriot, *The Biosocial Construction of Femininity: Mothers and Daughters in Nineteenth-Century America* (New York: Greenwood

Press, 1988), 123. On the sick role, see Talcott Parsons, *The Social System* (New York: Free Press of Glencoe, 1951), 428–47.

69. A useful overview of the role of technology in medicine is Stanley J. Reiser, *Medicine and the Reign of Technology* (Cambridge: Cambridge University Press, 1978). The advent of laboratory-based knowledge production and its consequences for our thinking about disease have been examined in Andrew Cunningham and Perry Williams, eds., *The Laboratory Revolution in Medicine* (Cambridge: Cambridge University Press, 1992). On the role of technology in hospitals during this period, see Joel Howell, *Technology and the Hospital* (Baltimore: Johns Hopkins University Press, 1995). See also Charles Rosenberg, *The Care of Strangers: The Rise of America's Hospital System* (New York: Basic Books, 1987); Morris Vogel, *The Invention of the Modern Hospital: Boston, 1870–1930* (Chicago: University of Chicago Press, 1980); David Rosner, *A Once Charitable Enterprise: Hospitals and Health Care in Brooklyn and New York, 1885–1915* (New York: Cambridge University Press, 1982); and Rosemary Stevens, *In Sickness and in Wealth: American Hospitals in the Twentieth Century* (New York: Basic Books, 1989).

70. Bloomfield credited Knud Faber with labeling "hypochromic anemia" as a disease in 1931. For other works on hypochromic anemia as a disease during this era, see William Dameshek, "Primary Hypochromic Anemia," *American Journal of Medical Science* 182 (October 1931): 520–33; G. Minot, *Idiopathic Hypochromic Anemia* (New York: International Press, 1932); M. Wintrobe and R. Beebe, "Idiopathic Hypochromic Anemia," *Medicine* 12 (May 1933): 187; and T. K. Waugh, "Hypochromic Anemia with Achlorhydria," *Archives of Internal Medicine* 47 (1931): 71.

71. These intellectual negotiations, engendered by social tensions between the laboratory and the clinic, are discussed in Russell Maulitz, "Physicians versus Bacteriologists: The Ideology of Science in Clinical Medicine," and Gerald Geison, "Divided We Stand: Physiologists and Clinicians in the American Context," in *The Therapeutic Revolution: Essays in the Social History of American Medicine*, ed. Morris Vogel and Charles Rosenberg (Philadelphia: University of Pennsylvania Press, 1979). See also Keith Wailoo, "A Disease *Sui Generis:* The Origins of Sickle Cell Anemia and the Emergence of Modern Clinical Research, 1904–1924," *Bulletin of the History of Medicine* 65 (1991): 185–208, and J. Wright, "The Development of the Frozen Section Technique, the Evolution of Surgical Biopsy, and the Origins of Surgical Pathology," *Bulletin of the History of Medicine* 59 (1985): 295–326.

72. Weber, "Two Diseases Due to Fashion," 961.

73. Ibid., 960. For replies to Weber, see Elder, "Diseases Due to Fashion," and Waterhouse, "Diseases Due to Fashion." This debate is discussed in Sir Humphry Davy Rolleston, *Aspects of Age, Life, and Disease* (London: Kegan Paul, Trench, Trubner, and Co., 1928), 88, 99.

74. A. Bloomfield, "Relations between Primary Hypochromic Anemia and Chlorosis," *Archives of Internal Medicine* 50 (1932): 328–36.

75. Ibid., 336.

76. Bloomfield acknowledged that, although the technical procedures used by doctors to define *chlorosis* in the past and to diagnose *hypochromic anemia* in the present were quite different, the modern technician's insight in no way supplanted the judgment of such masters as William Osler and T. Clifford Allbutt. Ibid., 328. Another discussion of the problematic relationship between the diagnosis of hypochromic anemia and chlorosis is K. Faber and H. Gram, "Relations between Gastrica Achylia and Simple and Pernicious Anemia," *Archives of Internal Medicine* 34 (1924): 658.

77. "Many older clinicians," Bloomfield wrote, "cling in an almost sentimental manner to the idea that chlorosis is a highly specific disease . . . This to a naive extreme." Bloomfield, "Primary Hypochromic Anemia and Chlorosis," 334.

78. Ibid., 329, 334.

79. Ibid., 336. Bloomfield argued that both hypochromic anemia and chlorosis would best be labeled "syndromes without fixed characteristics."

80. Fowler, "Chlorosis—An Obituary," *Annals of Medical History* 8 (1936): 176.

81. "Until the latter problem is solved," Fowler wrote, "the reasons for the disappearance of chlorosis will remain in darkness and with its disappearance the explanation of its etiology becomes increasingly difficult." Ibid., 176.

82. By the end of the 1930s, physicians were of several different minds about the supposed relationship between hypochromic anemia and chlorosis. Some thought that chlorosis had been redistributed into new categories and that, with "the introduction of more accurate diagnostic methods in the beginning of the 20th century . . . cases previously diagnosed as chlorosis were discovered to have [been] tuberculosis or some bleeding lesion in the gastrointestinal tract." Isadore Olef, "Chlorosis," *Annals of Internal Medicine* 10 (1937): 165. E. B. Krumbhaar simply stated that "the relationship . . . is not clear." Krumbhaar, "Modern Concepts of Anemia from the Clinical Standpoint," *Bulletin of the New York Academy of Medicine* 13 (1937): 508–9.

83. L. J. Witts, *Hypochromic Anaemia* (Philadelphia: F.A. Davis, 1961), 4.

84. Quotation from Emil Schwarz, *Chlorosis: A Retrospective Investigation* (Brussels, 1951), appears in W. Crosby, "Whatever Became of Chlorosis?" *Journal of the American Medical Association* 257 (1987): 2800.

85. Irvine Loudon, "The Diseases Called Chlorosis," *Psychological Medicine* 14 (1984): 27–36; Irvine Loudon, "Chlorosis, Anaemia, and Anorexia Nervosa," *British Medical Journal* 281 (1980): 1673.

86. Nicholas Jewson, "The Disappearance of the Sick-Man from Medical Cosmology," *Sociology* 10 (1976): 224–44. On the rise of laboratory medicine, see also Erwin Ackerknecht, *A Short History of Medicine* (Baltimore: Johns Hopkins University Press, 1952).

87. Loudon recognized in chlorosis two modern diseases, hypochromic anemia and anorexia nervosa. Loudon, "The Diseases Called Chlorosis."

88. Crosby, "Whatever Became of Chlorosis?" 2799.

89. Ralph Stockman, "The Causes and Treatment of Chlorosis," *British Medical Journal* 2 (1895): 1473–89.

90. "The History of Iron in Medicine," in *Clinical Disorders of Iron Metabolism*, 2d ed., ed. V. Fairbanks, J. Fahey, and E. Beutler (New York: Grune and Stratton, 1969), 21.

91. A noteworthy attempt to bring historical perspective to such modern ideas was P. Cranefield and C. McBrooks, eds., *The Historical Development of Physiological Thought* (New York: Hafner, 1959).

92. Delafield, "The Clinic—On Blood Diseases," 770–75.

93. Charles Rosenberg argued that nineteenth-century therapeutic practice was structured by a "liturgy of healing." He contrasted this to twentieth-century notions of specific cures. Charles Rosenberg, "The Therapeutic Revolution," in Vogel and Rosenberg, *The Therapeutic Revolution*.

94. Several historians have explored the nuances of this therapeutic skepticism. See John Harley Warner, *The Therapeutic Perspective: Medical Practice, Knowledge, and Identity in America, 1820–1885* (Cambridge: Harvard University Press, 1986).

95. Cabot, "Diseases of the Blood-forming Organs," 727. See also Henry Christian, "A Sketch of the History of the Treatment of Chlorosis with Iron," in *Medical Library and Historical Journal* 1 (1903): 176–80. Christian praised Thomas Sydenham for first demonstrating the value of iron in chlorosis. Even more important, he believed, were Pierre Blaud's invention of Blaud's iron pills in 1831 and Blaud's ingenious method of gradually increasing the dosage until recovery occurred and then gradually decreasing the dosage. Richard Cabot acknowledged that, other than the use of quinine in malaria and the prescription of mercury and iodide of potassium in syphilis, "there is no other drug [than iron in chlorosis] the beneficial effects of which we can trace with the accuracy of a scientific experiment." Cabot, "Diseases of the Blood-forming Organs," 727.

96. Cabot, "Diseases of the Blood-forming Organs," 727. See also Richard Cabot, *A Layman's Handbook of Medicine,* 301. William Osler, to the contrary, believed that iron could not be considered a specific: "Patients will recover fairly quickly as a result of the administration of iron without any changes in their habits, and . . . it is also true that patients will improve without administration of iron, provided we correct their constipation and improve their general hygiene." William Osler, "Chlorosis," in *Modern Medicine: Its Theory and Practice*, ed. William Osler and Thomas McCrae (Philadelphia: Lea and Febiger, 1908), 4:648.

97. "Now and then," noted Richard Cabot, some cases did not respond to "the combination of iron administered . . . with proper hygiene." Something stronger than iron was needed: "In some of these, recovery is hastened by the adminis-

tration of arsenic in the form of Fowler's solution." R. Cabot, "Pernicious and Secondary Anemia, Chlorosis, and Leukemia," in *Modern Medicine: Its Theory and Practice*, ed. William Osler, Thomas McCrae, and Elmer Funk (Philadelphia: Lea and Febiger, 1927), 5:66–67.

98. "In any case of chlorosis which does not yield readily to iron administered in the proper manner and in the proper doses," Cabot wrote, "we have reason for doubting the diagnosis." Ibid., 66.

99. Beifeld, "Chlorosis," 981.

100. On the "flowering of consumerism" in medicine in the 1920s, see Stevens, *In Sickness and in Wealth*, 105–39. Roland Marchand examined the complexities of advertising and consumer culture in the 1920s, arguing (in part) that health became one among the newly purchasable commodities. Roland Marchand, *Advertising the American Dream: Making Way for Modernity, 1920–1940* (Berkeley: University of California Press, 1985).

101. Russell Haden, "Historical Aspects of Iron Therapy in Anemia," *Journal of the American Medical Association* 111 (1938): 1061. See also Charles Williamson and Harold Ets, "The Value of Iron in Anemia," *Archives of Internal Medicine* 36 (1925): 333.

102. Maurice Strauss, "The Use of Drugs in the Treatment of Anemias," *Journal of the American Medical Association* 107 (1936): 1633, 1636.

103. Wintrobe noted in 1953: "There is no excuse nowadays . . . for a doctor who just picks a shotgun type of blood tonic from the medical advertisements and hopes for the best." "Blood and Iron," *Time* 62 (2 November 1953): 106.

104. Albert B. Hagedorn, "The Diagnosis and Treatment of Iron-Deficiency Anemia," in *Medical Clinics of North America* 40 (1956): 953.

105. "It is apparent," wrote Patek and Health, "that insufficient intake of iron, loss of iron by menstrual and other blood losses, and the demands for iron by a growing organism are three important factors in the production of chlorosis." Patek and Heath, "Chlorosis," 1465.

106. They concluded that "severely anemic mothers . . . then, seem to provide their infants with less iron than do normal mothers . . . Maternal iron depletion is an etiological factor in the development of hypochromic anemia of infancy." Ibid., 1465.

107. In 1941, Dorothy Wiehl concluded that, "for girls, the highest hemoglobin value is at age 12 years . . . other evidence suggests, however, that this early, but temporary, higher level may be typical." See Dorothy Wiehl, "Selecting Cases of Anemia among Adolescents," *American Journal of Public Health* 31 (1941): 1075. One photo essay in AMA's journal *Hygeia* portrayed two types of girl, one slouching in her chair with anemia and the other playing field hockey. The caption read: "The general lassitude of a child may not be a mere pose of adolescence but a symptom of a physical disorder. One of those could be anemia." "Anemia (a Photographic Record)," *Hygeia* 25 (1947): 435.

108. Harold Burn's 1962 book summarized much of this iron-centered thinking. Harold Burn, *Drugs, Medicines, and Man* (New York: Scribner's, 1962), 165.

109. Simone de Beauvoir, "The Data of Biology," in *The Second Sex*, trans. H. M. Parchley (New York: Modern Library, 1952), 50.

110. De Beauvoir wrote: "We must view the facts of biology in the light of an ontological, economic, social, and psychological context . . . the body of woman is one of the essential elements in her situation in the world. But that body is not enough to define her as woman." Ibid., 32, 54.

111. As one scholar of Simone de Beauvoir writes: "There is in *The Second Sex* a recognition that women will never be free unless they establish a sense of themselves as female, as well as human." Toril Moi, *Simone de Beauvoir: The Making of an Intellectual Woman* (Cambridge, Mass.: Blackwell, 1994), 210.

112. "Too Busy to Be Sick," *Time* 80 (16 November 1962): 67.

113. Shuang Ruy Huang, "Chlorosis and the Iron Controversy: An Aspect of Nineteenth Century Medicine" (Ph.D. diss., Harvard University, 1977), 204. The historical record provided plenty of evidence to contradict this revisionist interpretation of chlorosis. As A. L. Bloomfield noted in 1960, "It was not until recent years, that the idea that 'chlorosis' was simply a variety of hypochromic, iron deficiency anemia came to be generally recognized." A. L. Bloomfield, *A Bibliography of Internal Medicine: Selected Diseases* (Chicago: University of Chicago Press, 1960), 78–87. See also L. J. Witts, *Hypochromic Anaemia* (Philadelphia: F.A. Davis, 1969), and Fairbanks, Fahey, and Beutler, *Clinical Disorders of Iron Metabolism*, 54.

114. "According to Beutler," wrote Huang, "the term iron-deficiency anemia has replaced such terms as chlorosis, essential hypochromic anemia, hypochromic anemia, anemia of chronic blood loss, hookworm anemia, chronic chlorosis, late chlorosis . . . and many others. Before the common denominator of these conditions—iron deficiency—was recognized, these various clinical syndromes now considered under the unifying concept of iron-deficiency anemia, were often considered separate entities." Huang, "Chlorosis and the Iron Controversy," 221.

115. Hematologists like Ernest Beutler used updated tools of hemoglobin estimation and bone marrow analysis, echoing the conclusions of their late nineteenth-century predecessors. The new technology of bone marrow aspiration allowed Beutler to style himself as a reformer, to see clearly that these women were suffering both from anemia and from a subtle psychological abuse by other physicians. "In 1956," he later wrote to a colleague, "I turned my attention to a topic which had fascinated me for a number of years, iron deficiency . . . I saw many patients, particularly women, who had mild anemia associated with marked tiredness and weakness. It was fashionable, even then, to attribute such symptoms to psycho-neurosis. This was a diagnosis which required no objective support, and seemed all-too-readily accepted by most physicians . . . In examining the bone marrow [however] of one such patient, I noticed that iron was to-

tally absent." Ernest Beutler to Maxwell Wintrobe, no date, Maxwell Myer Wintrobe Papers, box 9, folder: "Beutler, Ernest," pp. 29–30, Marriott Library, University of Utah, Salt Lake City.

116. Hudson noted that, "while developing medical knowledge often clarifies previously puzzling aspects of disease, it must be remembered that today's medical understanding is itself a stand of sand." Robert Hudson, "The Biography of Disease: Lessons from Chlorosis," *Bulletin of the History of Medicine* 51 (1977): 460.

117. This fact, wrote Siddall, "offers the clue to follow . . . 'The diagnosis of anemia due to iron deficiency should signal a search for blood loss.' In retrospect, the most obvious excessive artificial blood loss endured by both mothers and daughters during the nineteenth century seems to have been overlooked by historians; namely, the depletion resulting from the popular remedy of bloodletting." A. Clair Siddall, "Chlorosis—Etiology Reconsidered," *Bulletin of the History of Medicine* 56 (1982): 254.

118. Though this hypothesis, like so many others about chlorosis, was highly speculative, Siddall echoed an emerging critique of technology and specialization. One of the most concerted assaults on medical technology, highlighting the problem of iatrogenic disease, was Ivan Illich, *Medical Nemesis: The Expropriation of Health* (New York: Pantheon Books, 1976).

119. Donna Haraway, "Situated Knowledges: The Science Question in Feminism and the Privilege of Partial Perspective," in *Technology and the Politics of Knowledge*, ed. Andrew Feenberg and Alastair Hannay (Bloomington: Indiana University Press, 1995), 175–94.

120. My analysis of chlorosis comes closest, perhaps, to that developed by historian Karl Figlio, who argued that "the distinction between natural and human should itself be treated as an historically rooted phenomenon, made by people in the service of interests." Figlio was not concerned (as I have been) with the role of technology in the process. Karl Figlio, "Chlorosis and Chronic Disease in Nineteenth-Century Britain: The Social Construction of Somatic Disease in Capitalist Society," *Social History* 3 (May 1978): 168.

Chapter 2   The Rise and Fall of Splenic Anemia: *Surgical Identity and Ownership of a Blood Disease*

1. Malcolm Harris and Maximilian Herzog, "Splenectomy in Splenic Anemia or Primary Splenomegaly," *Annals of Surgery* 34 (1901): 113.

2. Ibid.

3. Berkeley Moynihan, *The Spleen and Some of Its Diseases; Being the Bradshaw Lectures, 1920* (Philadelphia: W.B. Saunders, 1921), 4.

4. In the nineteenth-century tradition of physical diagnosis, splenic enlargement had a variety of meanings. During the late nineteenth century, physicians

could still quote the words of ancient scholars like Pliny (from *Natural History*): "For sure it is that intemperate laughers have always great Splenes." Quotation from Moynihan, *The Spleen and Its Diseases*, 4.

5. See, for example, Mary Dunham Hankinson-Jones, *The Spleen; or the Human Battery* (n.p.: Hankinson-Jones, 1904), and Lucretia Hubbell, *The Spleen, the Regulator of the Body and Preventer of Disease* (Norwich, Conn.: Hubbell, [1876?]). Both of these are discussed below.

6. The historical literature abounds in discussions of the role of antisepsis and asepsis in the transformation of surgery. See Christopher Lawrence, ed., *Medical Theory, Surgical Practice: Studies in the History of Surgery* (New York: Routledge, 1992), especially Christopher Lawrence, "Democratic, Divine, and Heroic: The History and Historiography of Surgery." See also Gert Brieger, "American Surgery and the Germ Theory of Disease," *Bulletin of the History of Medicine* 40 (1966): 135–45; Owen Wangensteen, *The Rise of Surgery: From Empiric Craft to Scientific Discipline* (Minneapolis: University of Minnesota Press, 1978); Frederick Cartwright, *The Development of Modern Surgery* (New York: T.Y. Crowell, 1968); Loyal Davis, *Fellowship of Surgeons: A History of the American College of Surgeons* (Springfield, Ill.: Charles C Thomas, 1960); and Mark Ravitch, *A Century of Surgery: The History of the American Surgical Association* (Philadelphia: Lippincott, 1981). For a contemporary's analysis, see Caleb Williams Saleeby, *Modern Surgery and Its Making: A Tribute to Listerism* (London: Herbert and Daniel, [1912?]), and American Surgical Association, *Minutes of the American Surgical Association, 1880–1968* (Dallas: reprinted for the association by Taylor Publishing, 1972).

7. Samuel Hopkins Adams, "Modern Surgery," *McClure's Magazine*, 26 March 1905, 482–92. Quotation is from p. 483.

8. William Osler and Thomas MacCrae, eds., *The Principles and Practice of Medicine*, 8th ed. (New York: Appleton, 1918), 886.

9. W. J. Mayo, "The Splenomegalies," *Surgical Clinics of North America* 1 (1921): 1306.

10. Harold Burrows, *The Pitfalls of Surgery* (London: Balliere, Tindall, and Cox, 1925), vii.

11. There is a historically enduring, and complex, relationship between exploratory surgery and cultural ideals of exploration. Rene Fox and Judith Swazey have noted how the language of space exploration informed the history of the Jarvik-7 heart experiments. Rene Fox and Judith Swazey, "Desperate Appliance: A Short History of the Jarvik-7 Artificial Heart," in *Spare Parts: Organ Replacement in American Society* (New York: Oxford University Press, 1992). For a history of the meaning of exploration in the nineteenth-century United States, see William Goetzmann, *Exploration and Empire: The Explorer and the Scientist in the Winning of the American West* (New York: Knopf, 1966).

12. See John Foker, "The Consequences of Splenectomy," in John Najarian and John Delaney, *Advances in Hepatic, Biliary and Pancreatic Surgery* (Chicago:

Year Book Medical Publishers). Also William Crosby, "The Spleen," in *Blood, Pure and Eloquent*, ed. Maxwell Wintrobe (New York: McGraw-Hill, 1980), and "Splenectomy vs. Splenorrhaphy," in *Surgical Debates*, ed. Alden Harken (Philadelphia: Hanley and Belfus, 1988).

13. A. H. T. Robb-Smith, "Osler's Influence on Hematology," *Blood Cells* 7 (1981): 513–33.

· 14. W. W. Keen, *Sixty Years of Surgery, 1862–1922* (Boston: n.p., 1922), 189.

15. J. Collins Warren, "The Surgery of the Spleen," *Annals of Surgery* 33 (1908): 513. See also G. B. Johnston, "Splenectomy," *Annals of Surgery* 48 (1908): 50, and J. Wesley Bovee, "Splenectomy for Congestive Hypertrophy," *Annals of Surgery* 31 (1900): 705–13.

16. Warren, "The Surgery of the Spleen," 513.

17. Dating the advent of modern surgery to the late nineteenth century, the British surgeon William Evans wrote that "the advantages of the antiseptic method in surgery have been nowhere more clearly seen than in surgery of the stomach, bowel, and the other abdominal organs." William Evans, *Medicine Science To-day: A Popular Account of the More Recent Developments in Medicine and Surgery* (Philadelphia: Lippincott, 1912), 170.

18. Ibid., 179.

19. W. W. Keen, "Recent Progress in Surgery," in Keen, *Addresses and Other Papers* (Philadelphia: W.B. Saunders, 1905), 97.

20. Ibid., 100.

21. Keen, *Sixty Years of Surgery*, 192.

22. For a synthetic assessment of "antimodernist" sentiment during this era, see T. J. Jackson Lears, *No Place of Grace: Antimodernism and the Transformation of American Culture, 1880–1920* (New York: Pantheon Books, 1981). See also Robert Weibe, *The Search for Order, 1877–1920* (Westport, Conn.: Greenwood Press, 1967).

23. Hubbell, *Spleen, Regulator of the Body*, 3.

24. Ibid., 3, 4–5.

25. Francis Markoe, "Two Cases of Successful Splenectomy," *Annals of Surgery* 20 (1894): 738. Markoe noted that "surgical interference had been decided legitimate at a consultation of the hospital staff. Consent had been readily obtained from both the patient and his father."

26. James P. Warbasse, "On the Surgery and Physiology of the Spleen," *Annals of Surgery* 20 (1894): 227.

27. Warbasse, "Surgery of the Spleen," 205–27. See also James Murphy (Sunderland), "A Successful Splenectomy for Chronic Inflammatory Hyperplasia," *Annals of Surgery* 21 (1895): 116–18.

28. Warbasse, "Surgery of the Spleen," 206.

29. Still, most surgeons admitted, as did J. Wesley Bovee, that "splenectomy is not an operation to be lightly entered upon with scarcely any knowledge of the conditions demanding it and of those absolutely contraindicating it." J. Wesley

Bovee, "Splenectomy for Congestive Hypertrophy," *Annals of Surgery* 31 (1900): 708.

30. See William Osler, "Splenic Anemia," *American Journal of Medical Sciences* 124 (1902): 751–70. Other notable writings on splenic anemia around the turn of the century include Aldred Warthin and George Dock, "Splenic Anemia," *American Journal of Medical Science* 127 (1904): 24–55; Alfred Stengel, "Diseases of the Spleen," in *Twentieth Century Practice,* ed. Thomas Stedman (New York: William Wood, 1903), 9:355–88; Alfred Stengel, "Varieties of Splenic Anemia," *American Journal of Medical Science* 128 (1904): 497–533; William Osler, "On Splenic Anemia," *American Journal of Medical Science* 119 (1900): 19; and William Osler, "Splenic Anemia," *Transactions of the Association of American Physicians* 17 (1902): 429–61. Other related writings from later periods include W. J. Mayo, "The Splenomegalies," *Surgical Clinics of North America* 1 (1921): 1306, and H. Z. Giffin, "Splenectomy in Pernicious Anemia," *Surgical Clinics of North America* 25 (1917): 157.

31. One physician tentatively noted, "From pernicious anemia[,] splenic anemia is distinguished by the enlargement of the spleen . . . though in a clinical sense the anemia is pernicious, being progressive and fatal." Samuel West, "Splenic Anemia," in *A System of Medicine by Many Writers,* ed. T. C. Allbutt, vol. 6 (New York: Macmillan, 1898).

32. For more on the rise of abdominal surgery and its politics, see the brief discussion in Rosemary Stevens, *American Medicine and the Public Interest* (New Haven: Yale University Press, 1971), 78–80, 333–39.

33. "Transactions of the Chicago Surgical Society," *Annals of Surgery* 34 (1901): 197.

34. Chicago Surgical Society, "Rupture of the Spleen," *Surgery, Gynecology, and Obstetrics* 4 (1907): 653 (abstract).

35. Ibid.

36. These comments are paraphrases of Jonnesco, appearing in "Abdomen: I. Splenectomy" (Proceedings of the Twelfth International Congress of Medicine, Moscow, 1897), *Annals of Surgery* 26 (1897): 724.

37. "Transactions of the Chicago Surgical Society," *Annals of Surgery* 34 (1901): 199.

38. Berkeley Moynihan, *Abdominal Operations,* 3d ed. (Philadelphia: W.B. Saunders, 1914), 462. An informative biography of Moynihan is Donald Bateman, *Berkeley Moynihan: Surgeon* (London: Macmillan, 1940). See also Osler Club of London, *Selected Writings of Lord Moynihan: A Centenary Volume* (London: Pitman Medical Publishing, 1967).

39. "The removal of the spleen," Moynihan wrote, "may be an operation of the greatest simplicity or of insuperable difficulty. Everything depends on absence of adhesions, which may bind the organ inseparably to the parts around it." Navigating around these ambiguous shores required "the utmost gentleness

and patience . . . Undue haste or carelessness," he concluded, "will court disaster." Berkeley Moynihan, *Abdominal Operations*, 3d ed. (Philadelphia: W.B. Saunders, 1914), 459.

40. Charles L. Bosk, *Forgive and Remember: Managing Medical Failure* (Chicago: University of Chicago Press, 1979).

41. Many were attracted to Rochester by the personalities of the Mayo brothers: "It is a common comment at Rochester that Dr. William J. Mayo is the dominating figure of the firm," wrote one contemporary, "and I have read the statement that those who know him best are inclined to rank him with such men as E. H. Harriman, J. Pierpont Morgan, J. J. Hill, Theodore Roosevelt, and other towering intellects who have so marvelously influenced their respective fields of activity." George Wiley Broome, *Rochester and the Mayo Clinic: A Fair and Unbiased Story Calculated to Aid Physicians to Greater Cures and Larger Incomes* (New York: Shakespeare Press, 1914), 13.

42. In an adulatory history of the Mayo brothers, Helen Clappesattle concluded that, before the Mayo Clinic, "the omissions and errors of medicine had accumulated a vast reservoir of uncured illness of long standing, to which the new surgery made it possible for qualified practitioners to bring relief. And the Mayo brothers began practice at just the right moment to be the first to tap that reservoir." Helen Clappesattle, *The Doctors Mayo* (Minneapolis: University of Minnesota Press, 1941), 338.

43. William Mayo, "The Splenomegalies," *Boston Medical and Surgical Journal* 190 (1924): 1–6. In 1913, he had simply argued that the spleen was "an agent of blood destruction." See also William Mayo, "Principles Underlying Surgery of the Spleen with a Report of Ten Splenectomies," *Journal of the American Medical Association* 54 (1910): 14; William Mayo, "The Relation of the Spleen to Certain Obscure Clinical Phenomena," *Collected Papers of the Mayo Clinic* 9 (1917): 357; William Mayo, "Surgery of the Spleen," *Surgery, Obstetrics, and Gynecology* 37 (1919): 234; William Mayo, "Results of Splenectomy in the Anemias," *Transactions of the American Surgical Association* 37 (1919): 483–93; and William Mayo, "The Splenomegalies," *Surgical Clinics of North America* 1 (1921): 1306. See also Berkeley Moynihan, "Surgery of the Spleen," in W. W. Keen, ed., *Surgery: Its Principles and Practice* (Philadelphia: W.B. Saunders, 1908), 3:1068.

44. According to Broome, writing in 1914, the public press promoted the idea that, at both Rochester and Lourdes, "there . . . seems to be no limitation to the kind of disease cured." Broome, *Rochester and the Mayo Clinic*, 25.

45. In Broome's view, "the astonishingly large number of about 2,000 persons passed thru the Mayo offices in the one month of August . . . [and] invalidism remained a dominating factor in their lives, and they now came to Rochester for relief." Ibid., 119. In Clappesattle's account, this largely beneficial trend was also fraught with dangers (especially when surgeons encountered so-called neurotic women). "When word spread of Dr. Will's work on ulcers, seldom a week went by without several neurotic women appearing to ask for stomach operation. A

little wearily Dr. Will warned his fellow surgeons against this 'vast army of neurasthenics' . . . Many have already had their movable organs fixed (kidneys and uterus) and the removable ones removed (ovaries and appendix) and now are anxious to secure relief by a further resort to the knife." Clappesattle, *The Doctors Mayo*, 322.

46. Broome, *Rochester and the Mayo Clinic*, 57.

47. Peter English, *Shock, Physiological Surgery and George Washington Crile: Medical Innovation in the Progressive Era* (Westport, Conn.: Greenwood Press, 1980). See also Mayo, "Splenectomy in the Anemias," 483.

48. Berkeley Moynihan, *Abdominal Surgery*, 3d ed. (Philadelphia: W.B. Saunders, 1914), 2:453.

49. For more specific assessments of the outcome of splenectomy, see Joseph Miller, "Pernicious Anemia," *Journal of the American Medical Association* 67 (1916): 729. "Regarding the mortality from splenectomy, the figures of Mayo have already been given, 11 per cent, in eighteen cases. This represents the lowest reported operative mortality in a relatively large series of cases." See also Charles Peck, "Splenectomy for Pernicious Anemia," *Journal of the American Medical Association* 67 (1916): 788–90. "The accumulating evidence of the results of splenectomy has proved the etiologic relation of the changes in the spleen to the disease . . . What the exact nature of the process may be is still more or less obscure, but the spleen plays the most important part is certain" (p. 788).

50. This reviewer noted: "W. J. Mayo has also thrown much light on diseases of the spleen . . . And now comes the leading English surgeon Moynihan with his recent book on the spleen." "Editorial: The Surgeon as Internist," *Northwest Medicine* 21 (1922): 192. See also "Review of *The Spleen and Some of Its Diseases*," *Northwest Medicine* 21 (1921): 64. Other significant works on the spleen included James Compton Burnett, *Diseases of the Spleen; and Their Remedies Clinically Illustrated*, American ed. (Philadelphia: Boericke and Tafel, 1917), and Eugene Hillhouse Pool and Ralph Stillman, *Surgery of the Spleen* (New York: Appleton, 1923).

51. By 1924, one reviewer could note that, "since the spleen is the graveyard of worn out red cells, enlargement of it leads to over-great destruction of red cells and anemia, hence the value of splenectomy . . . Mayo has utilized his enormous surgical, and therefore tactile and ocular experience, to enrich the technically medical side of practice . . . more than any internist has accomplished, by his articles on the liver, kidneys and spleen." "Review of 1924 Collected Papers of the Mayo Clinic and Mayo Foundation," in *Northwest Medicine* 24 (1924): 354.

52. Keen, *Sixty Years of Surgery*, 159.

53. Hankinson-Jones, *The Spleen; the Human Battery*, 9, 11.

54. Ibid., 5. "If the spleen retards progress in the science of medicine, which is obliged to go around it, because it [science] cannot run it down, or govern it, and is finally driven to desperation, because science does not know its use," she asked, "is it not time to give it the benefit of the doubt?"

55. Ibid., 7.

56. "While every surgeon . . . feels able to take to pieces any part of the human frame . . . blindly, yet to good purpose many have stayed their hand at the spleen." Ibid., 7–8.

57. Samuel Hopkins Adams, "Modern Surgery," *McClure's Magazine*, 26 March 1905, 483.

58. Weller Van Hook, "Editorial: Surgery, Past, Present and Future," *Surgery, Gynecology, and Obstetrics* 3 (1906): 816.

59. On the role of bureaucracy in Progressive Era reform, see Weibe, *The Search for Order*.

60. Richard Cabot, *A Guide to the Clinical Examination of the Blood for Diagnostic Purposes*, 5th ed. (New York: William Wood, 1904), 182. In Ann Arbor in 1901, George Dock lectured to his students on the differences between organic causation and association. "When we say that the patient has splenic leukemia at the present time, we mean that he has leukemia in which the spleen is enlarged. We do not mean to say that it is the primary seat of the disease . . . It might be said, why not remove this enormous force? The answer is, although the size of it seems very great and a very imposing site of disease . . . in the surgical aspect it is not so very promising, for it is a very dangerous operation . . . and the spleen therefore should not be removed." "Case of Leukemia," George Dock Notebooks: 1900–1901, no. 1, 98–99, Bentley Historical Library, University of Michigan, Ann Arbor.

61. Stengel, "Varieties of Splenic Anemia," 498.

62. On these debates and other tensions in the history of technology in the early twentieth-century hospital, see Joel Howell, *Technology and the Hospital* (Baltimore: Johns Hopkins University Press, 1995).

63. J. C. DaCosta, "Address on the Occasion of the Graduation Exercises at the Naval Medical School in Washington, March 30, 1907," in *The Trials and Triumphs of the Surgeon and Other Literary Gems* (Philadelphia: Dorrance, 1907), 394.

64. Ibid., 395–96.

65. Broome, *Rochester and the Mayo Clinic*, 58.

66. "$7,639 for Loss of Spleen," *New York Times*, 20 January 1912.

67. "What Does the Spleen Do?" *New York Times*, 22 January 1912.

68. "Whatever necessary functions it performed," they asserted confidently, "will be taken up and performed by other organs." "A Rare Operation on Mme. Dorrente," *New York Times*, 24 March 1909.

69. The American College of Surgeons became one of the dominant forces behind the hospital standardization movement in this era. For insight into this development, see Rosemary Stevens, *American Medicine and the Public Interest* (New Haven: Yale University Press, 1971), 119. See also Davis, *Fellowship of Surgeons*.

70. W. L. Babcock, "Simplification and Standardization of Surgical Technic in Hospitals," *Modern Hospital* 5 (December 1915): 7.

71. Stuart McGuire, *The Profit and Loss Account of Modern Medicine and Other Papers* (Richmond: C. H. Jenkins Publisher, 1915), 15, 18.

72. Comments by Beth Vincent appear after several conference papers, including Joseph Miller, "Splenectomy in Splenic Anemia," *Journal of the American Medical Association* 67 (1916): 728–29; D. Balfour, "Indications for Splenectomy in Certain Chronic Blood Disorders: The Technic of Operation," *Journal of the American Medical Association* 67 (1916): 791; and R. McClure, "Pernicious Anemia Treated by Splenectomy and Systematic Often-Repeated Transfusion of Blood," *Journal of the American Medical Association* 67 (1916): 797. Quotation appears on p. 797. On the other hand, as late as 1928, some surgeons attending the annual meetings of the American Surgical Association believed that splenectomy should continue to be a prevalent part of the surgical armamentarium. See Ravitch, *A Century of Surgery*, 661–62, 707.

73. Harvard's George Minot wrote that "there are certain cases grouped under the title splenic anemia . . . Removal of the spleen in such instances seems to inaugurate in some manner a stimulation of the bone marrow." George Minot, "Diminished Blood Platelets and Marrow Insufficiency," *Archives of Internal Medicine* 19 (1917): 1062.

74. Richard Mills Pearce, Edward Bell Krumbhaar, and Charles Harrison Frazier, *The Spleen and Anaemia: Experimental and Clinical Studies* (Philadelphia: Lippincott, 1918), v.

75. Ibid., 242.

76. "Statistical summaries, including valuable detailed information," wrote Frazier, "are thus frequently rendered useless when, on analysis, they are found to include several independent types of splenic disease." Ibid.

77. The reviewer noted that "surgery of the spleen has in the past occupied a restricted field. Now we are beginning to realize that this organ plays a considerable part in the etiology of diseases . . . This book should be carefully read by every surgeon who has not familiarized himself with this important subject." "Review of *The Spleen and Some of Its Diseases*," in *Northwest Medicine* 21 (1921): 64. See also "Editorial: The Surgeon as Internist," 192.

78. Moreover, Moynihan noted, "the results [of splenectomy] in splenic anemia, generally speaking have been good, but the operation is more difficult than in other conditions, and the mortality is considerable." Moynihan, *Spleen and Its Diseases*, 15.

79. James Carslaw, "Discussion on Surgical Treatment of Non-traumatic Affections of the Spleen," *British Medical Journal* 2 (1922): 1204.

80. Moynihan, *Spleen and Its Diseases*, 86.

81. Comment by Vincent followed Miller, "Splenectomy in Splenic Anemia," 728. A Baltimore surgeon, Edward Hanrahan, also proclaimed in 1925 that "splenic anemia is not a disease entity . . . it is a syndrome that may be brought about by various causes." Edward Hanrahan, "Splenic Anemia: A Study of End-Results with and without Splenectomy, Based on Thirty-five Cases," *Archives of Surgery* 10 (1925): 641. See also Edward Hanrahan, "Splenic Blood Disorders: A

Surgical Classification with Reference to Splenectomy," *Annals of Surgery* 81 (1925): 906–10.

82. One 1927 textbook of pathology concluded that "despite the improvement resulting from splenectomy . . . there has been much opposition directed of late against the consideration of Banti's disease as a distinct pathological entity." Francis Delafield and T. Mitchell Prudden, eds., *A Textbook of Pathology* (New York: William Wood, 1927), 548.

83. Moynihan, *The Spleen and Its Diseases*.

84. Franklin Martin, *Fifty Years of Medicine and Surgery: An Autobiographical Sketch* (Chicago: Surgical Publishing, 1934), 218.

85. H. Dale Collins, "Indications for Splenectomy," *Southern Medical Journal* 33 (1940): 659.

86. Harold Burrows, *The Pitfalls of Surgery* (London: Balliere, Tindall, and Cox, 1925), 505. The surgeon, Burrows believed, "does not measure correctly his own ignorance. None but the wisest can master such a difficult task as that" (p. 505).

87. Ibid. Burrows concluded: "Since the removal of the spleen is now being recommended in cases which are diagnosed as 'splenic anemia,' it is worth while mentioning that in the presence of the liver or ascites, the operation is likely to be disappointing in its results." See also Moynihan, *The Spleen and Its Diseases*, 15.

88. "It follows that cooperation between the internist, clinical lab worker, surgeon, and pathologist is essential." Isidore Cohn, "The Differential Diagnosis and Surgical Indications of Splenomegaly," *Southern Medical Journal* 31 (1938): 486.

89. L. F. Alrutz et al., "Thrombopenic Purpura," *Archives of Pathology and Laboratory Medicine* 1 (1926): 359.

90. Heneage Oglivie, in his 1929 book, noted that, "at the Mayo Clinic, it has been found that cases which have undergone splenectomy have lived on the average two and one half times as long as those in whom no operation was performed." Heneage Oglivie, *Recent Advances in Surgery* (Philadelphia: Blakiston, 1929), 312.

91. W. Crosby, "Splenectomy: In and Out of Fashion," *Archives of Internal Medicine* 145 (1985): 225. See also L. Weintraub, "Splenectomy: Who, When, and Why?" *Hospital Practice* 29 (15 June 1994): 27–34, and K. Marble et al., "Changing Role of Splenectomy for Hematologic Disease," *Journal of Surgical Oncology* 52 (1993): 169–71.

Chapter 3   Blood Work: *The Scientific Management of Aplastic Anemia and Industrial Poisoning*

1. For coverage of the George Mosher case, see the following issues and pages of the *New York Times* in 1929: 21 June, 19; 24 June, 14; 25 June, 35; 26 June, 17; 27 June, 2; 28 June, 7; 29 June, 14; 1 July, 29; 2 July, 14. Finally, see "Mosher Boy, 15,

Dies of Strange Malady," *New York Times,* 10 July 1929, 29, and autopsy reported 11 July, 25.

2. "Mosher Boy Dies," 29.

3. Ralph Larrabee, "Aplastic Anemia and Its Related Conditions," *Journal of the American Medical Association* 75 (1920): 1633.

4. Many elite physicians in the early twentieth century trained in pathology and thought of pathology as the "supreme court of diagnosis." See, for example, George Corner, *George Hoyt Whipple and His Friends: The Life Story of a Nobel Prize Pathologist* (Philadelphia: Lippincott, 1963); Harvey Cushing, *The Life of Sir William Osler* (Oxford: Clarendon Press, 1925); and Donald Fleming, *William Welch and the Rise of Modern Medicine* (Baltimore: Johns Hopkins University Press, 1954).

5. A specific study, focusing on the hospital in this era, is David Rosner, *A Once Charitable Enterprise: Hospitals and Health Care in Brooklyn and New York, 1885–1915* (New York: Cambridge University Press, 1982). On the general corporate industrial transformation of the early twentieth century, see Harry Braverman, *Labor and Monopoly Capital: The Degradation of Work in the Twentieth Century* (New York: Monthly Review Press, 1974), especially his discussion of scientific office management (pp. 305–12).

6. Daniel Nelson, *Managers and Workers: Origins of the New Factory System in the United States, 1880–1920* (Madison: University of Wisconsin Press, 1975), and David Montgomery, *Workers' Control in America: Studies in the History of Work, Technology, and Labor Struggles* (New York: Cambridge University Press, 1979). One of the most thoughtful studies of the ideology of "scientific management" is still Samuel Haber, *Efficiency and Uplift: Scientific Management in the Progressive Era, 1890–1920* (Chicago: University of Chicago, 1964). In medicine, the laboratory represented one arm of this bureaucratic trend. On the rise of the laboratory and its epistemological (rather than bureaucratic) implications, see Knud Faber, *Nosography: The Evolution of Clinical Medicine in Modern Times* (New York: Hoeber, 1922), and Stanley J. Reiser, *Medicine and the Reign of Technology* (New York: Cambridge University Press, 1978).

7. Keen insight into Hamilton's career and public health concerns is provided in Barbara Sicherman, *Alice Hamilton: A Life in Letters* (Cambridge: Harvard University Press, 1984).

8. David Linn Edsall, "The Transformation of Medicine: An Address Delivered at the Dedicatory Exercises of Duke University Medical School and Duke Hospital, Durham, N.C., April 20, 1931," *Southern Medical Journal* 24 (1931): 1103–13.

9. Paul Ehrlich, "Über einen Fall von Anamie mit Bemerkungen über regenerative Veranderungen des Knochenmarks," *Charite Ann* 13 (1888): 300. A useful discussion of Ehrlich and the history of bone marrow studies is Mehdi Tavasolli, "Bone Marrow: The Seedbed of Blood," in Wintrobe, *Blood, Pure and Eloquent.*

A traditional biography of Ehrlich is Martha Marquardt, *Paul Ehrlich* (New York: Shuman, 1951).

10. Quotation is attributed to Frank Billings, in Edward Hirsch, *Frank Billings: The Architect of Medical Education, an Apostle of Excellence in Clinical Practice, a Leader in Chicago Medicine* (Chicago: Hirsch, 1966), 13.

11. For a detailed analysis of the correlation of marrow with blood cell pathology by Rudolph Virchow, Julius Cohnheim, and other nineteenth-century hematological researchers, see Maxwell Wintrobe, *Hematology: The Blossoming of a Science* (Philadelphia: Lea and Febiger, 1985). On the emergence of the clinico-pathological tradition, see Erwin Ackeknecht, *Medicine at the Paris Hospital, 1784–1848* (Baltimore: Johns Hopkins University Press, 1967). See also Esmond Long, *A History of Pathology* (New York: Dover, 1965); Faber, *Nosography*; Michel Foucault, *The Birth of the Clinic: An Archeology of Medical Perception* (New York: Pantheon Books, 1973); and Russell Maulitz, *Morbid Appearances: The Anatomy of Pathology in the Early Nineteenth Century* (Cambridge: Cambridge University Press, 1987).

12. William Gardner and William Osler, "Case of Progressive Pernicious Anaemia," *Canada Medical and Surgical Journal* 5 (March 1877): 20.

13. Ralph Lavenson, "Aplastic Anemia, with Report of a Case," *Transactions of the Association of American Physicians* 21 (1907): 307–24. See also Ralph Lavenson, "The Nature of Aplastic Anemia and Its Relation to Other Anemias," *American Journal of Medical Sciences* 133 (1970): 100–113, and L. Crummer, "A Case of Aplastic Anemia," *Journal of the American Medical Association* 49 (1907): 2086. Another early report was G. Evans and M. Halton, "An Unusual Case of Anemia," *Journal of the American Medical Association* 46 (1905): 1195–97.

14. For insight on the role of pathology in medicine and the status of pathological science, see J. H. Means, *The Association of American Physicians: Its First Seventy-five Years* (New York: McGraw-Hill, 1961). See also Thomas Bonner, *American Doctors and German Universities* (Lincoln: University of Nebraska Press, 1963).

15. Aldred Warthin, *Practical Pathology for Physicians and Students* (Ann Arbor: George Wahr, 1897), 7. A comparison of the 1897 edition of this text with the 1911 edition makes clear that, while autopsy lay at the core of pathological practice in 1897, by 1911 laboratory diagnostics had become the centerpiece of pathology. See Aldred Warthin, *Practical Pathology: A Manual of Autopsy and Laboratory Technique for Students and Physicians* (Ann Arbor: University of Michigan Press, 1911). This transition is even more striking when one compares the 1897 and 1938 editions of Mallory and Wright's textbook of pathology. F. B. Mallory and J. H. Wright, *Pathological Technic* (Philadelphia: W.B. Saunders, 1897); F. B. Mallory, *Pathological Technique* (Philadelphia: W.B. Saunders, 1938).

16. Partly because pathology had no immediate economic value, it remained a small field. See Fleming, *William Welch*.

17. Quoted in Harvey Cushing, *The Life of Sir William Osler* (Oxford: Claren-

don Press, 1925), 237, 252. Also, historian Esmond Long noted that, "in Philadelphia, Osler was the doctor's pathologist . . . he was concerned primarily with the precise information each [postmortem] examination gave for understanding the course of the disease in the individual patient." Esmond Long, *A History of American Pathology* (Springfield, Ill.: Charles C Thomas, 1962), 160.

18. See William Osler, "Diseases of the Blood and Blood-Glandular System," in *A System of Practical Medicine*, ed. William Pepper (Philadelphia: Lea Brothers, 1885). See also William Osler, "Diseases of the Blood," in *Principles and Practice of Medicine* (New York: Appleton, 1894), 182–233, and William Osler, "[Treatment of] Diseases of the Blood and Ductless Glands," in *American Textbook of Applied Therapeutics*, ed. James Wilson and Augustus Eshner (Philadelphia: W.B. Saunders, 1896), 902–27. For one of his earliest writings on the bone marrow and disease, see Osler, "Fatty Degeneration of the Organs; Hyperplasia of the Bone-Marrow," *Montreal General Hospital Pathological Reports* 1 (1877): 94–97. (All reprints available in William Osler Library, McGill University, Montreal.)

19. Frank Billings recalled that, in St. Mary's Hospital in Chicago during the 1870s, autopsies were few because the nuns in the Catholic hospital objected to them. "Persistent efforts were required to convince some members of the medical staff and especially the Sisters, that necropsies, conducted scientifically, were absolutely necessary in order to improve the quality of medical and surgical services." Quoted in Hirsch, *Frank Billings*, 23.

20. On the increasing difficulty of obtaining bodies for pathological practice, the emergence of state regulations, and pathology's close association with the poorhouse, see David Humphrey, "Dissection and Discrimination: The Social Origins of Cadavers in America, 1760–1915," in *Essays on the History of Medicine*, ed. Saul Jarcho (New York: New York Academy of Medicine, 1976), 269–77; H. Montgomery, "A Body Snatcher Sponsors Pennsylvania's Anatomy Act," *Journal of Medical History* 21 (1966): 382–91; and G. B. Jenkins, "The Legal Status of Dissecting," *Anatomical Record* 7 (1913): 395. An excellent cultural history of the cadaver and dissection in nineteenth-century Britain is Ruth Richardson, *Death, Dissection and the Destitute* (New York: Penguin Books, 1988).

21. Warthin, *Practical Pathology* (1897), 7. Warthin believed that the information gained would provide a more complete chronicle of mortality trends and a valuable portrait of the public's health.

22. Charles Rosenberg has argued that, "from the patient's perspective, the [early twentieth-century] hospital seemed impersonal and bureaucratic . . . Specialists addressed themselves to a focus narrowed by their training." Charles Rosenberg, *The Care of Strangers: The Rise of America's Hospital System* (New York: Basic Books, 1987), 5. Also see Morris Vogel, *The Invention of the Modern Hospital: Boston, 1870–1930* (Chicago: University of Chicago Press, 1980).

23. See Rosner, *A Once Charitable Enterprise*. For a discussion of nursing in the American hospital, see Susan Reverby, *Ordered to Care: The Dilemma of American*

Nursing, 1850–1945 (Cambridge: Cambridge University Press, 1987). See also Rosenberg, *The Care of Strangers*.

24. William Osler, "On the Educational Value of the Medical Society," *Boston Medical and Surgical Journal* 148 (1903): 275.

25. Richard Cabot, "On the Relation between Laboratory and Clinical Work," *Boston Medical and Surgical Journal* 164 (1911): 884.

26. Richard Cabot, "Ether Day Address: Traditions, Standards, and Prospects on the Massachusetts General Hospital," *Boston Medical and Surgical Journal* 182 (1920): 292.

27. New textbooks highlighted the rise of a new laboratory expertise. See, for example, Richard Cabot, *A Guide to the Clinical Examination of the Blood for Diagnostic Purposes* (New York: William Wood, 1897). This was the first American textbook in hematology. On the conflict arising over this new mode of medical work, see Morris Vogel and Charles Rosenberg, eds., *The Therapeutic Revolution: Essays in the Social History of Medicine* (Philadelphia: University of Pennsylvania Press, 1979); especially Gerald Geison, "Divided We Stand: Physiologists and Clinicians in the American Context," 67–90, and Russell Maulitz, "'Physicians versus Bacteriologists': The Ideology of Science in Clinical Medicine," 91–108. Two contemporary accounts of these tensions are C. F. Hoover, "The Reputed Conflict between Laboratory and Clinical Medicine," *American Medical Association Bulletin* 25 (May 1930): 110–112, and Richard Cabot, "The Historical Development and Relative Value of Clinical Methods of Diagnosis," *Boston Medical and Surgical Journal* 157 (1907): 151. See also Joel Stanley Reiser, *Medicine and the Reign of Technology* (New York: Cambridge University Press, 1978), and Howell, *Technology and the Hospital*.

28. The AAP was an organization originally comprising 100 nationally known physicians. See J. H. Means, *The Association of American Physicians: Its First Seventy-Five Years* (New York: McGraw-Hill, 1961). The William Pepper laboratory had been founded specifically to define the relationship of laboratory-based analysis to traditional medical practice. See George Corner, *Two Centuries of Medicine: A History of the School of Medicine, University of Pennsylvania* (Philadelphia: Lippincott, 1965).

29. Lavenson, "Aplastic Anemia," 313.

30. Ibid. For a useful overview of hematological theory and practice around 1900, see James Ewing, *Clinical Pathology of the Blood* (Philadelphia: Lea and Brothers, 1901). See also Cabot, *Clinical Examination of the Blood*.

31. Cabot, quoted in Lavenson, "Aplastic Anemia," 314.

32. Richard Cabot, in Osler and McCrae, *Modern Medicine*, 637. "If this is yellow from end to end," Cabot wrote, "the case may be assigned to the aplastic type."

33. Estimated from *Index Catalogue of the Library of the Surgeon-General's Office* and *The Quarterly Cumulative Index to Current Medical Literature*. See, for example,

J. O'Malley and H. Conrad, "The Course of the Blood Changes in a Case of Aplastic Anemia," *Journal of the American Medical Association* 73 (1919): 1761; Isaac Abt, "Aleukemia, Leukemia with Clinical Symptoms of [A]plastic Anemia," *Medical Clinics of North America* 8 (1924): 427–36; A. Archibald, "Aplastic Anemia," *Medical Clinics of North America* 3 (1919): 759; W. B. Fontaine, "Aplastic Anemia," *Southern Medical Journal* 16 (1923): 495–500; S. W. Sappington, "A Note on Types of Aplastic Anemia," *Hahnemann Monthly* 58 (1923): 737–46; R. A. Glenn and C. L. McVey, "Aplastic Anemia with Report of a Case," *Northwest Medicine* 18 (1919): 65–67; H. E. Marsh, "Aplastic Anemia," *Annals of Clinical Medicine* 3 (August 1924): 162–164; and S. W. Hurwitz, "The Factors of Coagulation in Experimental Aplastic Anemia," *Johns Hopkins Hospital Bulletin* 26 (1915): 235.

34. See, for example, LeRoy Crummer, "A Case of Aplastic Anemia," *Journal of the American Medical Association* 49 (1907): 2086.

35. J. H. Musser, "Study of a Case of Aplastic Anemia," *Archives of Internal Medicine* 14 (1914): 275–88. Quotation appears on p. 275.

36. Frederick Henry, "Relations between Chlorosis, Simple Anemia, and Pernicious Anemia," *Transactions of the Association of American Physicians* 4 (1889): 163.

37. Lavenson, "Aplastic Anemia," 321–22.

38. Ibid., 322–23.

39. Ibid., 321–22.

40. On the passing of morbid anatomy, see Sir J. F. Goodhart, *The Passing of Morbid Anatomy: The Harveian Oration for 1912 Delivered at the Royal College of Physicians on St. Luke's Day, October 18, 1912* (London: Murray, 1912). Goodhart noted that "pathology not only changes but it shifts its ground . . . forty years ago . . . our meetings were crowded with [gross pathological] specimens of all kinds . . . Now I am told that morbid anatomy is much less in evidence—we have left all that behind" (p. 14). See also H. E. MacDermot, *Maude Abbott; A Memoir* (Toronto: Macmillan, 1941).

41. Crummer, "A Case of Aplastic Anemia," 2086.

42. C. G. Geary and N. G. Testa, "Pathophysiology of Marrow Hypoplasia," in *Aplastic Anemia*, ed. C. G. Geary (London: Balliere, 1979), 11. They felt that "the main reason for the confusion was the lack of a method for examining marrow cellularity during life."

43. Frederick Washburn and John Bresnahan, "Medical and Surgical Efficiency in Large General Hospitals," *Modern Hospital* 5 (December 1915): 427–29.

44. William MacCarty, "Relations of Laboratories to Hospitals," *Modern Hospital* 11 (1918): 381. The hospital provided an organizational rationale for the conceptualization of disease and diagnosis. For an astute analysis of divisions of labor and classifications of the natural world, see Mary Douglas, *How Institutions Think* (Syracuse, N.Y.: Syracuse University Press, 1986).

45. See, for example, George Swift, "Better Hospitals in Washington," *North-*

west Medicine 20 (May 1921): 121–25. For a recent analysis, see Andrew Cunningham and Perry Williams, eds., *The Laboratory Revolution in Medicine* (New York: Cambridge University Press, 1992). An excellent analysis of changes occurring elsewhere in America is Ellis Hawley, *The Great War and the Search for a Modern Order* (New York: St. Martin's Press, 1992).

46. W. W. Duke, "Aplastic Anemia," *Journal of the American Medical Association* 91 (1928): 720–22. Some measured the numbers of monocytes, others documented the rise and fall of the polymorphonuclears, others traced the fluctuation of platelets, and others looked for diminution of all of these blood constituents before diagnosing aplastic anemia. Using his own criteria, J. P. Schneider had argued that aplastic anemia was defined by a "striking leucopenia" and "an extraordinary reduction in the blood-platelet count." On this basis, he stated, "There is no question of the propriety of giving aplastic anemia a separate and distinct pigeon-hole among the anemias . . . it stands quite on its own legs." J. P. Schneider, "Aplastic Anemia," *American Journal of Medical Science* 156 (1918): 799–807.

47. On the declining number of autopsies in hospitals, Ludwig Hektoen, "Necropsy Percentage in Relation to Hospital Professional Efficiency," *Modern Hospital* 22 (1924): 491–93. See also I. F. Volini, "Advantages of Autopsies and Clinico-pathological Conferences," *Hospital Progress* 11 (1930): 304–6; C. C. Guy, "Difficulties in Obtaining Autopsies," *Hospital Progress* 11 (1930): 301–10; L. J. Frank, "Autopsy as Essential to the Progress of Diagnosis in Medicine," *Modern Hospital* 24 (1925): 148–50. The difficulty, one observer noted, was that "the bone marrow as a tissue presents unusual difficulties for study, particularly due to its inaccessibility, and wide distribution. Its cellular state varies widely in different bones, different levels of the same bone, and different areas of a cross-section through a given level." R. P. Custer, "Studies on the Structure and Function of Bone Marrow: I. Variability of the Haemopoietic Pattern and Consideration of Method for Examination," *Journal of Laboratory and Clinical Medicine* 17 (1932): 951–60.

48. Historian W. D. Foster wrote that the rising number of for-profit laboratory services in the late nineteenth century gave physicians a false sense of objective control over clinical diagnosis. He concluded, "It is not what is true that is important but rather what men believe to be true. For the medical profession, on virtually negligible evidence, believed . . . that the administration of vaccines was dangerous unless controlled by a special laboratory test—the opsonic index." Such was their faith in this technology that many wrongly proclaimed: "'Inoculate when the patient is in the negative phase and you kill; inoculate when the patient is in the positive phase and you cure.'" W. D. Foster, *Pathology as a Profession in Great Britain and the Early History of the Royal College of Pathologists* ([London]: The College, [1982?]), 13. See also John Hornsby and Richard Schmidt, *The Modern Hospital: Its Inspiration, Its Architecture, Its Equipment, Its Operation* (Philadelphia: W.B. Saunders, 1913), especially "Department of Pathology," 279–391.

49. MacCarty, "Relation of Laboratories to Hospitals," 381.

50. See discussion in Maxwell Finland, *The Harvard Medical Center at Boston City Hospital* (Boston: Harvard Medical School, 1982).

51. In the 1910s, Larrabee headed the blood ward at the Massachusetts General Hospital. Roger Lee later recalled that "Dr. Beth Vincent and I made a complete resurvey of the clotting of blood, preliminary to some work that Vincent did in blood transfusion . . . Dr. Vincent removed the spleen from a series of cases of pernicious anemia and we studied that disease intensely. George R. Minot . . . joined our informal group . . . Minot and I thought we solved the problem of hemophilia—I still think so, even if all the world is not completely . . . convinced yet." Roger Lee, *The Happy Life of a Doctor* (Boston: Little, Brown, 1956), 35.

52. See R. C. Larrabee, "Aplastic Anemia, with Report of a Case," *American Journal of Medical Science* 142 (1911): 57–68; G. R. Minot, "Diminished Blood Platelets and Marrow Insufficiencies," *Archives of Internal Medicine* 19 (1917): 1062. Enthusiasm for the laboratory tests indicating this disease was also voiced in Thomas Buchman, "Progress in Medicine: Recent Advances in the Treatment of Anemia," *Boston Medical and Surgical Journal* (1923): 201. Buchman wrote that "with the manufacture of a suitable preparation of brilliant cresyl blue in America the counting of reticulated erythrocytes again becomes a clinically possible procedure . . . A knowledge of the percentage of these cells in the peripheral blood is, of course, empirical evidence of much value in the diagnosis of primary aplastic anemia."

53. Francis Rackemann, *The Inquisitive Physician: The Life and Times of George Richards Minot* (Cambridge: Harvard University Press, 1956); see also Frederick Washburn, *The Massachusetts General Hospital: Its Development, 1900–1939* (Boston: Houghton Mifflin, 1939).

54. Rackemann, *The Inquisitive Physician*, 100.

55. Minot, "Diminished Blood Platelets," 1062. See also G. R. Minot, R. Lee, and B. Vincent, "Splenectomy in Pernicious Anemia," *Journal of the American Medical Association* 67 (1916): 719.

56. Paul DeKruif, *Men Against Death* (New York: Harcourt, Brace, 1932), 94.

57. "So Wright, getting sorer and sorer, kept showing Minot the exact look of this weird blood sickness through the microscope . . . 'Why can't these baby bone marrow cells turn into good full-grown cells?'" Ibid., 95.

58. As Morris Fishbein noted, "The emphasis on the laboratory and on the machinery in recent years has made the philanthropists, the sociologists and the economists think that the medical problem of the future will be answered by more and more organization and mechanization." Morris Fishbein, *Doctors and Specialists* (Indianapolis: Bobbs-Merrill, 1930), 28.

59. MacCarty, "Relation of Laboratories to Hospitals," 381.

60. Hektoen, "Necropsy Percentage," 491–93.

61. MacCarty, "Relation of Laboratories to Hospitals," 381. The American So-

ciety of Clinical Pathology was founded in 1921–1922. For more on this reorganization of pathology, see Long, *A History of American Pathology*.

62. Thomas Arthur Flood, "The Relationship between the Clinical Laboratory and the Physician," *North Carolina Medical Journal* 21 (1922): 437.

63. Fishbein, *Doctors and Specialists*, 87.

64. William German, *Doctors Anonymous: The Story of Laboratory Medicine* (New York: Duell, Sloan, and Pearce, 1941), 139. "Unlike other medical men," German pointed out, "the pathologist cannot hope to become independent in his own field. He cannot go out and set up shop in any community that needs his services, for he is a doctor's doctor. The only channels by which his services reach the patient are controlled by other doctors" (p. 290). See also M. T. McEachern, "Role of the Clinical Pathologist in Hospital Efficiency," *Journal of Laboratory and Clinical Medicine* 10 (1925): 898–905, and, later, I. Davidsohn, "Relationship of Hospital Management to the Hospital Laboratory," *Hospitals* 13 (September 1939): 44–48. Davidsohn noted that "the department of clinical and pathological laboratories occupies a special position in relation to the management of the hospital. It constitutes a medical as well as an administrative unit."

65. For a more extensive discussion of these tensions between clinical pathologists and other specialists, see J. H. Wright, "The Development of the Frozen Section Technique, the Evolution of Surgical Biopsy, and the Origins of Surgical Pathology," *Bulletin of the History of Medicine* 59 (1985): 295–326.

66. Alexander Maximow, "Relation of Blood Cells to Connective Tissues and Endothelium," *Physiological Review* 4 (1924): 533–63. A discussion of Maximow and tensions between clinicians and physiologists is mentioned in Tavasolli, "Bone Marrow," 71. In 1934, three authors acknowledged that "examination of the peripheral blood may be, at times, no index as to the condition of the blood forming organs [i.e. the marrow]." W. P. Thompson, M. N. Richter, and K. Edsall, "An Analysis of So-Called Aplastic Anemia," *American Journal of Medical Sciences* 187 (1934): 77–88. Quotation on p. 87.

67. E. Falconer and L. Morris, "A Clinical Comparison of Aplastic Anemia, Idiopathic Purpura Hemorrhagica, and Aleukemic Leukemia Based on Studies of the Bone-Marrow," *Medical Clinics of North America* 6 (1922): 353. See also Morris and Falconer, "Intravitam Bone Marrow Studies Preliminary Report: Part 1," *Archives of Internal Medicine* 30 (1922): 485–89, and Falconer and Morris, "Intravitam Bone Marrow Studies: Part II. Survey of the Clinical Field," *Archives of Internal Medicine* 30 (1922): 491–506. Another advocate and user of the technique was Bryce Fontaine, "Aplastic Anemia with Report of a Case—Differential Diagnosis of the Anemias Due to Hemolysis, and Due to Hematopoietic Degeneration," *Southern Medical Journal* 16 (1923): 495–500. See also L. F. Alrutz, J. T. Nortell, and E. C. Piette, "Thrombopenic Purpura," *Archives of Pathology and Laboratory Medicine* 1 (1926): 356–60.

68. J. B. McElroy, "The Differentiation of Aplastic Anemia and Essential

Thrombocytopenia: Its Importance from a Therapeutic Standpoint," *Southern Medical Journal* 19 (1926): 328.

69. An analysis of the changing economics of pathology in medicine is William White, *Public Health and Private Gain: The Economics of Licensing Clinical Laboratory Personnel* (Chicago: Maaroufa Press, 1979). Some pathologists recognized that a loss in status would accompany this new role as "scientific managers." See R. A. Kilduffe, "Editorial: The Choice of a Pathologist," *Journal of Laboratory and Clinical Medicine* 11 (1926): 694–96.

70. L. Selling, "Benzol as a Leucotoxin—Studies on the Degeneration and Regeneration of the Blood and Hematopoietic Organs," *Johns Hopkins Hospital Reports* 17 (1916): 83–136; L. Selling, "A Preliminary Report of Some Cases of Purpura Hemorrhagica Due to Benzol Poisoning," *Johns Hopkins Hospital Bulletin* 21 (1910): 33–37.

71. Selling concluded that the pathological result of benzol poisoning was essentially aplastic anemia.

72. See, for example, Leonard Parry, *The Risks and Dangers of Various Occupations and Their Prevention* (London: Scott, Greenwood, 1900). Exposure to benzol, Parry noted, caused "headache, giddiness, difficulty walking, breathing, sleeplessness, insensibility and finally death" (p. 17).

73. On the recognition of "silicosis" as a legitimate industrial disease in this era, see David Rosner and Gerald Markowitz, *Deadly Dust: Silicosis and the Politics of Occupational Disease in Twentieth-Century America* (Princeton: Princeton University Press, 1991). Quotation from p. 4.

74. The letterhead of the American Association for Labor Legislation, of which Hoffman was a member, proclaimed their goal to be the "Conservation of Human Resources." Frederick Hoffman to Alroy Phillips, 9 October 1914, Papers of Frederick Hoffman, 1908–1916, vol. 2, Hagley Museum and Library, Delaware.

75. For a description of Edsall's work in industrial disease, see Joseph Aub and Ruth Hapgood, *Pioneer in Modern Medicine: David Linn Edsall of Harvard* (Cambridge: Harvard Medical Alumni Association, 1970).

76. Ibid., 184. See also David Linn Edsall, "Medical-Industrial Relations of the War," *Johns Hopkins Hospital Bulletin* 29 (1918): 197.

77. Minot, "Diminished Blood Platelets," 1062.

78. Schneider, "Aplastic Anemia," 799–807. Other physicians also began to criticize the nomenclature of aplastic anemia. See Harry Greenwald, "Aplastic Anemia," *American Journal for the Diseases of Children* 47 (1934): 360–70, and Harry Greenwald, "Myelophthisis," *Journal of Pediatrics* 3 (1933): 117–31. Other skeptical discussions of the legitimacy of the term *aplastic anemia* appeared in Thompson, Richter, and Edsall, "Analysis of So-Called Aplastic Anemia"; E. Pernokis, "Aplastic Anemia," *Medical Clinics of North America* 17 (1933): 377–83; E. S. Mills, "Idiopathic Aplastic Anemia or Aleukia Hemorrhagica," *American Journal of Medical Science* 181 (1931): 521–23; and J. H. Root, "Idiopathic Aplastic Anemia: With

Report of a Case in a Child of 9 Years Having Usual Bone Pathology," *New England Journal of Medicine* 203 (1930): 1225–31.

79. Alice Hamilton, *Industrial Poisons in the United States* (New York: Macmillan, 1925), 1.

80. By 1914, Hamilton had begun to explore the effects of various agents and chemicals on the health of American industrial workers. Alice Hamilton, *Exploring the Dangerous Trades: The Autobiography of Alice Hamilton* (Boston: Little, Brown, 1943), 294–96, 388. Throughout the 1920s, other industrial hygienists and reformers at the state level would also pursue these themes, publicizing the effects of chemical agents on working men and women in America. Emory Roe Hayhurst, *A Survey of Industrial Health-Hazards and Occupational Disease in Ohio* (Columbus: F.J. Heer, 1915), 220–26, discusses the health effects of work in rubber-making plants, including benzol poisoning and aplastic anemia.

For literature in the twenties, see T. M. Legge, "Chronic Benzol Poisoning," *Journal of Industrial Hygiene* 1 (1920): 539–41; A. R. Smith, "Chronic Benzol Poisoning among Women Industrial Workers—a Study of the Women Exposed to Benzol Fumes in Six Factories," *Journal of Industrial Hygiene* 10 (1928): 73–93; L. Greenburg, "Benzol Poisoning as an Industrial Hazard: VII. Results of Medical Examinations and Clinical Tests Made to Discover Early Signs of Benzol Poisoning in Exposed Workers," *Public Health Reports* 41 (1926): 1526–39.

81. Alice Hamilton, "The Growing Menace of Benzene (Benzol) Poisoning in American Industry," *Journal of the American Medical Association* 78 (1922): 627, 630. See also T. F. Harrington, "Industrial Benzol Poisoning in Mass.," *Boston Medical and Surgical Journal* 177 (1917): 203–6, and Frederick Flinn, "Some of the Newer Industrial Hazards," *Boston Medical and Surgical Journal* 197 (1928): 1309–14.

82. Barbara Sicherman, *Alice Hamilton: A Life in Letters* (Cambridge: Harvard University Press, 1984).

83. Lead poisoning was for many years the most prominent concern. For an excellent analysis of Alice Hamilton and industrial medicine, from primary materials, see Sicherman, *Alice Hamilton*.

84. Hamilton, "Growing Menace of Benzene (Benzol)." This fact was also emphasized during World War II by J. J. Bloomfield, "War's Influence on Industrial Hygiene," in *Manual of Industrial Hygiene*, ed. William Gafafer (Philadelphia: W.B. Saunders, 1943), 7.

85. Hamilton, *Industrial Poisons*, v. Hamilton also praised the medical world for "an enormous increase in the interest . . . in industrial toxicology of late years, especially since our entrance into the war in 1917." Ibid., vii. Public health officials sought to use the laboratory as a tool for education, uplift, and moral reform. They began the fight against pellagra and hookworm in the South and the "campaign" against diseases like tuberculosis, venereal disease, and polio. Hamilton was only the most prominent among those who made a career of raising the public awareness of industrial diseases. Often she did so by telling stories of brave

working men who were suddenly and fatally struck down by an insidious poison during what had seemed like an average day at work.

86. Committee on Industrial Hygiene to Frederick Hoffman, 11 December 1913, Papers of Frederick Hoffman, 1908–1916, vol. 1.

87. "One cannot depend on the changes in the blood-forming organs alone for diagnosis of benzol poisoning." Alice Hamilton, *Industrial Toxicology* (New York: Harper and Brothers, 1934), 162–63.

88. A. K. Smith and L. A. DeBlois to J. J. Moosman, January 1923 Safety Bulletin: "Warning of Possible Fatal Poisoning,"p. 1, Joseph Moosman Papers, Hagley Museum and Library.

89. Safety bulletin, received 5 January 1923, letterhead of E.I. DuPont de Nemours and Co., Service Department, Wilmington, Delaware, Safety Division. The bulletin stated: "The recent case occurred after considerable improvement in the ventilation of the building . . . While blood transfusions were resorted to, [the workers] died . . . from profound changes in the blood brought about by the action of benzene."

90. The Barrett Company, Benzol Department to Alice Hamilton, 3 January 1924, Alice Hamilton Papers, series IV, box 2, folder 40: "Benzene, Aniline, Etc. Correspondence, 1913–1942," Schlesinger Library, Radcliffe College.

91. Alice Hamilton to the Barrett Company, 7 January 1924, Alice Hamilton Papers.

92. Hamilton also suggested a more "scientific" air analysis: "(2) the determination of quantitative air analyses of the safe limits of benzol vapor in the air which must be breathed by workers for 8 hours out of the 24." Alice Hamilton to Barrett Company, Benzol Department, 7 January 1924, Alice Hamilton Papers.

93. On "The Rise and Decline of Welfare Capitalism" in the 1910s and 1920s, see Howard Brody, *Workers in Industrial America: Essays on the Twentieth Century Struggle* (New York: Oxford University Press, 1980). Brody argues that "it is comforting to think that welfare capitalism never was a success, never persuaded workingmen that they were best off as wards of the employer . . . The facts, however, suggest otherwise." It collapsed because it could not survive the downturn in the business cycle. Hamilton's managerial paternalism was an academic support of the goals of welfare capitalism. For more on industrial hygiene and Hamilton during this period, see Christopher Sellers, "The Public Health Service's Office of Industrial Hygiene and the Transformation of Industrial Medicine," *Bulletin of the History of Medicine* 65 (1991): 42–73.

94. Quoted in Alice Hamilton, *Industrial Poisons in the United States* (New York: Macmillan, 1925), 400. The council also noted: "This would appear to confirm the conclusion of our previous report that the benzene hazard in industry is a real, but not a sensational, one."

95. John Martin Askey, M.D., to Alice Hamilton, 25 March 1930, Alice Hamilton Papers, series IV, box 2, folder 40.

96. Safety Bulletin from Medical Division, A. K. Smith, and Safety Division, L. A. DeBlois: "Our plants and laboratories should be on their guard, not only against benzene poisoning but also against the insidious chronic form."

97. Ibid., 4.

98. J. Moosman to C. M. Foss, General Motors Corp., New York, 21 May 1924, memorandum.

99. Hamilton, *Industrial Poisons*, 6.

100. There were, indeed, many other instances where hematologists like Minot called for such close blood monitoring of the workers. See Minot, "Blood Examination in Trinitrotoluene Workers," *Journal of Industrial Hygiene* 1 (1919): 301–18.

101. She noted in the preface to her 1925 book, *Industrial Poisons*, "Physicians in private practice have given me the greatest assistance yet there are limitations to the value of the information obtained in this way" (p. v). "Union physicians were so sympathetic to their men as to dull their critical faculties . . . [company doctors] often indulge in moral observations on the character of workingmen and the evils of trade-unionism . . . The statements of the men themselves should be treated with respect, and checked up, and often will prove to be founded on close observation" (p. vi).

102. Hamilton to Greenough, Lyman, and Cross, counselors at law, Providence, R.I., 6 April 1932, Alice Hamilton Papers, series IV, box 2, folder 40: "Benzene, Aniline, Etc."

103. She wrote, "The man had a susceptibility to benzol above the average." Hamilton to unknown recipient, 18 August 1933, Hamilton Papers.

104. Ibid., 1.

105. Hamilton, *Industrial Toxicology*, 165.

106. Writing in 1938, pathologist Madeleine Fallon noted that "it is the author's belief that there is no such thing as true essential aplastic anemia. All aplastic anemias are the result of some toxic damage to the marrow or an exhaustion phenomenon . . . [Moreover, she wrote,] aplastic anemia is a relative condition depending on how severely the bone marrow is involved." Fallon, "Classification of the Anemias," in *Handbook of Hematology*, ed. Hal Downey (New York: Hoeber, 1938), 2171.

107. R. Cabot, "Case 13101: An Obscure Anemia," *Boston Medical and Surgical Journal,* 196 (1927): 404–9.

108. "The difficulty is that one is at a great disadvantage in looking at blood unless one has stained it oneself." Ibid., 406.

109. Cabot concluded that the splenectomy was justified not because of any physiological rationale, but as a last resort. "Here is a man . . . whose diagnosis in spite of a great deal of study cannot be settled, and we are willing to take any chance. Yes, perfectly justified." Ibid., 409.

110. By 1927, in the minds of many other physicians, a diagnosis of aplastic

anemia would have necessitated acceptance of the etiological role of benzol poisoning.

111. She wrote: "Martland of Newark, who has seen more industrial benzol poisoning than any other man in this country, writes me that one cannot depend on the changes in the blood-forming organs alone for a diagnosis of benzol poisoning." Hamilton, *Industrial Toxicology*, 163.

Chapter 4   The Corporate "Conquest" of Pernicious Anemia:
Technology, Blood Researchers, and the Consumer

1. Lawrence Kass, *Pernicious Anemia*, Major Problems in Internal Medicine, vol. 7 (Philadelphia: W.B. Saunders, 1978), i. See also Arthur Bloomfield, *A Bibliography of Internal Medicine: Selected Diseases* (Chicago: University of Chicago Press, 1960).

2. J. H. Means and Wyman Richardson, "Impressions of the Nature of Pernicious Anemia in Light of Newer Knowledge," *Journal of the American Medical Association* 91 (1928): 923. They wrote: "Joslin, not many years ago, joyfully exclaimed 'Insulin is here' . . . In some respects the latter discovery [the discovery of an 'anti-pernicious anemia body'] is the greater of the two." Thomas Ordway and L. W. Gorham described the discovery as "epoch-making" in "The Treatment of Pernicious Anemia with Liver and Liver Extract," *Journal of the American Medical Association* 91 (1928): 928.

3. George Minot and Beth Vincent, "Splenectomy in Pernicious Anemia," *Journal of the American Medical Association* 67 (1916): 719. See also S. A. Levine and W. S. Ladd, "Pernicious Anemia: A Clinical Study of One Hundred and Fifty Consecutive Cases with Special Reference to Gastric Anacidity," *Bulletin of the Johns Hopkins Hospital* 32 (1921): 254.

4. George Minot and William Murphy, "Treatment of Pernicious Anemia by a Special Diet," *Journal of the American Medical Association* 87 (1926): 470; Minot and Murphy, "Observations on Patients with Pernicious Anemia Partaking of a Special Diet," *Transactions of the Association of American Physicians* 41 (1926): 72–73.

5. "Pernicious Anemia Cure Wins Our $10,000 Annual Award," *Popular Scientific Monthly*, February 1931, 30.

6. William Castle, "The Conquest of Pernicious Anemia," in Wintrobe, *Blood, Pure and Eloquent*. Another glowing account is Rackemann, *The Inquisitive Physician*. For recent accounts, see Allen Weisse, *Medical Odysseys: The Different and Sometimes Unexpected Pathways to Twentieth-Century Medical Discoveries* (New Brunswick, N.J.: Rutgers University Press, 1991); John Krantz, Jr., *Historical Medical Classics Involving New Drugs* (Baltimore: Williams and Wilkins, 1990); and Marcel Florkin, "The Nature and Therapy of Pernicious Anaemia," *Clio Medica* 8 (1973): 223–27.

7. Lionel Whitby, "Addisonian Anemia," *British Medical Journal* 1 (1955): 1403.

8. Minot continued: "We would not ordinarily utilize a patient for a test of an extract whose count was above 3 million." George Minot to Dr. Blankenhorn, 13 May 1929, George Minot Papers, box 5, file: Committee on Pernicious Anemia, Countway Library, Harvard University.

9. George Minot, "The Development of Liver Therapy in Pernicious Anemia (the Nobel Lecture Delivered at Stockholm on December 12, 1934)," *Les Prix Nobel en 1934* (Stockholm: Almquist and Wiksell, 1934).

10. William Needles, "Neurological Complications of Pernicious Anemia," *Archives of Neurology and Psychiatry* 26 (1930): 346–58. See also William Cadwalader, *Diseases of the Spinal Cord* (Baltimore: Williams and Wilkins, 1932).

11. Lee, *The Happy Life of a Doctor*, 225.

12. Ibid.

13. T. J. Jackson Lears, "From Salvation to Self-Realization: Advertising and the Therapeutic Roots of the Consumer Culture, 1880–1930," in *The Culture of Consumption: Critical Essays in American History, 1880–1980*, ed. Richard Wightman Fox and T. J. Jackson Lears (New York: Pantheon Books, 1983), 3.

14. A detailed reference to the emergence of clinical research in various institutions is A. McGehee Harvey, *Science at the Bedside: Clinical Research in American Medicine, 1905–1945* (Baltimore: Johns Hopkins University Press, 1981).

15. Among the abstracts and articles appearing in the *American Journal of Medical Science* were the following: William Pepper, "Progressive Pernicious Anaemia," *American Journal of Medical Science* 62 (1875): 313–47; Frederick Henry and William Osler, "Atrophy of the Stomach, with the Clinical Features of Progressive Pernicious Anaemia," *American Journal of Medical Science* 90 (1886): 498–511. For several years Osler edited the abstracts of foreign and domestic articles in medicine for this journal. Short notes on pernicious anemia appeared frequently. (For a few such abstracts, see "Pernicious Anaemia," April 1882, 551; "Pernicious Anaemia in a Child Five," January 1885, 253; "The Etiology and Curability of Pernicious Anaemia," October 1886, 531; "Pernicious Anaemia," November 1888, 618; "The Pathology of Pernicious Anaemia," April 1888, 398; "Pernicious Anaemia," August 1890, 185; "The Treatment of Pernicious Anaemia by Arsenic," May 1894, 575; and "The Treatment of Pernicious Anaemia," September 1896, 334.)

16. "Pernicious Anemia: A New Disease," *Medical Times Gazette* 2 (1876): 581. See also Thomas Addison, "Anaemia—Disease of the Suprarenal Capsules," *London Medical Gazette* 8 (1849): 517, and A. Biermer, "Progressive Pernicious Anemia," *Correspondenzbl. Schweitz. Aertz* 2 (1872): 15.

17. Addison quoted in William Osler, "Diseases of the Blood," in William Pepper, *A System of Practical Medicine* (Philadelphia: Lea and Brothers, 1894), 900.

18. Ibid.

19. Robert Edes, "Clinical Lecture on a Case of Idiopathic Anaemia," *Boston Medical and Surgical Journal* 106 (1882): 457–58. "On inspection the patient was

seen to be a muscular young man, not emaciated, but exceedingly pale, his skin being almost yellow and the mucous membranes almost white" (p. 457).

20. Editorial, "Progressive Pernicious Anaemia," *Boston Medical and Surgical Journal* 122 (1890): 306.

21. Frank Billings, "Report of the Progress of Cases of Pernicious Anemia Presented to the Association in 1900, and Report of a Case of Pernicious Anemia, with Diffuse Spinal-Cord Lesion and Postmortem Findings," *Transactions of the Association of American Physicians* 16 (1901): 291.

22. In the case of the idle gentleman, J. M. DaCosta noted that "I can recall a case of a gentleman who lived a club life—not a dissipated life, but an indolent one—who had a remission of eleven months, and in that time had absolutely no treatment. Then came a relapse in which he died." DaCosta, commenting after Billings, "Progress of Pernicious Anemia."

23. Alexander McPhedran, "Observations on the Nature and Treatment of Pernicious Anemia," *Transactions of the Association of American Physicians* 16 (1901): 422.

24. On this view of the natural history of disease, see Owsei Temkin, "The Scientific Approach to Disease: Specific Entity and Individual Sickness," in *The Double Face of Janus and Other Essays in the History of Medicine* (Baltimore: Johns Hopkins University Press, 1977). For more on the nineteenth-century physician as naturalist, see John Haller, *American Medicine in Transition, 1840–1910* (Urbana: University of Illinois Press, 1981), 204–9; see the chapter by that name in John A. Ryle, *The Natural History of Disease* (London: Oxford University Press, 1936); and Henry Cohen, "The Evolution of the Concept of Disease," in *Concepts of Medicine*, ed. Brandon Lush (New York: Pergamon Press, 1961).

25. Most physicians found no pathological basis for the definition of pernicious anemia, death (for the most part) being the best diagnostic evidence. Osler assumed that the bone marrow was the "source and origin of the evil." Osler, "Diseases of the Blood," 905. But this view was not widely held.

26. In 1884, Osler regretted that "many a man, pitchforked, so to speak, by local exigencies . . . cannot break the invidious bar of defective training which effectually shuts him off from the latter [original work and investigation] and the higher duties of his position." It was largely in response to such constraints that the Association of American Physicians was formed. William Osler, "Commentary," *Canadian Medical and Surgical Journal* 12 (1884): 3–7. On the AAP's history, see J. H. Means, *The Association of American Physicians: Its First Seventy-Five Years* (New York: McGraw-Hill, 1961). In 1886, the AAP's first president, Francis Delafield, emphasized that "we all like to give instruction and to gain reputation, and both of these we can do in the societies already existing. But we also want a society in which we can learn something." Francis Delafield, "Opening Remarks," *Transactions of the Association of American Physicians* 1 (1886): 1.

27. One article noted that the British clinician William Hunter was "one of

those who regards pernicious anemia as a distinct and separate entity, not mere-ly an extreme form of anaemia or chlorosis." "Editorial: The Urine in Pernicious Anaemia," *Boston Medical and Surgical Journal* 121 (1889): 344–45. See also "Edi-torial: Progressive Pernicious Anaemia," *Boston Medical and Surgical Journal* 122 (1890): 306–7. See also J. P. Crozer Griffith, "The Pathology of Pernicious Ane-mia," *Transactions of the Association of American Physicians* 6 (1891): 239–50.

28. William Osler, "Chauvinism in Medicine," address before the Canadian Medical Association, Montreal, 17 September 1902, William Osler Papers, William Osler Library, McGill University, Montreal, Canada.

29. Delafield, "The Clinic—On Blood Diseases," 775.

30. Noting the prevailing atmosphere of skepticism during one AAP discus-sion, Hobart Hare commented that, "in regard to what Dr. Cabot said about the use of arsenic, I would like to know why he believes this drug to be useless. Cer-tainly, wonderful improvement takes place under its use, and when we again and again get good results we must attribute it to the drug." Frederick Henry, "Clin-ical Notes of Cases of Pernicious Anemia," *Transactions of the Association of Amer-ican Physicians* 15 (1900): 346–66; quotation on p. 362. Others responded that ar-senic might coincide with a remission, but it was nearly impossible to prove that arsenic had caused the response. See also Byron Bramwell, "Clinical Lectures on a Case of Progressive Pernicious Anaemia Cured by Arsenic," *Medical Times Gazette* 1877 (15 September): 323–24.

31. Billings, "Progress of Pernicious Anemia," 280–99.

32. McPhedran, "Observations on Pernicious Anemia," 422.

33. Osler, "Diseases of the Blood," 905–6.

34. R. Cabot, "Pernicious Anaemia: A Study of 50 Cases," *Boston Medical and Surgical Journal* 135 (1896): 104–7.

35. Osler, "Diseases of the Blood," 902.

36. Osler (1894), in Pepper *Text-book of Medicine*, 2:205–6. "Pernicious anemia may be readily distinguished from chlorosis, by the clinical examination of the blood, which will reveal in the former disease the increased globular richness in haemoglobin and the presence of Erhlich's gigantoblasts" (pp. 205–6).

37. The term *poikilocytosis* (from Greek) meant, according to Osler, "various-ly shaped."

38. Henry had earlier insisted that "the symptoms of pernicious anemia are those of a simple anemia aggravated and intensified." Frederick Henry, *Anaemia* (Philadelphia: Blakiston, 1887), 55.

39. Delafield, "The Clinic—On Blood Diseases," 775.

40. See J. P. Crozer Griffith and Charles Burr, "The Pathology of Pernicious Anemia," *Transactions of the Association of American Physicians* 6 (1891): 239–50.

41. Frederick Henry, "Relations between Chlorosis, Simple Anaemia and Per-nicious Anaemia" *Journal of the American Medical Association* 13 (1889): 500, and Frederick Henry, "Relations between Chlorosis, Simple Anaemia and Pernicious

Anemia, including Leucocythemia and Hodgkin's Disease," *Transactions of the Association of American Physicians* 4 (1889): 160–73.

42. Henry, "Chlorosis, Simple Anaemia and Pernicious Anemia, including Leucocythemia"(*Trans AAP*), 160.

43. Osler "took issue with Dr. Henry in regard to chlorosis. He [Osler] held that chlorosis was absolutely distinct from pernicious anaemia, for the following reasons: 1. the sex; he had never seen chlorosis in a male. 2. The pathological condition . . . 3. The character of the blood. He considered the diminution of the percentage of haemoglobin a distinctive feature of chlorosis. 4. Curability. Although in chlorosis there is a tendency to relapse, each given attack can be cured if sufficiently large doses of iron are employed." Henry, "Chlorosis, Simple Anaemia and Pernicious Anaemia" (*JAMA*), 501. Kinnicutt of New York and William Pepper of Philadelphia "agreed with Dr. Osler" (pp. 501–2).

44. See Russell Maulitz, "Physicians versus Bacteriologists: The Ideology of Science in Clinical Medicine," and Gerald Geison, "Divided We Stand: Physiologists and Clinicians in the American Context," in *The Therapeutic Revolution*, ed. Morris Vogel and Charles Rosenberg (Philadelphia: University of Pennsylvania Press, 1979).

45. "The diagnosis [of pernicious anemia] is made," said Hewes, "simply by the examination of the stained specimen [of blood] where we can determine the excess of megaloblasts." Henry Hewes, "Practical Blood Examination," *Boston Medical and Surgical Journal* 145 (1901): 121, 123.

46. In 1896, Cabot had written the first American textbook on hematology.

47. Cabot noted that "I have repeatedly failed to find any megaloblasts at the first examination, yet had no difficulty discovering them a day or two later." Richard Cabot, "Pernicious Anaemia: A Study of One Hundred and Ten Cases," *Transactions of the Association of American Physicians* 15 (1900): 346.

48. Billings, "Progress of Pernicious Anemia," 330. Many physicians, when confronted with the question of megaloblastic diagnosis, hedged. Alfred Stengel wrote, "I agree with Dr. Dock that no sharp line can be drawn between the different types of red blood corpuscles. They seem to be variations which merge into each other without any sharp distinctions." In George Dock, "A Case of Fatal Epistaxis (from Endothelioma of the Nose) with a Study of the Blood," *Transactions of the Association of American Physicians* 14 (1899): 136.

49. George Dock Notebooks, 1899–1900, p. 219, 5 December 1899, Bentley Historical Society, University of Michigan, Ann Arbor.

50. "All other blood changes in this disease . . . are from the practical standpoint of diagnosis, of subordinate importance." Henry, "Clinical Notes of Pernicious Anemia" (*Trans AAP*), 362.

51. Frederick Henry, "Further Notes of a Case of Pernicious Anemia Reported at the Meeting of the Association of American Physicians in 1900," *Transactions of the Association of American Physicians* 16 (1901): 301.

52. Ibid., 302.

53. John Lovett Morse, "Some Cases Which Were Not Pernicious Anemia," *Boston Medical and Surgical Journal* 147 (1902): 587.

54. J. B. Herrick, "The Relation of the Clinical Laboratory to the Practitioner of Medicine," *Journal of the American Medical Association* 48 (1907): 1916.

55. For discussions concerning membership in the AAP, see J. H. Means, *The Association of American Physicians: Its First Seventy-Five Years* (New York: McGraw-Hill, 1961). See also George Dock, "Address of the President," *Transactions of the Association of American Physicians* 32 (1917): 1.

56. S. Coupland, "Pernicious Anaemia," in Allbutt, *A System of Medicine*, 519.

57. Ibid., 534.

58. R. Larrabee, "The Treatment of Pernicious Anemia," *Boston Medical and Surgical Journal* 176 (1917): 553; Morse, "Cases Which Were Not Pernicious Anemia," 587. Larrabee noted: "This occurs frequently enough to demand that before the diagnosis of pernicious anemia is definitely made, every case should be thoroughly studied for evidences of a causative condition . . . Never make the diagnosis on the blood alone."

59. For a discussion of these tensions in the history of sickle cell anemia, see Keith Wailoo, "A Disease *Sui Generis:* The Origins of Sickle Cell Anemia and the Emergence of Modern Clinical Research, 1904–1924," *Bulletin of the History of Medicine* 65 (1991): 185–208, and Herrick, "Relation of the Clinical Laboratory." See also C. N. B. Camac, "Hospital and Ward Clinical Laboratories," *Journal of the American Medical Association* 35 (1900): 219–27.

60. Mayo, "Splenectomy in the Anemias," 581.

61. Samuel West, in Allbutt's *A System of Medicine,* "From pernicious anemia splenic anemia is distinguished by the enlargement of the spleen, as well as by the condition of the blood" (p. 547).

62. Mayo, "Splenectomy in the Anemias,"581.

63. E. B. Krumbhaar, "Late Results of Splenectomy in Pernicious Anemia," *Journal of the American Medical Association* 67 (1916): 740.

64. G. R. Minot and R. Lee, "Treatment of Pernicious Anemia—Especially by Transfusion and Splenectomy," *Boston Medical and Surgical Journal* 187 (1917): 770.

65. W. W. Roblee, "Splenectomy in Primary Pernicious Anemia," *Journal of the American Medical Association* 64 (1915): 796.

66. T. L. Szlapka, "Splenectomy in Pernicious Anemia," *Medical Clinics of North America* 3 (1920): 773–82. Szlapka noted, prematurely, that splenectomy for pernicious anemia has been a "disappointment and . . . has now largely been abandoned." A more positive assessment of splenectomy appeared in N. M. Percy, "Pernicious Anemia: Splenectomy, Blood Transfusion," *Surgical Clinics of North America* 1 (1917): 251–70.

67. Thomas Buckman, "Progress in Medicine: Recent Advances in the Treatment of Anemia," *Boston Medical and Surgical Journal* (1923): 203.

68. Julius Friedenwald, "The Gastro-intestinal Disturbances Observed in Pernicious Anemia," *Boston Medical and Surgical Journal* 147 (1912): 160–62.

69. Many of the first generation of authors had emphasized the gastric aspects of pernicious anemia. See William Osler and Frederick Henry, "Atrophy of the Stomach, with Clinical Features of Progressive Pernicious Anemia," *American Journal of Medical Sciences* 91 (1886): 498–511; F. P. Kinnicutt, "Atrophy of the Gastric Tubules: Its Relation to Pernicious Anemia," *American Journal of Medical Sciences* 94 (1887): 419; and F. P. Kinnicutt, "Atrophy of the Gastric Tubules; Its Relation to Pernicious Anemia," *Transactions of the Association of American Physicians* 2 (1887): 179.

70. Friedenwald, "Gastro-intestinal Disturbances in Pernicious Anemia," 160.

71. "Two conditions must be classified as a result of a common cause," Friedenwald noted. Ibid.

72. See Joseph Kirsner, "One Hundred Years of Gastro-enterology," in *Grand Rounds: One Hundred Years of Internal Medicine*, ed. Russell Maulitz and Diana Long (Philadelphia: University of Pennsylvania Press, 1988). See also Bryce Fontaine, "A Study of the Symptoms of Achylia Gastrica," *Southern Medical Journal* 17 (July 1924): 466–69.

73. George Dock Notebooks, 1899–1900, 5 December 1899, p. 223, Bentley Historical Library, University of Michigan, Ann Arbor.

74. S. A. Levine and W. S. Ladd, "Pernicious Anemia: A Clinical Study of One Hundred and Fifty Consecutive Cases with Special Reference to Gastric Anacidity," *Bulletin of the Johns Hopkins Hospital* 32 (1921): 254. See also A. F. Hurst, "Achlorhydria; Its Relation to Pernicious Anemia and Other Diseases," *Lancet* 1 (1923): 111.

75. S. E. Durst, "Familial Pernicious Anemia: A Discussion of an Unusual Group of Cases with a Consideration of Achlorhydria as the Dominant Etiological Factor," *American Journal of Medical Science* 172 (1926): 173–74.

76. Ibid., 184.

77. H. W. Woltmann, "The Nervous System in Pernicious Anemia: An Analysis of One Hundred and Fifty Cases," *American Journal of Medical Science* 157 (1918): 408. See also H. W. Woltmann, "Brain Changes Associated with Pernicious Anemia," *Archives of Internal Medicine* 21 (1918): 791–836.

78. Richard Harvey, "Combined System Disease," *Medical Clinics of North America* 6 (1922): 371–76. For early descriptions of the neurological symptoms of pernicious anemia, see C. E. Riggs, "Some Nervous Symptoms of Pernicious Anemia," *Journal of the American Medical Association* 61 (1913): 481.

79. Harvey, "Combined System Disease," 371–75.

80. Larrabee, "The Treatment of Pernicious Anemia," 553.

81. Ibid., 553.

82. Minot and Lee, "Treatment of Pernicious Anemia," 770.

83. R. M. Pearce, E. B. Krumbhaar, and C. Frazier, *The Spleen and Anemia* (Philadelphia: W.B. Saunders, 1913). See also Llewelys Barker and Thomas Sprunt, "The Treatment of Some Cases of So-called Pernicious Anemia," *Journal of the American Medical Association* 69 (1917): 1919–27.

84. E. B. Krumbhaar, "Late Results of Splenectomy in Pernicious Anemia," *Journal of the American Medical Association* (1916): 724.

85. The words of Johns Hopkins' William Thayer exemplified the situation in 1916. He recalled a patient whose spleen he had ordered removed: "She made what appeared to be a complete recovery from the standpoint of her anemia and remained well for a year and a half. Her [spinal] cord changes failed to progress. Then, in about two or three months, she rapidly went down hill with a relapse and died from a characteristic pernicious anemia." His comment appears following R. McClure, "Pernicious Anemia Treated by Splenectomy and Systematic Often-Repeated Transfusion of Blood," *Journal of the American Medical Association* 67 (1916): 797. Two other authors wrote in 1917, "Benzol, roentgen ray, faradization, transfusion, and splenectomy, may produce fluctuations in the blood picture, and these fluctuations may be interpreted as improvements if one so desires; but the essential disease of the blood-forming organs still run their usual course." E. Butterfield and R. Stillman, "The Broader Aspects of Hematological Diagnosis," *American Journal of Medical Science* 154 (1917): 796.

86. G. Minot and J. Sampson, "Germanium Oxide as a Remedy for Anemia," *Boston Medical and Surgical Journal* 189 (1923): 629–32.

87. William Osler, "The Hospital Unit in University Work," *Lancet* 1 (1911): 211–13 (delivered before the Northumberland and Durham Medical Society).

88. Harvey, *Science at the Bedside*.

89. The emergence of academic and industrial research in other disciplines has been discussed by John Servos, "Industrial Research and Science: Chemical Engineering and MIT, 1900–1939," *ISIS* 71 (1991): 531–49, and Robert Kargon, "Temple to Science: Cooperative Research and the Birth of the California Institute of Technology," *Historical Studies in the Physical Sciences* 8 (1977): 3–31.

90. "There is no known treatment that cures pernicious anemia," wrote Lee and Minot in 1917. "Occasionally, one finds reports of cures, but such instances apparently represent either very long remissions or incorrect diagnoses." Minot and Lee, "Treatment of Pernicious Anemia," 764.

91. As Minot wrote to a fellow doctor, "Very few cases were diagnosed until the disease existed for several months." Minot to Blankenhorn, 13 May 1929, George Minot Papers.

92. George Whipple, "Abstract of Discussion," *Journal of the American Medical Association* 91 (1928): 932–34.

93. Minot had also noted that "cases that have developed spinal cord changes as a rule do not do well with splenectomy, and it is thus not indicated in such cases. Neither splenectomy nor transfusion checks these changes, though some ben-

efit from them may be seen with a rising red count from any cause." Minot and Lee, "Treatment of Pernicious Anemia," 770.

94. Quoted in L. Kass, *Pernicious Anemia* (Philadelphia: W.B. Saunders, 1978), 26. [From an interview with Murphy appearing in "Recollections of J. B. Murphy," *Medical World News* (1972)].

95. Kass, *Pernicious Anemia*, 26.

96. G. R. Minot and W. P. Murphy, "Treatment of Pernicious Anemia by a Special Diet," *Journal of the American Medical Association* 87 (1926): 470–76.

97. A useful overview of academic-pharmaceutical relations in the 1920s and 1930s is John Swann, *Academic Scientists and the Pharmaceutical Industry: Cooperative Research in Twentieth-Century America* (Baltimore: Johns Hopkins University Press, 1988).

98. Ibid., 153–69. The chapter, "The Scientist as Project Researchers," focuses on Harvard–Eli Lilly research collaboration on pernicious anemia.

99. J. H. Means and Wyman Richardson, "Impressions of the Nature of Pernicious Anemia in Light of Newer Knowledge," *Journal of the American Medical Association* 191 (1928): 923. See also L. Gorham, "Treatment of Pernicious Anemia by the Minot-Murphy Method," *Transactions of the Association of American Physicians* 43 (1929): 112–23.

100. Means and Richardson, "Nature of Pernicious Anemia," 923.

101. Edward Mason, "Pernicious Anemia: Report of a Case Treated with a High Liver Diet for Approximately Four Years," *Journal of the American Medical Association* 90 (1928): 1527–29; H. M. Bubert, "Subacute Combined Sclerosis," *Journal of the American Medical Association* 90 (1928): 903–6; E. McPeak and DeW. Neighbors, "Minot-Murphy Diet in Pernicious Anemia," *Southern Medical Journal* 20 (1927): 926–31.

102. Armand Cohen, "Subacute Combined Sclerosis Progressive during Remission of Pernicious Anemia," *Journal of the American Medical Association* 90 (1928): 1787; see also William Cadwalader, *Diseases of the Spinal Cord* (Baltimore: Williams and Wilkins, 1932). Cadwalader cited several other authors who found that spinal cord symptoms continued even during treatment with liver. Cadwalader noted: "liver therapy alone is not always reliable in permanently arresting the progress of objective spinal symptoms" (p. 159). See also C. C. Ungley and M. M. Suzman, "Subacute Combined Degeneration of the Cord: Symptomatology and Effects of Liver Therapy," *Brain* 52 (1929): 271–94.

103. R. Isaacs, C. Sturgis, and M. Smith, "Limitations of the Liver Treatment in Pernicious Anemia," *Transactions of the Association of American Physicians* 43 (1928): 127–31; see also R. Isaacs, C. Sturgis, and M. Smith, "Treatment of Pernicious Anemia," *Journal of the American Medical Association* 91 (1928): 1687.

104. Douglas MacAlpine, "Nervous and Mental Aspects of Pernicious Anemia," *Lancet* 2 (1929): 643–47. Quotation on p. 646.

105. H. Z. Giffin considered using liver as a diagnostic tool on borderline pa-

tients: "In such cases the question might arise whether or not it will be possible to use the liver diet as a diagnostic test." H. Z. Giffin, "Abstract of Discussion [at 1928 meetings]," *Journal of the American Medical Association* 91 (1928): 1690.

106. Isaacs, Sturgis, and Smith noted that "our experience has been, therefore, that the treatment of patients with uncomplicated pernicious anemia is very satisfactory . . . In a certain number of patients who are receiving this treatment the associated lesions of the spinal cord may not improve or may progress rapidly." Isaacs, Sturgis, and Smith, "Limitations of the Liver Treatment in Pernicious Anemia," 131.

107. W. S. Middleton, "Erythropoietic Response of Various Anemias to Liver Therapy," *Journal of the American Medical Association* 91 (1928): 863.

108. Cyrus Sturgis and Raphael Isaacs, "The Gastrointestinal Tract in Anemia Pernicious," *American Journal of Surgery* 11 (January 1931): 31.

109. Middleton, "Erythropoietic Response of Various Anemias," 863.

110. William Needles, "Neurologic Complications of Pernicious Anemia," *Archives of Neurology and Psychiatry* 26 (1930): 346–58. Needles argued that he and several others "had never seen a case of pernicious anemia in which the spinal cord signs . . . were favorably affected by liver treatment" (p. 347).

111. Ibid.

112. "In praising the value of liver as a means of therapy," Needles concluded, "neither complete pessimism nor complete optimism if justified." Ibid., 357.

113. T. Ordway and L. W. Gorham, "Treatment of Pernicious Anemia with Liver and Liver Extract," *Journal of the American Medical Association* 91 (1928): 925.

114. A consensus formed around validating the obvious benefits of liver therapy, while maintaining a well-grounded skepticism about a cure for pernicious anemia. See also G. Whipple, "Experimental Anemias, Diet Factors and Related Pathologic Changes of Human Anemias," *Journal of the American Medical Association* 91 (1928): 863–67, and R. West and E. Nichols, "Liver Fractions in Pernicious Anemia," *Journal of the American Medical Association* 91 (1928): 867–68. In his 1929 book, Paul Clough wrote that "liver must be kept up indefinitely . . . These facts would indicate that a radical 'cure' has not been achieved. Liver probably produces merely a symptomatic arrest of the disease usually amounting to a symptomatic cure." Paul Clough, *Diseases of the Blood* (New York: Harper and Brothers, 1929), 148.

115. Ordway and Gorham, "Treatment of Pernicious Anemia," 925.

116. E. B. Krumbhaar, "Thoughts on the Morbid Processes Active in Pernicious Anemia," *American Journal of Medical Science* 175 (1928): 525.

117. Paul Clough stated that "in many cases the patients acquire a craving for liver, and may eat it ravenously. The capacity of consuming with relish such large quantities of liver over long periods of time seems almost a specific characteristic of the disease." Clough, *Diseases of the Blood*, 145. Clough also noted that "they [Minot and Murphy] regard a failure to secure improvement after 6 weeks treat-

ment as nearly always indicating either mistaken diagnosis or an insufficient amount of liver" (p. 148).

118. Lee, *The Happy Life of a Doctor*. See Rosemary Stevens, "Hospitals in the 1920s: The Flowering of Consumerism," in *In Sickness and in Wealth: American Hospitals in the Twentieth Century* (New York: Basic Books, 1989), ch. 5; see also William Leuchtenberg, *The Perils of Prosperity, 1914–1932* (Chicago: University of Chicago Press, 1958).

119. T. J. Jackson Lears, "From Salvation to Self-realization: Advertising and the Therapeutic Roots of the Consumer Culture, 1880–1930," in Fox and Lears, *The Culture of Consumption*; see also Roland Marchand, *Making the American Dream: Advertising and Modernity* (Berkeley: University of California Press, 1986).

120. Walter W. R. May, "A Newspaper Man's Impression of the Medical Profession," *Northwest Medicine* 28 (1929): 35–37.

121. Ibid., 36.

122. See, for example, M. M. Suzman, "The Basal Metabolism in Pernicious Anemia and Subacute Combined Degeneration of the Spinal Cord," *American Journal of Medical Science* 184 (1932): 682. "This investigation is part of an attempt to ascertain more about the nature of subacute combined degeneration of the cord and its relation to pernicious anemia" (p. 682). See also L. F. Barker, "Neuro-anemic Syndromes," *Southern Medical Journal* 25 (1932): 687–91.

123. W. B. Castle and W. C. Townsend, "Observations on the Etiologic Relationship of Achylia Gastrica to Pernicious Anemia: II. The Effect of the Administration to Patients with Pernicious Anemia of Beef Muscle after Incubation with Normal Human Gastric Juice," *Journal of the American Medical Association* 178 (1929): 764–77; see also William Dameshek, "Some Types of 'Primary' Anemia and Their Treatment," *New England Journal of Medicine* 205 (1931): 1093–1104. He wrote that "this patient, then, had all the typical symptoms of pernicious anemia, and most of the signs of that disease . . . There was no response to liver extract but striking response to large doses of iron . . . The condition might be considered as an unusual type of pernicious anemia . . . Recently twelve patients with a very similar clinical syndrome have been observed" (p. 1098).

124. See, for example, Richard Cabot, "Progressive Neurological Symptoms with Liver and Brain Therapy," *New England Journal of Medicine* (1931): 303–5.

125. George Minot, "The Treatment of Pernicious Anemia with Liver or an Effective Liver Fraction," The Mary Scott Newbold Lecture, Lecture XVIII, *Transactions of the College of Physicians of Philadelphia* 49 (1927): 145.

126. He stated that "failure of liver therapy in a case diagnosed pernicious anemia implies inadequate treatment, an incorrect diagnosis, or the existence of complication." Minot, "Liver Therapy in Pernicious Anemia (Nobel Lecture)," 4. For other physicians, however, strict adherence to the Minot-Murphy liver diet was not necessary. "A balanced, liberal, general diet plus sufficient liver is equally effective." Gorham, "Treatment by the Minot-Murphy Method," 112–23. Com-

menting on Minot and the shifting definition of pernicious anemia in 1931, J. H. Musser noted that "Minot in one of his early papers said that his treatment had no effect on cord symptoms. Later he changed his mind. It so happens that I have seen patients who have improved markedly . . . and others who have not shown much improvement. I think there is often temporary improvement, but the cord symptoms return and the patient ultimately expires." J. H. Musser, "Three Types of Anemia," *Southern Medical Journal* 24 (1931): 106.

127. New research questions emerged. Some focused on creating the most effective liver extract administration. Castle and Morris Bowie, "A Domestic Liver Extract for Use in Pernicious Anemia: Method of Preparation," *Journal of the American Medical Association* 92 (1929): 1830–32; William Castle and F. H. Taylor, "Intravenous Use of Liver Extract for Use in Pernicious Anemia," *Journal of the American Medical Association* 96 (1932): 1198–1201.

128. William Dameshek, "Anemia," *Hygeia* 1947: 432.

129. Indeed, the association of anemia with diet had been, arguably, commonplace in the late nineteenth century. See A. L. Skoog, "Liver Therapy Advocated during the Last Century for the Anemias," *Journal for the History of Medicine* 19 (1946): 233–35.

130. James Madison, *Eli Lilly: A Life, 1885–1977* (Indianapolis: Indiana Historical Society, 1989), 66–67.

131. Ibid., 83.

132. Madeleine Fallon, "Classification of the Anemias, Blood Pictures in the Anemias, and Anemias in Infants and Children," in *Handbook of Hematology*, ed. Hal Downey (New York: Hoeber, 1938), 2170.

133. Wyndham Lloyd, *A Hundred Years of Medicine* (London: Duckworth, 1939), 222–23. For an excellent study involving insight into a similar disease history, see Chris Feudtner, "Bitterseet: The Transformation of Diabetes into a Chronic Illness in Twentieth-Century America" (Ph.D. diss., University of Pennsylvania, 1995).

134. An Alabama researcher named Tom Spies would argue in 1946 that folic acid was effective in treating anomalous cases of pernicious anemia. After extensive studies, it became clear that spinal cord changes became abruptly *worse* under the influence of folic acid. Tom Spies, *Experiences with Folic Acid* (Chicago: Year Book Medical Publishers, 1947). Later, with the discovery and refinement of vitamin B_{12} in the late 1940s, it appeared that the true "magic bullet" for pernicious anemia had been discovered. But, as Harold Burn noted in 1962, "Vitamin B_{12} cures pernicious anemia only when it given by injection, and not when it is given by mouth." Burn, *Drugs, Medicine, and Man* (New York: Scribner's, 1962), 168. On complications arising from liver extract therapy, see Steven Schwartz and Helen Legere, "Treatment of Liver Extract Sensitivity," *Blood* 1 (1946): 307–16; S. Feinberg, H. Alt, and R. Young, "Allergy to Injectable Liver Extract: Clinical and Immunological Observations," *Annals of Internal Medicine* 18 (1943): 311; and Clement Krantz, "Anaphylactic Reactions following Medication with Parenter-

al Liver Extract," *Journal of the American Medical Association* 110 (1938): 802.

135. In the words of one historian, "In support of his theory he performed the following experiment. He gave some steak to a normal person to eat; then when it was partly digested, he took it out of the normal person's stomach, and gave it to a patient with pernicious anemia [actually combine system degeneration]!" It was not the steak alone but the steak which had been digested by normal gastric juice that was effective. Burn, *Drugs, Medicine, and Man*, 168.

Castle, whose 1930 work was not recognized by the Nobel Committee, thus introduced a more complex model of the diseases. Castle and Taylor, "Intravenous Use of Liver Extract"; W. B. Castle and W. C. Townsend, "Observations on the Etiologic Relationship of Achylia Gastrica to Pernicious Anemia: II. The Effect of the Administration to Patients with Pernicious Anemia of Beef Muscle after Incubation with Normal Human Gastric Juice," *Journal of the American Medical Association* 178 (1929): 764–77; William Castle and Morris Bowie, "A Domestic Liver Extract for Use in Pernicious Anemia: Method of Preparation," *Journal of the American Medical Association* 92 (1929): 1830–32. The disease was the product of the interaction of an abnormal physiology with absence of a key nutritional element.

136. "Liver Preparations," *Bulletin of the Council on Pharmacy and Chemistry* 63 (1935): 788.

137. Ibid., 858.

138. Ibid., vol. 35A, new series, discussion 4. It was nearly impossible to find patients who had not "received arsenic and blood transfusions within a month" or who were "free of certain complications." Ibid., 858. Harry Marks brought this material to my attention.

139. Lloyd, *A Hundred Years of Medicine*, 222.

140. Lee, *The Happy Life of a Doctor*, 225.

141. For this and other insights on the historical meanings of health and disease, see Owsei Temkin, "Health and Disease," in *The Double Face of Janus*, 437.

142. C. Heath, "A Broadcast Message by the State Department of Public Health—the Use and Abuse of Liver Diet," *New England Journal of Medicine* 204 (1931): 1171–73. Quotation on p. 1173.

143. Elmer Miner, *Living the Liver Diet* (St. Louis: C.V. Mosby, 1931); Dorothy Stewart, *The Liver Cookery Book, Containing Recipes for Cooking Liver without the Addition of Fat, and Menus for Fourteen Days* (London: J. Wright Bristol and Sons, 1933).

Chapter 5   Detecting "Negro Blood": *Black and White Identities and the Reconstruction of Sickle Cell Anemia*

1. James Herrick, "Peculiar Elongated and Sickle-shaped Red Blood Corpuscles in a Case of Severe Anemia," *Transactions of the Association of American Physicians* 25 (1910): 553–61; idem, "Peculiar Elongated and Sickle-shaped Red Blood

Corpuscles in a Case of Severe Anemia," *Archives of Internal Medicine* 6 (1910): 517–21. See also T. Savitt and M. Goldberg, "Herrick's 1910 Report of Sickle Cell Anemia: The Rest of the Story," *Journal of the American Medical Association* 261 (1989): 266–71; C. Lockhard Conley, "Sickle Cell Anemia: The First Molecular Disease," in Wintrobe, *Blood, Pure and Eloquent*; and Keith Wailoo, "A Disease *Sui Generis:* The Origins of Sickle Cell Anemia and the Emergence of Modern Clinical Research, 1904–1924," *Bulletin of the History of Medicine* 65 (1991): 185–208. An excellent overview article is Todd Savitt, "The Invisible Malady: Sickle Cell Anemia in America, 1910–1970," *Journal of the National Medical Association* 73 (1981): 739–46.

2. Verne Mason, "Sickle Cell Anemia," *Journal of the American Medical Association* 79 (1922): 1318–19; W. Taliaferro and J. Huck, "The Inheritance of Sickle Cell Anemia in Man," *Genetics* 8 (1923): 594–98.

3. Thomas Cooley and Pearl Lee, "The Sickle Cell Phenomenon," *American Journal of the Diseases of Children* 32 (1926): 340; see also Cooley and Lee, "Observations of the Sickle Cell Phenomenon," *Transactions of the American Pediatric Society* 38 (1926): 58–59.

4. The sickle cell trait is referred to as an autosomal recessive trait.

5. In a 1947 paper on the issue, Neel wrote, "If the homozygous-heterozygous hypothesis is correct, then both parents of any patient with sickle cell anemia should always sickle . . . If, on the other hand, the disease is due to a dominant gene with variable expression, only one parent need sickle." J. V. Neel, "The Inheritance of Sickle Cell Anemia," *Science* 40 (1949): 64.

6. For scholarship on this theme, see Kenneth Ludmerer, *Genetics and American Society* (Baltimore: Johns Hopkins University Press, 1972); see also Daniel Kevles, "Blood, Big Science, and Biochemistry," in his *In the Name of Eugenics: Genetics and the Uses of Human Heredity* (New York: Knopf, 1985), 223–37; see also Judith Swazey and Karen Reeds, "The Lesson of Rare Maladies: Sickle Cell Anemia and the Genetic Control of Protein Structure," in *Today's Medicine, Tomorrow's Science: Essays on the Paths of Discovery in the Biomedical Sciences*, ed. Judith Swazey and Karen Reeds, Public Health Service Publ. 78-244 (Washington, D.C.: GPO, 1978), 73–92.

7. For a discussion of this refutation of past hematological thought, see Bernard Seeman, *The River of Life: The Story of Man's Blood from Magic to Science* (New York: W.W. Norton, 1961).

8. The flaw in the hemoglobin was caused by an incorrectly substituted amino acid. Sickle hemoglobin differs from normal hemoglobin because valine has replaced glutamic acid at two points on the molecule.

9. Linus Pauling, Harvey Itano, S. J. Singer, and Ibert Wells, "Sickle Cell Anemia: A Molecular Disease," *Science* 110 (1949): 543–48.

10. George Gray, "Sickle Cell Anemia," *Scientific American* 185 (August 1951): 56–59, 59.

11. For more on thinking about heredity and society in the early twentieth century, see Peter Bowler, *The Mendelian Revolution: The Emergence of Hereditarian Concepts in Modern Science and Society* (London: Athlone, 1989); Charles Rosenberg, "The Bitter Fruit: Heredity, Disease, and Social Thought," in his *No Other Gods: On Science and American Social Thought* (Baltimore: Johns Hopkins University Press, 1976); and Martin Pernick, *The Black Stork: Eugenics and the Death of "Defective" Babies in American Medicine and Motion Pictures since 1915* (New York: Oxford University Press, 1996). On the relations of Mendelian genetic thought and medicine, see Ludmerer, *Genetics and American Society*. A useful review of the relation between genetic thought and the eugenics social movement is Kevles, *In the Name of Eugenics*.

12. See, for example, F. Clarke, "Sickle Cell Anemia in the White Race with Report of Two Cases," *Nebraska Medical Journal* 18 (1923): 376–79; Thomas Cooley and Pearl Lee, "Sickle Cell Anemia in a Greek Family," *American Journal of Diseases of Children* 38 (1929): 103–6; S. Rosenfeld and J. Pincus, "The Occurrence of Sicklemia in the White Race," *American Journal of Medical Science* 184 (1932): 674–82; W. P. Sights and S. D. Simon, "Marked Erthrocytic Sickling in a White Adult, Associated with Anemia, Syphilis and Malaria," *Journal of Medicine* 12 (1931): 177–81; Russell Haden and Ferris Evans, "Sickle Cell Anemia in the White Race—Improvement in Two Cases following Splenectomy," *Archives of Internal Medicine* 60 (1937): 133–42; J. Cooke and J. Mack, "Sickle Cell Anemia in a White American Family," *Journal of Pediatrics* 5 (1934): 601.

13. M. A. Ogden, "Sickle Cell Anemia in the White Race," *Archives of Internal Medicine* 71 (1943): 164–182.

14. "Sickle Cell Anemia, a Race Specific Disease," *Journal of the American Medical Association* 133 (1947): 33–34.

15. See, for example, George Frederickson, *Black Image in the White Mind: The Debate on Afro-American Character and Destiny, 1817–1914* (New York: Harper and Row, 1971); Nancy Stepan, *The Idea of Race in Science: Great Britain, 1800–1960* (Hamden, Conn.: Archon Books, 1982); Elazar Barkan, *The Retreat of Scientific Racism: Changing Concepts of Race in Britain and the United States between the World Wars* (Cambridge: Cambridge University Press, 1992).

16. F. James Davis, *Who is Black? One Nation's Definition* (State College: Pennsylvania State University, 1991); see also Barbara Fields' essay, "Ideology and Race in American History," in J. Morgan Kousser and James M. McPherson, *Region, Race, and Reconstruction: Essays in Honor of C. Vann Woodward* (Oxford: Oxford University Press, 1982), 143–78; Winthrop Jordan, *White over Black: American Attitudes towards the Negro, 1550–1812* (New York: Penguin, 1969); Reginald Horsman, *Race and Manifest Destiny: The Origins of American Racial Anglo-Saxonism* (Cambridge: Harvard University Press, 1981).

17. "Our pollution behaviour is the reaction which condemns any object or idea likely to confuse or contradict cherished classifications" (p. 36). "We find in

any culture worthy of the name various provisions for dealing with ambiguous or anomalous events" (p. 39). Mary Douglas, *Purity and Danger: An Analysis of Concepts of Pollution and Taboo* (New York: Ark Paperbacks, 1966).

18. Some physicians wrote about sickle cell anemia from different clinical standpoints without engaging in discussions about the meaning of Negro blood. Consider, for example, E. W. Page and M. Z. Silton, "Pregnancy Complicated by Sickle Cell Anemia," *American Journal of Obstetrics and Gynecology* 37 (1939): 53; Wallace Yater and Mario Mollari, "The Pathology of Sickle Cell Anemia: Report of a Case with Death during an 'Abdominal Crisis,'" *Journal of the American Medical Association* 96 (1931): 1671–75; W. Willis Anderson, "Sickle Cell Anemia," *Journal of the American Medical Association* 99 (1932): 905.

19. See John Haller, *Outcasts from Evolution: Scientific Attitudes of Racial Inferiority, 1859–1900* (Urbana: University of Illinois Press, 1971); Frederickson, *Black Image in the White Mind*; and William Stanton, *The Leopard's Spots: Scientific Attitudes towards Race in America, 1815–1859* (Chicago: University of Chicago Press, 1960). See also Samuel Cartwright, "Report on the Diseases and Physical Peculiarities of the Negro Race," *New Orleans Medical and Surgical Journal* 7 (1851): 707–9.

Recently, several historians have explored racial inequalities in health and access to health care. See, for example, Vanessa Gamble, *Making a Place for Ourselves: The Black Hospital Movement, 1920–1945* (New York: Oxford University Press, 1995); David McBride, *From TB to AIDS: Epidemics among Urban Blacks since 1900* (Albany: State University of New York Press, 1991); David McBride, *Integrating the City of Medicine: Blacks in Philadelphia Health Care, 1910–1965* (Philadelphia: Temple University Press, 1989); Todd Savitt, *Medicine and Slavery: Health Care and Diseases of Blacks in Antebellum Virginia* (Urbana: University of Illinois Press, 1978); and Kenneth Kiple, *Another Dimension to the Black Diaspora: Diet, Disease, and Racism* (Cambridge: Cambridge University Press, 1981). Two excellent studies of black health and medical research on venereal disease are James Jones, *Bad Blood: The Tuskegee Syphilis Experiments* (New York: Free Press, 1981), and Allan Brandt, "Racism and Research: The Case of the Tuskegee Syphilis Study," in *Sickness and Health in America: Readings in the History of Medicine and Public Health*, ed. Judith Leavitt and Ronald Numbers (Madison: University of Wisconsin Press, 1985). A fine bibliography of medical writings on black health is Mitchell Rice and Woodrow Jones, *Health of Black Americans from Post-reconstruction to Integration, 1871–1960* (New York: Greenwood Press, 1990).

20. One contemporary regarded the Great Migration as "probably next to emancipation the most noteworthy event which has happened to the Negro in America." Ray Standard Baker, "The Negro Goes North," *World's Work* 34 (July 1917): 315. See also Haller, "The Politics of 'Natural Extinction,'" in Haller, *Outcasts from Evolution*.

21. C. Vann Woodward, *The Strange Career of Jim Crow*, 3d rev. ed. (New York:

Oxford University Press, 1974); William Cohen, *At Freedom's Edge: Black Mobility and the Southern White Quest for Racial Control, 1861–1915* (Baton Rouge: Louisiana State University Press, 1991).

22. John Higham, *Strangers in the Land: Patterns of American Nativism, 1860–1925* (New York: Athenaeum, 1963). For an excellent study of the migration and urban life, see James Grossman, *Land of Hope: Chicago, Black Southerners, and the Great Migration* (Chicago: University of Chicago Press, 1989); see also Ira Katznelson, *Black Men/White Cities: Race, Politics, and Migration in the United States, 1900–1930, and Britain, 1948–1968* (Chicago: University of Chicago Press, 1976).

23. Thomas Murrell, "Syphilis and the American Negro: A Medico-legal Study," *Journal of the American Medical Association* 54 (1910): 848.

24. F. Petersen and W. Haines, *A Textbook of Legal Medicine and Toxicology* (Philadelphia: W.B. Saunders, 1903), 433.

25. "Negro and Migration," *Southern Medical Journal* 17 (1923): 230–31.

26. Curtice Rosser, "Rectal Pathology in the Negro," *Journal of the American Medical Association* 84 (1926): 93.

27. An illuminating discussion of this disease discourse in Atlanta, Georgia, is Tera Hunter, chapter 1 of *To "Joy My Freedom": Southern Black Women's Lives and Labors after the Civil War* (Cambridge: Harvard University Press, forthcoming). See also David McBride, *From TB to AIDS: Epidemics among Urban Blacks since 1900* (Albany: State University of New York Press, 1991); James Jones, *Bad Blood: The Tuskegee Syphilis Experiments* (New York: Free Press, 1981); John Haller, *Outcasts from Evolution*; Frederickson, *Black Image in the White Mind*; Grossman, *Land of Hope*; Higham, *Strangers in the Land*.

28. C. Jeff Miller, "Special Problems of the Colored Woman," *Southern Medical Journal* 25 (1932): 734. For an even more visceral statement of the "Negro problem," see also Marvin Graves, "The Negro as a Menace to the White Race," *Southern Medical Journal* 9 (1916): 407–13.

29. In the early twentieth century, many physicians used this assumption (as many had in the previous century) to sanction what historian John Haller called an "ideology of separation and disenfranchisement." John S. Haller, "The Physician versus the Negro: Medical and Anthropological Concepts of Race in the Late Nineteenth Century," *Bulletin for the History of Medicine* 44 (1970): 154–67.

30. See George Dock and C. C. Bass, *Hookworm Disease* (St. Louis: C.V. Mosby, 1910), and John Ettling, *The Germ of Laziness: Rockefeller Philanthropy and Public Health in the New South* (Cambridge: Harvard University Press, 1981).

31. As late as 1931, one of the leaders of attempts to eradicate the hookworm from the South recalled this economic feature of disease: "Any 'old timer' in hookworm work is a firm believer in the doctrine that this disease is an important factor in the backwardness of certain children in their school work." C. W. Stiles, "Hookworm Disease in Certain Parts of the South: A New Plan of Attack," *Southern Medical Journal* 25 (1931): 191. Other Southern physicians called hook-

worm an "economic disease monstrosity." J. H. Musser and Willard Wirth, "Anemia in the South," *Annals of Clinical Medicine* 5 (1927): 861–64.

32. W. G. Smillie and D. L. Augustine, "Vital Capacity of the Negro Race," *Journal of the American Medical Association* 87 (1926): 2055–58.

33. The problem of institutionally induced anemias provided a focal point for many discussions of social reform. See, for example, Lewis Terman, "The Effects of School Life upon the Nutritive Processes, Health, and the Composition of the Blood," *Popular Science Monthly* 84 (1914): 257. Terman cites several authors who argue that "the underlying cause of school anemia . . . is to be sought in the influence of excessive accumulations of toxic products of fatigue" (p. 259). See also C. W. Stiles, "Is the So-Called 'Cotton Mill Anemia' of the Gulf-Atlantic States due to Lint or to Hookworms?" *Southern Medical Journal* 4 (1911): 508–13; Maxwell Wintrobe and M. W. Miller, "Normal Blood Determinations in the South," *Archives of Internal Medicine* 43 (1929): 96; and J. H. Musser and W. R. Wirth, "Anemia in the South," *Annals of Clinical Medicine* 5 (1927): 861.

34. C. W. Stiles, "Hookworm Disease in Its Relation to the Negro," *Southern Medical Journal* 2 (1909): 1125–26. For more on Stiles and hookworm, see Ettling, *Germ of Laziness*. See also James Cassedy, "The Germ of Laziness in the South, 1900–1915: Charles Wardell Stiles and the Progressive Paradox," *Bulletin of the History of Medicine* 45 (1971): 159–69; William Bowers, "Country Life Reform: A Neglected Aspect of Progressive Era History," *Agricultural History* 45 (1971): 211–21; and Alan Marcus, "The South's Native Foreigner: Hookworm as a Factor in Southern Distinctiveness," in *Disease and Distinctiveness in the American South*, ed. Todd Savitt and James Harvey Young (Knoxville: University of Tennessee Press, 1988).

35. Stiles, "Hookworm in Relation to the Negro," 1126.

36. V. Sydenstricker, "Sickle Cell Anemia," *Southern Medical Journal* 17 (1924): 177–83. W. A. Mulherin quoted from p. 182–83.

37. Earl Browne, "Sickle Cell Anemia," *Medical Clinics of North America* 9 (1926): 1191–97. Quotation on p. 1192.

38. Horace Anderson, "Sickle Cell Anemia," *American Journal of Medical Science* 171 (1926): 641–48. See also A. R. Moser and W. J. Shaw, "Sickle Cell Anemia in a Northern Negro," *Journal of the American Medical Association* 84 (1925): 507.

39. Stanley Reiser, *Medicine and the Reign of Technology* (New York: Cambridge University Press, 1978).

40. Jerome Cook and Jerome Meyer, "Severe Anemia with Sickle Shaped and Elongated," *Archives of Internal Medicine* 16 (1915): 644–51; R. E. Washburn, "Peculiar and Elongated Sickle-shaped Red Blood Corpuscles in a Case of Severe Anemia," *Virginia Medical Semi-monthly* 15 (1911): 490–93.

41. Emmel, "A Study of the Erythrocytes in a Case of Severe Anemia with Elongated Sickle-shaped Red Blood Corpuscles," *Archives of Internal Medicine* 20 (1917): 592.

42. Ibid., 594.

43. Ibid. For a full discussion of Emmel's work, see Keith Wailoo, "'A Disease *Sui Generis'*: The Origins of Sickle Cell Anemia and the Emergence of Modern Clinical Research, 1904–1924," *Bulletin of the History of Medicine* 65 (1991): 185–208.

44. The total number of reported cases of sickle cell anemia during this period is quite small, approximately one hundred case reports in the American medical literature from 1920 to 1940. But the pattern of defining sickle cell anemia as a "potential disease" was evident everywhere. Two representative articles from the 1920s are S. Jamison, "Sickle Cell Anemia, a Case Report," *Southern Medical Journal* 18 (1925): 795, and J. Levy, "The Origin and Fate of Sickle-shaped Red Blood Cells," *Archives of Pathology* 7 (1929): 820.

45. Physicians chose to think of the sicklemia condition as a latent disease phase, rather than as a benign condition. Cooley and Lee, "The Sickle Cell Phenomenon."

46. V. P. Sydenstricker, "Sickle Cell Anemia," *Southern Medical Journal* 17 (1924): 177; idem, "Further Observations on Sickle Cell Anemia," *Journal of the American Medical Association* 83 (1924): 12. Mason's hypothesis was put forth in his 1922 article: "It is of particular interest that up to the present the malady has been seen only in the Negro, and so far as could be ascertained, it is the only disease peculiar to that race." Verne Mason, "Sickle Cell Anemia," *Journal of the American Medical Association* 79 (1922): 1318–19.

47. For more on the 1920s and physical anthropology, see George Stocking, "The Scientific Reaction against Cultural Anthropology, 1917–1920," in his *Race, Culture, and Evolution: Essays in the History of Anthropology* (New York: Free Press, 1968).

48. John Huck, "Sickle Cell Anemia," *Bulletin of the Johns Hopkins Hospital* 34 (1923): 335–44; see also Taliaferro and Huck, "Inheritance of Sickle Cell Anemia," 598.

49. Huck's work followed the noted work of Archibald Garrod who, in the first decade of the century, had demonstrated the Mendelian nature of such diseases as alkaptonuria. See Archibald E. Garrod, "The Croonian Lectures on Inborn Errors of Metabolism," *Lancet* 2 (1908): 1–7, 73–79, 142–48, 214–20. Quotation from Taliaferro and Huck, "Inheritance of Sickle Cell Anemia," 597.

50. See chapters 3 and 4 of this book. The career of Florence Sabin at the Rockefeller Institute also exemplifies this trend. See George Corner, *A History of the Rockefeller Institute for Medical Research, 1901–1953: Origins and Growth* (New York: Rockefeller Institute Press, 1964).

51. Peter Bowler, *The Mendelian Revolution: The Emergence of Hereditarian Concepts in Modern Science and Society* (Baltimore: Johns Hopkins University Press, 1989), 158. For a useful primary source on eugenics and the uses of hereditary knowledge, see Ellsworth Huntington, *Tomorrow's Children: The Goals of Eugenics* (New York: Wiley, 1935).

52. Kevles, *In the Name of Eugenics.*

53. Cooley and Lee, "The Sickle Cell Phenomenon," 340; see also Cooley and Lee, "Observations of the Sickle Cell Phenomenon," 58–59.

54. For a few observes, the "latency" of most cases was reassuring. Edward Steinfeld and Joseph Klauder, "Sickle Cell Anemia," *Medical Clinics of North America* 10 (1927): 1563. For others, the relationship between the trait and the latent disease was simply puzzling. See Francis Wood, ed., *A Textbook of Pathology*, 14th ed. revised of F. Delafield and T. M. Prudden, *A Textbook of Pathology* (New York: Wood, 1927).

55. G. M. Brandau, "Incidence of Sickle-Cell Trait in Industrial Workers," *American Journal of Medical Science* 180 (1930): 814–15.

56. It was not uncommon to select workers for tasks on the basis of their race. Different races possessed different susceptibilities and immunities to chemical exposure, fatigue, and infections. In her *Industrial Poisons in the United States* (New York: Macmillan, 1925), for example, Alice Hamilton included a section on race, in which she noted: "In making of dye intermediates and coal tar dyes it is said to be desirable to employ Negroes in the preparation and handling of such substances as paranitralin and dinitrochlorobenzene because they are not subject to the distressing dermatoses from which white men suffer when they do work of this sort" (p. 6).

57. G. S. Graham and S. H. McCarty, "Sickle Cell (Meniscocytic) Anemia," *Southern Medical Journal* 23 (1930): 598–607; H. Weiner, "Sickle Cell Anemia in Italian Child," *Journal of Mount Sinai Hospital* 4 (1937): 88–91. Weiner noted that, "although all authors have emphasized the fact, it is not generally appreciated that a wet preparation should be observed for twenty four hours before being sure that the case is not sickle cell anemia."

58. See Swazey and Reeds, *Today's Medicine, Tomorrow's Science*, 79. For more on the relationship between latent and active disease, see I. J. Sherman, "The Sickling Phenomenon—Anemia vs. Trait," *Bulletin of the Johns Hopkins Hospital* 67 (1940): 309.

59. In the 1920s, the "one-drop rule" came to define an individual as Negro. For more on this definition of race according to "blood," see Joel Williamson, *New People: Miscegenation and Mulattoes in the United States* (New York: Free Press, 1980); F. James Davis, *Who Is Black?*; and also Lawrence Wright, "One Drop of Blood," *New Yorker* 70 (1994): 46–55.

60. One of the few exceptions to this was E. Vernon Hahn and Elizabeth Gillespie, "Sickle Cell Anemia: Report of a Case Greatly Improved by Splenectomy, Experimental Study of Sickle Cell Formation," *Archives of Internal Medicine* 39 (1927): 233–54.

61. These cases made up a minority of the total cases reported, but cases of sickle cell anemia in white patients served an important role in rationalizing the disease as a Negro disease. See, for example, F. Clarke, "Sickle Cell Anemia in the

White Race with Report of Two Cases," *Nebraska Medical Journal* 18 (1923): 376–79; W. P. Sights and S. D. Simon, "Marked Erythrocytic Sickling in White Adult, Associated with Anemia, Syphilis, and Malaria, Case" *Journal of Medicine* 12 (June 1931): 177–78; J. Cooke and J. Mack, "Sickle Cell Anemia in a White American Family," *Journal of Pediatrics* 5 (1934): 601; R. G. Archibald, "Sickle Cell Anemia in the Sudan," *Transactions of the Royal Society for Tropical Medicine and Hygiene* 19 (1926): 389; S. Moore, "The Bone Changes in Sickle Cell Anemia with a Note on Similar Changes Observed in Skulls of Ancient Mayan Indians," *Journal of the Missouri Medical Association* 26 (1929): 561; W. B. Stewart, "Sickle Cell Anemia: Report of a Case with Splenectomy," *American Journal for the Diseases of Children* 34 (July 1927): 72–80; S. Rosenfeld and J. Pincus, "The Occurrence of Sicklemia in the White Race," *American Journal of Medical Science* 184 (1932): 674–82; Thomas Cooley and Pearl Lee, "Sickle Cell Anemia in a Greek Family," *American Journal for the Disease of Children* 38 (July 1929): 103–6; J. S. Lawrence, "Human Elliptical Erythrocytes," *American Journal of Medical Science* 181 (1931): 240; J. S. Lawrence, "Elliptical and Sickle-shaped Erythrocytes in the Circulating Blood of White Persons," *Journal of Clinical Investigation* 5 (1927): 31; Haden and Evans, "Sickle Cell Anemia in the White Race"; L. Pollock and W. Dameshek, "Elongation of the Red Blood Cells in a Jewish Family," *American Journal of Medical Science* (1935): 822–34.

For literature in later decades, see also "Sickle Cells in Whites," *Scientific American* 185 (August 1951): 58; Louis Greenwald and John Burrett, "Sickle Cell Anemia in a White Family," *American Journal of Medical Science* 199 (1940): 768; R. A. Guyton and R. W. Heinle, "Sickle Cell Anemia in the White Race," *American Journal of Medical Science* 220 (1950): 272; John Hodges, "The Effect of Racial Mixtures upon Erythrocytic Sickling," *Blood* 5 (1950): 805–10; Weiner, "Sickle Cell Anemia in Italian Child."

62. Blood provided a key symbol for framing and legitimating such cultural anxieties about interracial mixing. Joel Williamson has argued that "it is not too much to say that Southern whites in the early twentieth century became paranoid about invisible blackness. In their minds blood, not environment, carried civilization and one wrong drop meant contamination of the whole." Williamson, *New People*, 103.

63. Cooley and Lee, "Sickle Cell Anemia in a Greek Family," 106. And see Cooley and Lee, "Series of Cases of Splenomegaly in Children with Anemia and Peculiar Bone Changes," *Transactions of the American Pediatric Society* 37 (1925): 37.

64. John Lawrence, "Elliptical and Sickle-shaped Erythrocytes in the Circulating Blood of White Persons," *Journal of Clinical Investigation* 5 (December 1927): 31–49. Quotation on p. 44.

65. Ibid., 46.

66. "It seems reasonable," Lawrence wrote, "to assume there may be some relationship between two conditions [elliptical erythrocytes and sickle cells] which have so many points in common." J. S. Lawrence, "Human Elliptical Erythro-

cytes," *American Journal of Medical Science* 181 (1931): 240.

67. Sights and Simon, "Marked Erythrocytic Sickling in a White Adult," 177–78.

68. Rosenfeld and Pincus, "Sicklemia in the White Race," 682.

69. Ibid., 675.

70. In a case documented by Weiner in 1937, "both [the parents] appear to be normal, healthy white adults, with no Negro features . . . [As they were from Mistretta, Italy] they say that Negroes were unknown in this town and were only seen with the circus. The parents are certain that there is no Negro blood in the family." Weiner, "Sickle Cell Anemia in Italian Child," 88.

71. Ibid., 91. See also "Sickle Cell Anemia: A Race Specific Disease," *Journal of the American Medical Association* 133 (1947): 34, and Rosenfeld and Pincus, "Sicklemia in the White Race," 674.

72. A. Ogden, "Sickle Cell Anemia in the White Race, with Report of Cases in 2 Families," *Archives of Internal Medicine* 71 (1943): 164.

73. See discussion of the Moorish origins of sickled cells in C. S. Sturgis, *Hematology* (Springfield, Ill.: Charles S Thomas, 1948), 330; see also Greenwald and Burrett, "Sickle Cell Anemia in a White Family."

74. Two Dallas physicians claimed to have found a case of sicklemia in a Mexican patient that could not be explained by admixture with Negro blood. They suggested that "perhaps the wide prevalence of sickle cell anemia of the blood played a part in the downfall of Mayan civilizations" (p. 1215). S. A. Wallace and W. P. Killingsworth, "Sicklemia in the Mexican Race," *American Journal of the Diseases of Children* 50 (1935): 1208.

75. For a historical overview of population genetics, physical anthropology, and disease ideology in this era, see Kenneth M. Weiss and Ranajit Chakraborty, "Genes, Populations, and Disease: 1930–1980: A Problem-oriented Review," in *A History of American Physical Anthropology: 1930–1980*, ed. Frank Spencer (New York: Academic Press, 1982).

76. Segregation policies were, of course, among the prominent issues that emerged in American race relations—segregation in federally run institutions (military and hospitals), segregation of the civilian blood supply, and segregation in other aspects of social life. See, for example, William J. Wilson, "Competitive Race Relations and the Proliferation of Racial Protests: 1940–1980," in *Power, Racism, and Privilege*, ed. William Julius Wilson (New York: Free Press, 1973).

77. Bauer also pointed out that "it has been demanded that all Negro patients in both medical and surgical services be tested routinely for sicklemia." Julius Bauer and Louis Fisher, "Sickle Cell Disease, with Special Regard to Its Nonanemic Variety," *Archives of Surgery* 47 (1943): 553–63; see also J. Bauer, "Sickle Cell Disease," *Archives of Surgery* 41 (1940): 1344.

78. Bauer, "Sickle Cell Disease," 544.

79. Bauer stridently claimed that "it is to be expected that not infrequently this

abnormal gene is only one among many other pathological genes; in other words, that sicklemia is one of numerous constitutional deviations of a person from the normal average . . . [and] that the well defined genopathy predisposing to sickle cell disease may be indicative of farther reaching chromosomal abnormalities known as status degenerativus." Ibid., 558.

80. Julian Herman Lewis, *The Biology of the Negro* (Chicago: University of Chicago Press, 1942), 233.

81. Ogden, "Sickle Cell Anemia in the White Race," 164.

82. "Once we are able to write about the racial behavior of disease without undue emotional influences and to scientifically consider it as a natural phenomenon, Negro physicians will be able to make momentous contributions to what has been called anthropathology (comparative racial pathology) . . . Particularly challenging to Negro physicians is sickle cell anemia . . . Fame and distinction await the man who can solve the problem of this malady." "Editorial: Race and Disease," *Journal of the National Medical Association* 40 (1948): 259.

83. "Sickle Cell Anemia, a Race Specific Disease," *Journal of the American Medical Association* 133 (1947): 33–34.

84. Ibid., 34. Extreme views on miscegenation and race mixing also appeared in the writings of some South African researchers and in explicitly eugenic publications. See, for example, A. B. Raper, "Sickle Cell Disease in Africa and America—a Comparison," *Journal of Tropical Medicine* 53 (1950): 49–53. In 1940, Greenwald and Burrett wondered about a "greater likelihood of the admixture of Negroid blood in geographical locations, where inbreeding is obviously quite common." Greenwald and Burrett, "Sickle Cell Anemia in a White Family," 769. See also John Hodges, "The Effect of Racial Mixtures upon Erythrocytic Sickling," *Blood* 5 (1950): 805–10. Hodges noted that "an attempt was made to arrive at a conclusion as to the purity or degree of racial admixture of Negroes and to determine the incidence of sickling in relation to racial admixture" (p. 805). He concluded that "the incidence of erythrocytic sickling is less in 'pure' Negroes than in those with small admixtures of white and American Indian ancestry" (p. 810). Such studies underline the continuing interest in determining the relation of the disease to the purity of the racial group.

85. Montague Cobb, review of Lewis's *Biology of the Negro*, in *Crisis* 49 (1942): 394. See also C. G. Woodson's review in *Journal of Negro History* 27 (1943): 359–61.

86. See Roy Kracke, *Diseases of the Blood and Atlas of Hematology* (Philadelphia: Lippincott, 1941), 331; see also W. P. Killingsworth and S. A. Wallace, "Sicklemia in the Southwest," *Southern Medical Journal* 29 (1936): 941.

87. Cooley, who had worked on sickle cell anemia for decades, raised the question: "Is there such a thing as a race-limited disease? My opinion is that there is no such thing." Thomas Cooley, "Hereditary Factors in the Blood Dyscrasias (President's Address)," *American Journal of the Diseases of Children* 62 (July 1941): 1–7. Cooley suggested that, "when a disease-producing mutation takes place, it

is evident that it will recur first in the neighborhood of its origin . . . In view of the present knowledge about the repeated appearance of mutations, it is only common sense to explain such occurrences as new appearances of the mutations, which may, of course, set up new foci of the disease."

88. "'Aryan' Blood Demand Handicaps Nazi Wounded," *New York Times*, 1 March 1942).

89. "Blood and Prejudice—Segregation of White and Negro Donations Brings a Protest," *New York Times*, 14 June 1942. The debate over Red Cross policy continued for some years. See "Red Cross Plans Big Blood Supply—New Program for Country Stirs Row over Supply from Various Races," *New York Times*, 10 July 1947). For a brief discussion of this issue from the perspective of the late 1950s, see Charles Hurd, *The Compact History of the American Red Cross* (New York: Hawthorn Books, 1959), 419–23. As late as 1959, a physician (Lydia Allen DeVilbiss) called for mandatory testing of Negroes seeking to marry and for control of the blood supply because of her concern about sickle cell anemia: "Premarital tests for sickled cells and the inherited trait would be of value in preventing sickle cell anemia in future generations . . . [She also emphasized that] the use of Negro blood in transfusions with white patients can result in unpleasant reactions." Lydia Allen DeVilbiss, "Sickle Cell Anemia," *American Mercury* 89 (1959): 130.

90. For more on the scholarship of anthropologists like Margaret Mead, Melville Herskovits, and others, see George Stocking, "The Scientific Reaction against Cultural Anthropology, 1917–1920," in his *Race, Culture, and Evolution.* See, for example, Margaret Mead, Theodosius Dobzhansky, et al., eds., *Science and the Concept of Race* (New York: Columbia University Press, 1968). By the early 1950s, biologists had begun using data on the biological diversity of the gene pool to argue that the notion of a Negro race in America was scientifically problematic. See, for example, B. Glass and C. C. Li, "The Dynamics of Racial Mixture: An Analysis Based on the American Negro," *American Journal of Human Genetics* 5 (1953): 1–20. They argued that the "gene pool of the North American Negro (socially defined) is now approximately 30 percent derived from white ancestry."

91. Gunnar Myrdal, *An American Dilemma*, vol. 1, *The Negro in a White Nation* (New York: McGraw-Hill Paperback Ed., 1964), 100.

92. Ibid. Myrdal was certainly not alone in pointing to the fallacies of racial thinking in America. Much of his discussion in this section was drawn from Lewis's *Biology of the Negro*, from the work of C. Montague Cobb, and from critical works of Herskovits and others in cultural and physical anthropology.

93. Bernard Seeman, *The River of Life: The Story of Man's Blood from Magic to Science* (New York: W.W. Norton, 1961), 12.

94. To some, *race* seemed a meaningless explanation for the disease. By the early 1940s, some physicians were ready to admit that the disease might have an existence independent of the Negro race. One Boston physician noted in 1941 that "the occurrence of sickle cell anemia in white persons has been reviewed recent-

ly, with the report of 13 cases occurring in persons from Mediterranean countries, especially Italy. This patient was Italian." Tracy B. Mallory, ed., "Case Records of the Massachusetts General Hospital: Case No. 27421," *New England Journal of Medicine* (1941): 626–30.

95. See Sturgis, *Hematology*. See also J. Holmes Smith, Jr., "Sickle Cell Anemia," *Medical Clinics of North America* 11 (1928): 1171–90; Earl Browne, "Sickle Cell Anemia," *Medical Clinics of North America* 9 (1926): 1191–97; and E. W. Page and M. Z. Silton, "Pregnancy Complicated by Sickle Cell Anemia," *American Journal of Obstetrics and Gynecology* 37 (1939): 53.

96. As late as 1938, some writers called "attention to the fact that patients with sickle cell anemia present evidence of acute abdominal disease, which may be confused with acute cholecystitis, acute appendicitis, acute salpingitis, peptic ulcer, and splenic infarcts." E. H. Campbell in "Acute Abdominal Pain in Sickle Cell Anemia," *Archives of Surgery* 31 (1935): 607, cited by A. Oschner and S. Murray, "Pitfalls in the Diagnosis of Acute Abdominal Conditions," *American Journal of Surgery* 41 (1938): 343–69.

97. W. B. Stewart, "Sickle Cell Anemia: Report of a Case with Splenectomy"; Hahn and Gillespie, "Sickle Cell Anemia"; V. P. Sydenstricker, "Sickle Cell Anemia," *Medical Clinics of North America* 12 (1929): 1451–57; Haden and Evans, "Sickle Cell Anemia in the White Race." For a discussion of the prevalence of splenectomy in sickle cell anemia, see Mark Ravitch, *A Century of Surgery, 1880–1980: The History of the American Surgical Association* (Philadelphia: Lippincott, 1981), 662. See also A. J. Bell, R. H. Cotte, and A. G. Mitchell, "Sickle Cell Anemia: Report of a Case in Which Splenectomy Was Performed," *Medical Bulletin of the University of Cincinnati* 5 (1928): 21–24; K. F. Bolard, "Discussion—Surgery of the Spleen," *Annals of Surgery* 88 (1928): 439–40; R. H. Jaffe and L. R. Hill, "Splenic Mycosis," *Archives of Pathology* 6 (1928): 196–209; M. Wollstein and K. V. Kriedel, "Sickle Cell Anemia," *American Journal of the Diseases of Children* 36 (1928): 998–1011; A. R. Rich, "Splenic Lesion in Sickle Cell Anemia," *Bulletin of the Johns Hopkins Hospital* 43 (1928): 398–99; W. D. Haggard, "Discussion—Surgery of the Spleen," *Annals of Surgery* 88 (1928): 440–41. On rheumatic fever, Max Wintrobe wrote in 1946: "It is sometimes impossible to distinguish sickle cell anemia from acute rheumatic fever, or its cardiac manifestations from those of rheumatic heart disease." Maxwell Wintrobe, "The Cardiovascular System in Anemia with a Note on the Particular Abnormalities in Sickle Cell Anemia," *Blood* 1 (1946): 127.

98. Yater and Mollari, "Pathology of Sickle Cell Anemia"; Louis Hamman, "Clinico-pathological Conference: I. A Case of Severe Anemia with Cardiac Manifestations; II. A Case of Obscure Infection," *Southern Medical Journal* 26 (1933): 666–68.

99. T. Winsor and G. Burch, "Sickle Cell Anemia: A Great Masquerader," *Journal of the American Medical Association* 129 (1946): 793–96. These authors suggested two new diagnostic techniques—a tourniquet test and a carbon dioxide test—

which resulted, they claimed, in "an unexpected discovery of 27 patients with active sickle cell anemia . . . Needless to say many clinical difficulties, errors in diagnosis and unnecessary special laboratory procedures were avoided" (p. 795). Even Bauer and Fisher found that "in many of the patients the disease was either subtle or strongly suggested clinical syndromes other then sickle cell anemia." Bauer and Fisher, "Sickle Cell Disease," 553.

100. As one pathologist later noted, some pediatricians "wouldn't even accept the diagnosis—a professor of pediatrics said [of one sickle cell patient] 'Why he's got rheumatic fever.'" Interview with Lemuel Diggs, Cordova, Tenn., 14 April 1993. Diggs also confirmed that surgeons often diagnosed appendicitis in these cases.

101. One author wrote, "It behooves us to study carefully the blood of young Negro patients for evidence of sickle cell anemia before subjecting them to surgical operation for the relief of abdominal pain." James Paullin in the discussion following James P. Baker, "Sickle Cell Anemia," *Virginia Medical Monthly* 69 (1942): 212.

102. One author predicted that "sickle cell anemia will become a common diagnosis when clinicians become more sickle cell anemia minded . . . and make moist preparations routine." Lemuel Diggs, "The Blood Picture in Sickle Cell Anemia," *Southern Medical Journal* 25 (1932): 619.

103. Steinfeld and Klauder, "Sickle Cell Anemia," 1566.

104. Frank Bethell, Cyrus Sturgis, Robert Hettig, and Otto Mallery, "Progress in Internal Medicine: Blood—a Review of Recent Literature," *Archives of Internal Medicine* (1942): 902; see also J. H. Connell, "Cerebral Necrosis in Sickle Cell Disease," *Journal of the American Medical Association* 118 (1942): 893.

105. There had always been cases of sickled cells in the context of other illnesses, such as pneumonia. Hugh Josephs, "The Johns Hopkins Medical Research Club—Clinical Aspects of Sickle Cell Anemia," *Bulletin of the Johns Hopkins Hospital* 43 (December 1928): 197–98.

106. Discussion by Cooley in Anderson, "Sickle Cell Anemia," *Journal of the American Medical Association* 99 (1932): 905.

107. Sydney Halpern, *American Pediatrics: The Social Dynamics of Professionalism, 1880–1980* (Berkeley: University of California Press: 1988), 96.

108. Cooley in Anderson, "Sickle Cell Anemia."

109. Among the authors writing on sickle cell anemia who were pediatricians were Cooley, Stewart, Cooke, Mack, Wallace, and Killingsworth. For more on pediatrics and child health in the 1920s, see Richard Meckel, *Save the Babies: American Public Health Reform and the Prevention of Infant Mortality, 1850–1929* (Baltimore: Johns Hopkins University Press, 1990).

110. Lemuel Diggs, C. Ahmann, and J. Bibb, "The Incidence and Significance of Sickle Cell Trait," *Annals of Internal Medicine* 7 (1935): 769–78. Quotation from

Diggs, "The Blood Picture" (1932), 615. See also Lemuel Diggs and Juanita Bibb, "The Erythrocyte in Sickle Cell Anemia," *Journal of the American Medical Association* 112 (1939): 695.

111. Diggs, "The Blood Picture," 615.

112. Lemuel Diggs, "The Sickle Cell Crisis," *American Journal of Clinical Pathology* 26 (1956): 1109–18; idem, "Treatment of the Sickle Cell Crisis," *Southern Medical Journal* 56 (1963): 472–74; Wallace Yater and Mario Mollari, "Sickle Cell Crisis" *Journal of the American Medical Association* 96 (1931): 1671–75; Frank Leivy and Truman Schnabel, "Abdomen Crises," *American Journal of Medical Science* 183 (1932): 381–89; Edward Torrance and Truman Schnabel, "Potassium Sulphocyanate: A Note on Its Use for the Painful Crises in Sickle Cell Anemia," *Annals of Internal Medicine* 6 (1932): 782–88.

113. Moses J. Newsom, "Malady Afflicts Race," *Memphis Commercial Appeal*, 1962, Folder: "Sickle Cell Anemia," Newspaper Collection, Memphis and Shelby County Public Library.

114. "Grant Renewed to Trace Strange Malady's Secret—Herff Foundation Will Again Help U-T Seek Facts of Sickle Cell Anemia," *Memphis Press-Scimitar*, May 1954, folder: "Herff Foundation" (Newspaper Collection, Memphis and Shelby County Public Library).

115. Sturgis, *Hematology*, 330.

116. Bowler, *Mendelian Revolution*, 167.

117. Thoughtful discussions of the rise of molecular biology include Garland Allen, *The Life Sciences in the Twentieth Century* (Cambridge: Cambridge University Press, 1978); John Servos, *Physical Chemistry from Ostwald to Pauling: The Making of a Science in America* (Princeton: Princeton University Press, 1990); Lily Kay, *The Molecular Vision of Life: Caltech, the Rockefeller Foundation, and the Rise of the New Biology* (New York: Oxford University Press, 1993); Jan Sapp, *Where the Truth Lies: Franz Moewus and the Origins of Molecular Biology* (Cambridge: Cambridge University Press, 1990); Robert Olby, *The Path to the Double Helix* (Seattle: University of Washington Press, 1974).

118. Linus Pauling, "The Normal Hemoglobins and the Hemoglobinopathies: Background," in "Hemoglobins and Hemoglobinopathies: A Review to 1931," ed. Rose Schneider, Samuel Charache, and Walter Schroeder, *Texas Reports on Biology and Medicine* 40 (1980–1981): 4.

119. Ibid., 5.

120. Ibid.

121. In the medical writings of this period, very little information on the personal or experiential aspect of the disease had emerged, except through commentaries on the patient's ability to work.

122. Following on the heels of the anthropologists, Switzer studied the converse problem: sickle cell anemia in the more isolated and "homogeneous" group

of Negroes on the Sea Islands in South Carolina. P. Switzer, "The Incidence of Sickle Cell Trait in Negroes from the Sea Island Area of South Carolina," *Southern Medical Journal* 43 (1950): 48–49.

123. See R. Isaacs, "Sickling: A Property of All Red Blood Cells," *Science* 112 (1950): 716–18.

124. According to Neel's revision of the Mendelian dominant argument, "Taliaferro and Huck suggested that a single dominant gene was involved, but the distinction between sicklemia and sickle cell anemia was not clearly understood at the time." Neel, "Inheritance of Sickle Cell Anemia," 64–66. See also Linus Pauling, Harvey Itano, S. J. Singer, and Ibert Wells, "Sickle Cell Anemia, a Molecular Disease," *Science* 110 (1949): 543–48.

125. L. S. Penrose, *Outline of Human Genetics* (New York: Wiley, 1959), 39.

126. Ibid.

127. Amoz Chernoff, "On the Prevalence of Hemoglobin D in the American Negro," *Blood* 10 (1956): 907–9. See also William Denny, Thomas Finn, and Robert Bird, "Clinical Diagnosis of Sickle-C Disease," *Archives of Internal Medicine* 99 (1957): 214–17; R. Myerson, E. Harrison, and H. Lohmuller, "Incidence and Significance of Abnormal Hemoglobins: Reports of a Series of 1,000 Hospitalized Negro Veterans," *American Journal of Medicine* 26 (1959): 543–46. These authors determined that 10.6 percent of 1,000 hospitalized Negroes had the "abnormal hemoglobins."

128. A. Atamer, "Hereditary Hemoglobinopathies," in *Blood Disease* (New York: Grune and Stratton, 1963), 175.

129. "Sickle Cells in Whites," *Scientific American* 185 (August 1951): 58, reported a case (reported in *Nature* by F. Dreyfuss and M. Benyesch of Jerusalem) in which patients "neither bear any resemblance to Negroes nor is heavy admixture of Negro blood at all probable." Conversely, some cases of thalassemia in Negroes emerged. O. Banks and R. Scott, "Thalassemia in Negroes: A Report of a Case of Cooley's Anemia in a Negro Child," *Pediatrics* 6 (1953): 622–27.

130. Harvey Itano, "Clinical States Associated with Alterations of the Hemoglobin Molecule," *Archives of Internal Medicine* 97 (1955): 136.

131. Quotation from John Moseley and John Manly, "Sickle Cell Disease: An Analysis of Recent Advances," *Journal of the National Medical Association* 46 (1954): 181. For examples of the new era, see E. W. Smith and C. L. Conley, "Clinical Features of the Genetic Variants of Sickle Cell Disease," *Bulletin of the Johns Hopkins Hospital* 94 (1954): 289; E. D. Thomas, A. G. Motulsky, and D. H. Walters, "Homozygous Hemoglobin C Disease," *American Journal of Medicine* 18 (1955): 832; Myerson et al., "Incidence and Significance of Abnormal Hemoglobin"; P. A. Galbraith and P. T. Green, "Hemoglobin C Disease in an Anglo Saxon Family," *American Journal of Medicine* 28 (1960): 969; Edward Hook and Gerald Cooper, "The Clinical Manifestations of Sickle Cell-Hemoglobin C Disease and Sickle Cell Anemia," *Southern Medical Journal* 51 (1958): 610; G. M. Eddington and H. Lehmann,

"Distribution of Hemoglobin C in West Africa," *Man* 36 (1956): 1.

132. Kenneth Walker, *The Story of Blood* (London: Herbert Jenkins, 1958), 28.

133. Owsei Temkin, "The Scientific Approach to Disease: Specific Entity and Individual Sickness," in *The Double Face of Janus*, 444–45.

134. Isaacs, "Sickling: A Property of All Red Blood Cells"; M. Murayama, "Molecular Mechanism of Red Cell 'Sickling,'" *Science* 153 (1966): 145–49; R. Bookchin, R. Davis, and H. Ranney, "Clinical Features of Hemoglobin C-Harlem, A New Sickling Hemoglobin Variant," *Annals of Internal Medicine* 68 (1968): 8–18; Rose Schneider, Jack Alperin, and Hermann Lehmann, "Sickling Tests: Pitfalls in Performance and Interpretation," *Journal of the American Medical Association* 202 (1967): 119 21.

135. Michael Michaelson, "Sickle Cell Anemia: An Interesting Pathology," *Ramparts* (October 1971): 52–58.

136. Schneider et al., "Sickling Tests," 119. "The diagnosis of sc disease cannot be established by means of the sickling test alone, but must be substantiated by electrophoretic and genetic data" (p. 119).

137. J. V. Neel, "Inheritance of the Sickling Phenomenon; with Special Reference to Sickle Cell Disease," *Blood* 6 (1951): 389.

138. Linus Pauling, *Molecular Architecture and the Processes of Life: The Twenty-First Sir Jesse Boot Foundation Lecture* (Nottingham: Sir Jesse Boot Foundation, 1949), 1, 12–13.

139. "The results indicate that a significant difference exists between the electrophoretic mobilities of hemoglobin derived from the erythrocytes of normal individuals and from those of sickle cell anemia individuals." Ibid., 54.

140. George Gray, "Sickle Cell Anemia," *Scientific American* 185 (August 1951): 56–59. Quotation on p. 59.

141. The proliferation of electrophoresis facilitated the diagnosis of abnormal hemoglobins—and contributed to the reductionist notion of a "hemoglobinopathy" (a pathology rooted in the hemoglobin). See H. Itano, "Human Hemoglobin," *Science* 117 (1953): 89; F. Livingstone, *Abnormal Hemoglobins in Human Populations: A Summary and Interpretation* (Chicago: Aldine Press, 1967).

142. On sickle cell anemia as the first "molecular disease," see Linus Pauling, Harvey Itano, S. J. Singer, and Ibert Wells, "Sickle Cell Anemia, a Molecular Disease," *Science* 110 (1949): 543–48; Gray, "Sickle Cell Anemia." See also C. Lockhard Conley, "Sickle Cell Anemia: The First Molecular Disease."

143. L. C. Dunn, *Heredity and Evolution in Human Populations* (Cambridge: Harvard University Press, 1959), 58.

144. A. C. Allison, "Protection Afforded by Sickle-Cell Trait against Subtertian Malarial Infection," *British Medical Journal* 1 (1954): 290–94.

145. See "Helpful Defects," *Scientific American* 190 (April 1974): 52.

146. William Levin, "Editorial: 'Asymptomatic' Sickle Cell Trait," *Blood* 13 (1958): 904–7. Quotation on pp. 905–6.

147. Ibid., 906.

148. See R. M. Nalbandian, ed., *Molecular Aspects of Sickle-Cell Hemoglobin: Clinical Applications* (Springfield, Ill.: Charles C Thomas, 1971).

149. S. Charache, "The Treatment of Sickle Cell Anemia," *Archives of Internal Medicine* 133 (1974): 698–705; Orah Platt, "Is There a Treatment for Sickle Cell Anemia?" *New England Journal of Medicine* 319 (1988): 1479–80.

150. Suggestive discussions of narrative and its relation to medicine and history include Kathryn Montgomery Hunter, *Doctors' Stories: The Narrative Structure of Medical Knowledge* (Princeton: Princeton University Press, 1991); Arthur Kleinman, *The Illness Narratives: Suffering, Healing and the Human Condition* (New York: Basic Books, 1988); see also Howard Brody, *Stories of Sickness* (New Haven: Yale University Press, 1987), and Hayden White, *The Content of the Form: Narrative Discourse and Historical Representation* (Baltimore: Johns Hopkins University Press, 1987).

Chapter 6 "The Forces That Are Molding Us": *The National Politics of Blood and Disease after World War II*

1. "Retrospectively this climate, full of glow, glitter and dynamism reminds me of the atmosphere of an amusement park rather than a golden age of science." Mehdi Tavassoli to Maxwell Wintrobe, 3 January 1983, Maxwell Myer Wintrobe Papers, box 25, folder: "Tavassoli, Mehdi," Marriott Library, University of Utah.

2. Ibid., 1.

3. Phillip Allen, president of the New York County Medical Society, in "To Your Health: Blood," NBC, 1957 (produced by NBC and the Medical Society of the County of New York), Museum of Television and Radio, New York.

4. Bernard Seeman, *The River of Life: The Story of Man's Blood from Magic to Science* (New York: W.W. Norton, 1961), 235.

5. Ibid., 234.

6. Christopher Feudtner, "The Want of Control: Ideas, Innovations, and Ideals in the Modern Management of Diabetes Mellitus," *Bulletin of the History of Medicine* 69 (1995): 66–90; see also idem, "Bittersweet: The Transformation of Diabetes into a Chronic Illness in Twentieth-Century America" (Ph.D. diss., University of Pennsylvania, 1995).

7. L. S. Penrose, *Outline of Human Genetics* (New York: Wiley, 1959), 125.

8. Garland Allen, *Life Sciences in the Twentieth Century* (New York: Cambridge University Press, 1979).

9. "[A] whole range of anemias arise from nutritional and metabolic disturbances." Seeman, *The River of Life*, 223.

10. The decline of "the anemias" signaled a new stage in disease identity, medical identity, and patient identity. Writing on *Drugs, Medicine, and Man* in 1962, physician Harold Burn suggested that "the problem of anemia is . . . one

which is not yet solved." Harold Burn, *Drugs, Medicine and Man* (New York: Scribner's, 1962), 170. In the case of pernicious anemia, the proliferation of new drugs, including the synthesis of vitamin B_{12}, had further fragmented its identity, suggesting that a variety of biomolecular mechanisms fully explained the disease. Burn observed that, with the discovery of vitamin B_{12} in 1948, the degenerative spinal cord changes so common after liver treatment vanished, "but they become abruptly worse under the influence of folic acid" (169). Even B_{12} had its limitations: "When there is excessive growth of bacteria high up in the intestines, the effectiveness of vitamin B_{12} given by mouth is low" (171).

11. William Dameshek, "'Boards' in Hematology?" *Blood* 31 (1968): 685.

12. Maxwell Wintrobe, "The American Society of Hematology: III. Posture of the American Society of Hematology in the Future," Maxwell Myer Wintrobe Papers, box 43, folder: "Past, Present, and Future," p. 3.

13. Ibid.

14. Maxwell Wintrobe, "Past, Present, and Future," Maxwell Myer Wintrobe Papers, box 43, folder: "Past, Present, and Future," part II, pp. 2–3.

15. Leon Jacobsen, "Autobiography of Leon Jacobsen," Maxwell Myer Wintrobe Papers, box 17, pp. 36, 37.

16. Ibid., 40.

17. "[This] was a patient with lymphatic leukemia who had failed to respond adequately to radiophosphorus and X-ray therapy." Ibid., 44.

18. Ibid., 51.

19. Alvin Mauer, Director of St. Jude's Children's Research Hospital, to Maxwell Wintrobe, 30 November 1982, Maxwell Myer Wintrobe Papers, box 20, folder: "Biographies, M–Mi," p. 3.

20. Mauer noted that "these studies were possible because of the availability of research grants from the National Cancer Institute." Ibid., 3–4.

21. "The Leukemic Terror," *Newsweek* 33 (7 March 1949): 54.

22. William Dameshek, "Editorial: Is Leukemia Increasing?" *Blood* 2 (1947): 101. Dameshek concluded that "the increased diagnostic acumen of the modern practitioner . . . seems hardly great enough to account for the spectacular jump" (p. 101).

23. Ibid., 54.

24. Sir MacFarlane Burnet, "The Research Frontier: Where is Science Taking Us?" *Saturday Review* 41 (2 August 1958): 38–39.

25. Dameshek, "Editorial: Is Leukemia Increasing?" 101.

26. What accounted for this increased incidence? One author wondered whether there was an "absolute increase in the rate, . . . whether it reflects more effective diagnosis and reporting, . . . [or whether the rise of leukemia reflected] excessive exposure to . . . radioactive contaminants in our atmosphere." See Seeman, *The River of Life*, 224.

27. Simpson's widow had dedicated $400,000 to the University of Michigan

for a pernicious anemia and blood disease research institute. Chris J. D. Zara-fonetis, "The Thomas Henry Simpson Memorial Institute for Medical Research," Maxwell Myer Wintrobe Papers, box 24, folder: "Simpson Memorial," pp. 1, 5.

28. "Research News: Part I. The Institute and Research on Pernicious Ane-mia," Maxwell Myer Wintrobe Papers, box 24, folder: "Simpson Memorial," p. 19.

29. "Research News," a publication of the Thomas Henry Simpson Memori-al Institute for Medical Research, Maxwell Myer Wintrobe Papers, box 24, fold-er: "Simpson Memorial," pp. 5, 6. Entire institutions, like the St. Jude's Children's Research Hospital, were created for leukemia research, organized around the promise of radiation and chemotherapy for a deadly childhood disease. St. Jude's was founded in 1958 and opened its doors in 1962.

30. Ibid., 8.

31. Alvin Mauer concluded, "the leukemia cell populations served as a rela-tively easily studied population for learning about the characteristics of prolifer-ation in cancer in general." Alvin Mauer, Director of St. Jude's Children's Re-search Hospital, to Maxwell Wintrobe, 30 November 1982, Maxwell Myer Wintrobe Papers, box 20, folder: "Biographies, M–Mi," p. 4. Useful studies of can-cer in twentieth-century politics and culture include James Patterson, *The Dread Disease: Cancer and Modern American Culture* (Cambridge: Harvard University Press, 1987); Robert Proctor, *Cancer Wars: How Politics Shapes What We Know and Don't Know about Cancer* (New York: Basic Books, 1995); and Stephen Strickland, *Politics, Science, and Dread Disease: A Short History of United States Medical Research Policy* (Cambridge: Harvard University Press, 1972).

32. E. Donnall Thomas, "Rays and Bone Marrow," *Time* 73 (13 April 1959): 72.

33. "Leukemia May Not Be Cancer," *Science Digest* 26 (July 1949): 50.

34. "The Institute and Leukemia," *Research News* (a publication of the Thomas Henry Simpson Institute for Medical Research), Maxwell Myer Wintrobe Papers, box 24, folder: "Simpson Memorial," p. 3.

35. Dameshek, "'Boards' in Hematology?" 683.

36. Joe Ross, "Biographical Statement," Maxwell Myer Wintrobe Papers, box 23, folder: "Joe F. Ross," p. 19.

37. Ibid.

38. Thomas, "Rays and Bone Marrow," 71–72.

39. Dameshek, "'Boards' in Hematology?"

40. David Prager, "Correspondence," *Blood* 47 (1976): 165–66.

41. Helen Ranney, "Survey of Staff Positions in Academic Hematology in 1971," *Blood* 40 (1972): 574–84.

42. Ross, "Biographical Statement," Maxwell Myer Wintrobe Papers, p. 20.

43. Wintrobe, "Past, Present, and Future," part II, Maxwell Myer Wintrobe Papers, box 43, folder: "Past, Present, and Future," pp. 2–3.

44. The sub-board in pediatric hematology/oncology of the American Board

of Pediatrics began to have regular meetings in 1972. The first certifying examination was given in 1974. On the emerging voice and identity of this pediatric focus, see Carl Pochedly, "From the Editor," *American Journal of Pediatric Hematology/Oncology* 1 (spring 1979): 1, and idem, "From the Editor," *American Journal of Pediatric Hematology/Oncology* 2 (spring 1980): 3. See also idem, "Emergence of Pediatric Hematology/Oncology as an Independent Specialty," *American Journal of Pediatric Hematology/Oncology* 7 (summer 1985): 183–90.

45. A thorough journalistic overview of this story is Thomas Maeder, *Adverse Reactions* (New York: William Morrow, 1994).

46. Thomas E. Woodward, "Chloramphenicol, Kuala Lumpur, and the First Therapeutic Conquest of Scrub Typhus and Typhoid Fever," in Carol L. Moberg and Zanvil A. Cohn, eds., *Launching the Antibiotic Era: Personal Accounts of the Discovery and Use of the First Antibiotics* (New York: Rockefeller University Press, 1990), 44; J. Ehrlich et al., "Chlormycetin, a New Antibiotic from a Soil Actinomycete," *Science* 106 (1947): 417.

47. Richard Harris, *The Real Voice* (New York: Macmillan, 1964), 100. Harris' book is an account of an investigation of the drug industry by Senator Estes Kefauver, Subcommittee on Antitrust and Monopoly. See also "Ad Hoc Conference on Chloramphenicol," National Research Council, *Division of Medical Services Bulletin,* 6 August 1952, Maxwell Myer Wintrobe Papers, box 70, folder: "Chloramphenicol," p. 2.

48. Ibid., 5. The sales data refer to Kapseals of 250 mg each.

49. Maxwell Wintrobe, "Testimony by Max Wintrobe in C.E. Case," Maxwell Myer Wintrobe Papers, box 70, folder: "Wintrobe Testimony," p. 15.

50. Other commentators on chloramphenicol include Francis Gilman Blake, *The Present Status of Antibiotic Therapy, with Particular Reference to Chloramphenicol, Aureomycin, and Terramycin* (Springfield, Ill.: Charles C Thomas, 1952).

51. "Ad Hoc Committee on Chloramphenicol," *National Research Council, Division of Medical Sciences Bulletin,* 6 August 1952, Maxwell Myer Wintrobe Papers, box 70, folder: "Chloramphenicol," p. 2.

52. Ibid., 6.

53. Ibid., 8. Quotations from Irving Kerlan and William Dameshek.

54. The figure of eight million was cited in the Federal Security Agency press release of 14 August 1952. "Ad Hoc Committee on Chloramphenicol," minutes, appendix B, p. 2, Maxwell Myer Wintrobe Papers.

55. Ibid., 8. William Dameshek asked "whether the increased incidence of the so-called idiopathic type may actually be due to increased exposure of the population to many chemicals" (p. 10).

56. Ibid., 10, 12. But Dr. Gilbert Beebe "reported that in the new International Classification refractory anemia is in a separate rubric entitled 'nonregenerative anemias.'"

57. Ibid., 14, 16.

58. Ibid., 9, 15. Keefer believed that "there was not enough evidence to warrant taking the drug off the market."

59. Ibid., 17. All of the conference participants concurred with the value of blood tests. Dameshek suggested that "peripheral blood studies might give some indication of the onset of blood dyscrasia." Smadel agreed that "blood counts would be indicated when the drug was given for longer than two weeks."

60. According to the Federal Security Agency press release of 14 August 1952, the label would read: "Warning: Blood dyscrasias may be associated with intermittent or prolonged use. It is essential that adequate blood studies be made."

61. See, for example, I. H. Krakoff, D. A. Karnofsky, and D. H. Burchenal, "Effect of Large Doses of Chloramphenicol on Human Subjects," *New England Journal of Medicine* 253 (1955): 7–10.

62. "Chlormycetin," *Medical Letter on Drugs and Therapeutics* 1 (3 April 1959): 21.

63. William Kessenich, Medical Director of the Food and Drug Administration, to Dr. Keith Cannan, Chairman, Division of Medical Sciences, National Research Council, 28 November 1960, Maxwell Myer Wintrobe Papers, box 70, folder: "Chloramphenicol," p. 1.

64. Ibid., 2.

65. "Chlormycetin and Aplastic Anemia," *Medical Letter on Drugs and Therapeutics* 3 (6 January 1961): 2. The article noted that William Dameshek "reports that of 30 patients with aplastic anemia he had seen in the past three years, eight had received significant amounts of chloramphenicol." It concluded, however, that "chloramphenicol is a valuable antibiotic when used with proper indications. Even though serious reactions are infrequent, there is little point in risking its toxic . . . potential in . . . infections for which equally effective and safer antibiotics are available."

66. Ibid., 3.

67. See Rachel Carson, *Silent Spring* (Boston: Houghton Mifflin, 1962), and Alan Marcus, *Cancer from Beef: DES, Federal Food Regulation, and Consumer Confidence* (Baltimore: Johns Hopkins University Press, 1994).

68. According to Brian Inglis, "in 1963 a survey revealed that more people were dying from the drug's side-effects than were being saved from death in the rare conditions for which it was recommended." Brian Inglis, *The Diseases of Civilization* (London: Hodder and Stoughton, 1981), 134.

69. Harris, *The Real Voice*, 96.

70. Maxwell Wintrobe, "Testimony by Wintrobe in the C.E. Case from 1979" (regarding the use of chloramphenicol in a case in Georgia), Maxwell Myer Wintrobe Papers, box 70, folder: "Wintrobe testimony," p. 14.

71. See, for example, W. R. Best, "Chloramphenicol-associated Blood Dyscrasias: A Review of Cases Submitted to the American Medical Association Registry," *Journal of the American Medical Association* 201 (1967): 181–88; R. O. Waller-

stein, P. K. Condit, and C. K. Caspter, "Statewide Study of Chloramphenicol Therapy and Aplastic Anemia," *Journal of the American Medical Association* 208 (1969): 2045–50; T. J. Fink and D. W. Gump, "Chloramphenicol: An Inpatient Study of Use and Abuse," *Journal of Infectious Disease* 138 (1978): 690–94; M. Silverman and P. R. Lee, *Pills, Profits, and Politics* (Berkeley: University of California Press, 1974); and Henry Feder, Carl Osier, and Eufronio Maderazo, "An Audit of Chloramphenicol Use in a Large Community Hospital," *Archives of Internal Medicine* 141 (1981): 597–98.

72. For one example, see Maxwell Myer Wintrobe Papers, box 70, folder: "Wintrobe Testimony." Wintrobe testified in a variety of cases of aplastic anemia, where patients and workers were exposed to chemicals and later developed the disease. His testimony frequently highlighted the lack of information on the connections between various chemicals and the disease.

73. A. J. Trevett and S. Naraqi, "Saint or Sinner? A Look at Chloramphenicol," *Papua New Guinea Medical Journal* 35 (1992): 210–16.

74. Haakon B. Benestad, "Drug Mechanisms in Marrow Aplasia," in *Aplastic Anemia*, ed. C. G. Geary (London: Balliere Tindall, 1979), 26.

75. "Chloramphenicol: Are Concerns about Aplastic Anemia Justified?" *Drug Safety* 7 (May–June 1992): 167–69; "Chloramphenicol: A Dangerous Drug?" *Acta Hematologica* 85 (1991): 171–72.

76. C. G. Geary, *Aplastic Anemia*, 1.

77. Richard Riegelman, "What to Do until the FDA Arrives," *Postgraduate Medicine* 70 (December 1981): 103–8.

78. *Occupational Exposure to Benzene*, U.S. Department of Health, Education, and Welfare, Public Health Service, Centers for Disease Control, National Institute for Occupational Safety and Health (Washington, D.C.: GPO, 1974). See also R. L. Verwilghen, "Indigenised Pharmaceuticals and Aplastic Anemia," *Lancet* 2 (1988): 1019 (letter). On chemical residues in meat and peach orchards from South Carolina causing aplastic anemia, see "Cluster of Aplastic Anemia," *Archives of Internal Medicine* 145 (1985): 635–640; Paul Lietman, "Chloramphenicol and the Neonate—1979 View," *Clinics in Pharmacology* 6 (March 1979): 151–61; Theodore J. Fink and Dieter W. Gump, "Chloramphenicol [sic]: An Inpatient Study of Use and Abuse," *Journal of Infectious Disease* 138 (1978): 690–94; and H. M. Feder and C. Osier, "An Audit of Chloramphenicol Use in a Large Community Hospital," *Archives of Internal Medicine* 141 (1981): 597–98.

79. For a history of electrophoresis, see Lily Kay, "Laboratory Technology and Biological Knowledge: The Tiselius Electrophoresis Apparatus, 1930–1945," *Pubblicazioni della Stazione Zoologica di Napoli—Section Ii: History and Philosophy of the Life Sciences* 10 (1988): 51–72.

80. Hermann Lehmann, "Newsletter: A Symposium on the Hemoglobinopathies," *Blood* 13 (March 1958): 302–3.

81. See, for example, E. W. Smith and C. L. Conley, "Clinical Features of the

Genetic Variants of Sickle Cell Disease," *Bulletin of Johns Hopkins Hospital* 94 (1954): 289; E. D. Thomas, A. G. Motulsky, and D. H. Walters, "Homozygous Hemoglobin C Disease," *American Journal of Medicine* 18 (1955): 832; Myerson et al., "Incidence and Significance of Abnormal Hemoglobin," 543; P. A. Galbraith and P. T. Green, "Hemoglobin C Disease in an Anglo Saxon Family," *American Journal of Medicine* 28 (1960): 969; Edward Hook and Gerald Cooper, "The Clinical Manifestations of Sickle Cell-Hemoglobin C Disease and Sickle Cell Anemia," *Southern Medical Journal* 51 (1958): 610; G. M. Eddington and H. Lehmann, "Distribution of Hemoglobin C in West Africa," *Man* 36 (1956): 1.

82. On population genetics and the evolutionary explanation of sickle cell anemia, see A. C. Allison, "Sickle Cell Anemia and Evolution," *Scientific American* 195 (August 1956): 87–88; "Sickle Cells in Whites: Editorial Note," *Scientific American* 185 (August 1956): 58; S. Weisenfeld, "Sickle Cell Trait in Human Biological and Cultural Evolution," *Science* 157 (8 September 1967): 1134–40; R. Singer, "The Sickle Cell Trait in Africa," *American Anthropologist* 55 (1953): 634–48; L. Mednick and M. Orans, "The Sickle-Cell Gene: Migration versus Selection," *American Anthropologist* 58 (1958): 293–95.

An important predecessor to these anthropomedical studies was A. B. Raper and W. J. Tomlinson, "Incidence of Sicklemia and Sickle Cell Anemia in 1,000 Canal Zone Examinations upon Natives of Central Africa," *American Journal of Medical Science* 209 (1945): 181.

83. "Helpful Defect," *Scientific American* 190 (April 1954): 52.

84. See B. Glass, "Malaria and Sickle Cell Anemia," *Science* 195 (5 October 1956): 619, and "Sickle Cell Anemia and Malaria," *Chemistry* 63 (June 1970): 22.

85. The term *balanced polymorphism* was first used by Neel in "Data Pertaining to Population Dynamics of Sickle Cell Disease," *American Journal of Human Genetics* 5 (1953): 154. Echoing this explanation, one physician wrote in 1963 that "sickle cell trait is protected against plasmodium falciparum infection, the mechanism being unknown." A. Atamer, "Hereditary Hemoglobinopathies," in *Blood Disease* (New York: Grune and Stratton, 1963), 177.

86. See also V. M. Ingram, "Gene Evolution and the Haemoglobins," *Nature* 189 (1961): 704–8.

87. L. S. Penrose, *Outline of Human Genetics* (New York: Wiley, 1959), 124.

88. See Peter Bowler, *Evolution: The History of an Idea* (Berkeley: University of California Press, 1984), for more on the evolutionary synthesis.

89. F. Livingstone, "The Origins of the Sickle-Cell Gene," in *Reconstructing African Culture History*, ed. Gabel and Bennett (Boston: Boston University Press, 1967), 139–66.

90. Weisenfeld, "Sickle Cell Trait in Evolution," 1136.

91. This counterthesis on the cultural origins of sickle cell anemia was, of course, one-half of the nature-nurture debate. In the early 1970s, this style of ecological history began to influence medical history. William McNeill, *Plagues and*

Peoples (Garden City, N.Y.: Anchor Press and Doubleday, 1972); William Crosby, *The Columbian Exchange: Biological and Cultural Consequences of 1492* (Westport, Conn.: Greenwood Press, 1972).

92. See M. F. Ashley Montagu, *Man's Most Dangerous Myth: The Fallacy of Race* (New York: Columbia University Press, 1942), and Jacques Barzun, *Race: A Study in Superstition* (New York: Harper and Row, 1965).

93. Stuart Edelstein, *The Sickled Cell: From Myths to Molecules* (Cambridge: Harvard University Press, 1986), 1.

94. This general issue of access to health care services became a key political focus in these years. Beginning in the late 1950s, the patient who was "living on borrowed blood" emerged as a social type. "The Sickle Threat," *Time* 73 (19 January 1959): 42. By 1966, *Ebony*—a new magazine aimed at black readers—could present dramatic stories of the "incurable 'Negro disease.'" "Incurable 'Negro Disease' Strikes Five in Family," *Ebony* 21 (May 1966): 154–56. Significantly, most of the cases profiled were of the sickle cell *trait*, rather than anemia, and the article presented the trait as a disaster waiting to strike the "carrier." These patient-centered portraits often focused on the pain of the disease.

95. In the late 1950s and 1960s, a "patient's perspective" emerged in articles such as "The Sickle Threat," *Ebony*. Other writings with this theme include Dick Campbell, "Sickle Cell Anemia and Its Effect on Black People," *Crisis* 78 (January–February 1971): 7–9; Joseph Phillips, "How I Cope with Sickle Cell Anemia," *Ebony* 31 (February 1976): 104–6; Dion Daniels, "Sickle Cell Anemia: A Patient's Tale," *British Medical Journal* 301 (1990): 673; and L. W. Diggs and E. Flowers, "Sickle Cell Anemia in the Home Environment: Observations on the Natural History of the Disease in Tennessee Children," *Clinical Pediatrics* 10 (1971): 697–700.

96. "Sickle Cell Anemia," Department of Health, Education and Welfare, Public Health Service Publ. 1341, Health Information Series, no. 119, 23 November 1965 (prepared by the Information Office, National Institute of Arthritis and Metabolic Disease, NIH).

97. "Sickle Cell Anemia," Department of Health, Education and Welfare, 15 December 1969 (prepared by the Information Office, National Institute of Arthritis and Metabolic Disease, NIH).

98. Roland Scott (a physician and outspoken author on sickle cell anemia) argued that, despite all the intense study and interest, the real importance of the disease was as a community health problem. R. B. Scott, "Sickle Cell Anemia: High Prevalence and Low Priority," *New England Journal of Medicine* 282 (1970): 164–65; idem, "A Commentary on Sickle Cell Disease," *Journal of the National Medical Association* 63 (1971): 1–2, 60. A thoughtful overview of Scott and his work is C. Pochedly, "Dr. Roland Scott: Crusader for Sickle Cell Disease and Children," *American Journal of Pediatric Hematology-Oncology* 7 (fall 1985): 265–69.

99. Legislation included the National Heart, Blood Vessel, Lung, and Blood Act of 1972 (Public Law 92-423), the Sickle Cell Anemia Control Act of 1972 (Pub-

lic Law 92-294); and Public Law 93-603 on renal disease and dialysis.

100. "Statement of John Henry Johnson, Former Pro Football Player, in behalf of the Black Athletes Foundation for Research in Sickle Cell Disease," in House Committee on Interstate and Foreign Commerce, Subcommittee on Public Health and Environment, *Bills to Provide for the Prevention of Sickle Cell Anemia and to Amend the Public Health Service Act to Provide for the Establishment of a National Sickle Cell Anemia Institute (HR 11742, HR 7654, and HR 11171)*, Serial no. 92-57, 92d Cong., 1st sess., 1971, 86.

101. "Statement of Hon. Dan Kuykendall, a representative from the state of Tennessee," House Committee, *Bills to Provide for the Prevention of Sickle Cell Anemia*, 46. The pain and the patient's desire to escape it, noted the law-and-order Republican Kuykendall, translated sickle cell anemia into a drug problem. "One of the byproducts . . . is the tendency to turn to narcotics . . . Sickle cell anemia victims turn to drugs not for the reasons that other young persons do, but simply to get relief from excruciating pain."

102. Ibid., 48.

103. Arno Motulsky, "The Heterozygote in Perspective," in *Cystic Fibrosis and Related Human and Animal Diseases*, ed. S. Jakowska (New York: Gordon and Breach, 1970), 86–87.

104. Senate Committee on Labor and Public Welfare, *Hearing before the Subcommittee on Health: To Provide for the Prevention of Sickle Cell Anemia (S. 2676)*, 92d Cong., 1st sess., 1971, 33.

105. *National Sickle Cell Anemia Control Act*, Public Law 92-294, 92d Cong., 2d sess. (16 May 1972).

106. Barbara Culliton, "Sickle Cell Anemia: The Route from Obscurity to Prominence," *Science* 178 (20 October 1972): 138–42; idem, "Sickle Cell Anemia: National Program Raises Problems as Well as Hopes," *Science* 178 (1972): 283–86; R. E. Jackson, "A Perspective of the National Sickle Cell Disease Program," *Archives of Internal Medicine* 183 (1974): 533; S. Charache, "Sickle-Cell Anemia: The Known and the Unknown," *Annals of Internal Medicine* 77 (1972): 148–49.

107. See, for example, R. M. Nalbandian et al., "Mass Screening for Sickle Cell Hemoglobin: Is There an Optimal Method?" *Journal of the American Medical Association* 234 (1975): 832–35. By the early 1970s, however, for African Americans sickle cell anemia had been framed as a civil rights issue. See "The Row over Sickle-Cell," *Newsweek* 81 (12 February 1973): 63–65; "Problems Seen in Genetic Tests: Mass Screenings Are Called Psychological Danger," *New York Times*, 25 May 1972, p. 1; "Sickle Cell: Resentment Complicates the Case," *New York Times*, 5 November 1972, p. 4; J. S. Keck, "Sickle Cell Legislation of 'The New Ghetto Hustle,'" *Journal of Family Law* 13 (1973–74): 278–310.

108. See, for example, "AMA Journal Publishes Recommendations for Mass Screening Programs for Sickle Cell Anemia," *New York Times*, 13 December 1971,

28, and "Screening for Disease in Blacks Questioned," *Los Angeles Times*, 14 October 1971, 2.

109. Dorothy Wilkinson, "Politics and Sickle Cell Anemia," *Black Scholar* 5 (May 1974): 26.

110. Michael Michaelson, "Sickle Cell Anemia: An 'Interesting Pathology,'" *Ramparts* 10 (October 1971): 52–58; Tabitha Powledge, "The New Ghetto Hustle," *Saturday Review of the Sciences* 1 (February 1973): 38–40; see also Jackson, "National Sickle Cell Disease Program," 533. Jackson notes: "Sickle cell counseling programs were highly criticized in some areas; accusations by various public groups were made that the program involved black genocide, job and insurance discrimination, and a confusion of health priorities."

111. Wilkinson, "Politics and Sickle Cell Anemia," 30. See Powledge, "The New Ghetto Hustle."

112. John Henry Johnson, House Committee, *Bills to Provide for the Prevention of Sickle Cell Anemia*, 86.

113. Moreover, particular electrophoretic tests were better than others. See, for example, Nalbandian et al., "Mass Screening for Sickle Cell Hemoglobin."

114. Robert Scott and Robert Gilbert, "Genetic Diversity in Hemoglobins: Disease or Nondisease," *Journal of the American Medical Association* 239 (1978): 137.

115. Ibid.

116. Ernest Beutler highlighted "the fact that 13% of physicians answering the questionnaire believed that sickle cell trait could be responsible for sickness with no other obvious explanation." Ernest Beutler, "Physicians Attitudes about Sickle Cell Disease and Sickle Cell Trait," *Journal of the American Medical Association* 224 (1974): 71.

117. F. I. D. Konotney-Ahulu, *Medical Considerations for Legalizing Voluntary Sterilization: Sickle Cell Disease as a Case in Point*, Law and Population Monography Series, no. 13 (1973), Law and Population Programme: The Fletcher School of Law and Diplomacy, Tufts University. See also Konotney-Ahuli, "Sickle Cell Trait and Altitude," *British Medical Journal* 1 (1972): 177–78.

118. Helen Ranney, "Editorial: Sickle Cell Disease," *Blood* 39 (1972): 436.

119. On this issue of screening and stigma, see Jane Brody, "Problems Seen in Genetic Tests—Mass Screenings Are Called a Psychological Danger," *New York Times*, 25 May 1972; "Sickle Cell—Resentment Complicates the Case," *New York Times*, 5 November 1972; C. Whitten, J. Thomas, and E. Nishiura, "Sickle Cell Trait Counseling—Evaluation of Counselors and Counselees," *American Journal of Human Genetics* 33 (1981): 802–16.

120. Is sickle cell trait, for example, a disease or a nondisease? Physicians and policymakers struggled with this question in the 1970s and still do today. In 1973 the Air Force Academy established a ban on sickle cell carriers. The ban was removed eight years later. "Critics say the health problems associated with sickle

cell trait have been exaggerated to the point that they restrict opportunities for blacks . . . The Air Force itself will continue to prohibit those with sickle cell trait from training as pilots or copilots." "Air Academy Drops Ban of Sickle Carriers," *Science* 211 (1981): 719. See also C. Holden, "Air Force Challenged on Sickle Trait Policy," *Science* 211 (1981): 257; Richard Serevo, "Blacks Only Need Apply: Genetic Screening at DuPont," *Nation* 23 (1980): 243–45.

121. The term was first used by G. H. Whipple and W. L. Bradford in 1936: "Mediterranean Disease—Thalassemia," *Journal of Medicine* 9 (1936): 279–311. See Barbara Culliton, "Cooley's Anemia: Special Treatment for Another Ethnic Disease," *Science* 178 (1972): 540–93.

122. L. C. Dunn, *Heredity and Evolution in Human Populations* (Cambridge: Harvard University Press, 1959), 52.

123. David Prager, "Correspondence," *Blood* 47 (1976): 165–66.

Conclusion: *Disease Identity in the Age of Technological Medicine*

1. Bernard Seaman, *The River of Life: The Story of Man's Blood from Magic to Science* (New York: W.W. Norton, 1961), 238.

2. Andrew Feenberg and Alastair Hannay, eds., *Technology and the Politics of Knowledge* (Bloomington: University of Indiana Press, 1995).

3. Contributors to this discussion have included Ludwig Fleck, who argued, in 1935, that "the relation between the Wassermann reaction and syphilis" was not biologically obvious, but rather was an "event in the history of thought." Ludwig Fleck, *Genesis and Development of a Scientific Fact* (Basel: Benno Schwabe, 1935; Chicago: University of Chicago Press, 1979), 97. See also Bruno Latour and Steven Woolgar, *Laboratory Life: The Construction of Scientific Facts* (Princeton: Princeton University Press, 1986). But consider the "backlash" against this kind of scholarship in the form of a diatribe against the history and sociology of science and against cultural studies of science by Paul Gross and Norman Levitt, *Higher Superstition: The Academic Left and Its Quarrels with Science* (Baltimore: Johns Hopkins University Press, 1994).

4. B. D. Cohen, *Hard Choices: The Mixed Blessings of Modern Medical Technology* (New York: G.P. Putnam's Sons, 1986); Louise B. Russell, *Educated Guesses: Making Policy about Medical Screening Tests* (Berkeley: University of California Press, 1994). See also Alonzo Plough, *Borrowed Time: Artificial Organs and the Politics of Extending Lives* (Philadelphia: Temple University Press, 1986).

5. Howard Segal, *Technological Utopianism in American Culture* (Chicago: University of Chicago Press, 1985); idem, *Future Imperfect: The Mixed Blessings of Technology in America* (Amherst: University of Massachusetts, 1994); Yaron Ezrahi, Everett Mendelsohn, and Howard Segal, eds., *Technology, Pessimism, and Postmodernism* (Boston: Kluwer Academic Publishers, 1994); and, defining technology more broadly, Michel Foucault, "The Political Technology of Individuals," in

Technologies of the Self: A Seminar with Michel Foucault, ed. Luther Martin, Huck Gutman, and Patrick Hutton (Amherst: University of Massachusetts Press, 1988). For a collection of recent works on technology in American society, see Randall Stross, ed., *Technology and Society in Twentieth Century America: An Anthology* (Chicago: Dorsey Press, 1989).

6. Dorothy Nelkin, *Dangerous Diagnostics: The Social Power of Biological Information* (New York: Basic Books, 1989).

7. Peter Kramer, *Listening to Prozac: A Psychiatrist Explores Antidepressant Drugs and the Remaking of the Self* (New York: Penguin Books, 1993). Citing the findings of one sociobiologist, Kramer noted "in each troop there was one male monkey in whose bloodstream there was a distinctly elevated level of serotonin, the mood-setting amine whose uptake is blocked by Prozac. The level of serotonin in this male was about one and a half times that in other males, and in every instance the high-serotonin male was the dominant male in the troop" (p. 212).

8. The pioneering work of E. Donnall Thomas on bone marrow transplantation in leukemia earned him the Nobel Prize in 1990. Max Wintrobe, *Hematology: The Blossoming of a Science* (Philadelphia: Lea and Febiger, 1985), 349.

9. "Bone Marrow Transplantation for Genetic Disorders," *Oncology (Huntington)* 3 (6 March 1992): 51–58, 63–66.

10. I. Roberts, "Bone Marrow Transplantation in Children: Current Results and Controversies; Meeting, Hilton Head Island, S.C., March 1994," *Bone Marrow Transplantation* 2 (1994): 197–99.

11. A recent debate, for example, about HLA matching, race, and organ transplantation has reopened the medical discussion on racial identity and biology.

12. C. Vermylen and G. Cornu, "Bone Marrow Transplantation for Sickle Cell Disease: The European Experience," *American Journal of Pediatric Hematology-Oncology* 1 (16 February 1994): 18–21.

13. J. F. Apperley, "Bone Marrow Transplantation for the Haemoglobinopathies: Past, Present, and Future," *Baillieres Clinical Haematology* 1 (1993): 299–325.

14. Ibid., 18–21. See also F. Bernaudin et al., "Bone Marrow Transplantation (BMT) in 14 Children with Severe Sickle Cell Disease (SCD): The French Experience," *Bone Marrow Transplantation* 12, Suppl. 1 (1993): 118–21. In this study, one patient of the fourteen developed aplastic anemia; ten were cured; and three were unassessed.

15. G. L. Bray et al., "Assessing Clinical Severity in Children with Sickle Cell Disease: Preliminary Results from a Cooperative Study," *American Journal of Pediatric Hematology-Oncology* 1 (16 February 1994): 50–54.

16. I. A. Roberts and S. C. Davies, "Sickle Cell Disease: The Transplant Issue," *Bone Marrow Transplantation* 4 (11 April 1993): 253–54; S. C. Davies, "Bone Marrow Transplant for Sickle Cell Disease—the Dilemma," *Blood Review* 1 (7 March

1993): 4–9; S. Piomelli, "Bone Marrow Transplantation in Sickle Cell Disease: A Plea for a Rational Approach," *Bone Marrow Transplantation* 10, Suppl. 1 (1992): 58–61.

17. "To Test or Not to Test," *Newsweek* 122 (27 December 1993): 42–43.

18. "The Killer We Don't Discuss," *Newsweek* 122 (27 December 1993): 40. This *Newsweek* magazine article suggested that "one of the freedoms most ardently sought by the women's movement was the freedom to talk openly about their bodies" (p. 40). See also "The Private Pain of Prostate Cancer," *Time* 140 (5 October 1992): 77.

19. D. S. Smith and W. J. Catalona, "The Nature of Prostate Cancer Detected through Prostate Specific Antigen-based Screening," *Journal of Urology* 152 (1994): 1732–36.

20. See, for example, E. J. Small, "Prostate Cancer: Who to Screen, and What the Results Mean," *Geriatrics* 48 (December 1993): 28–30, 35–38.

21. "Prostate Cancer," 40.

22. A. L. Potosky et al., "The Role of Increasing Detection in the Rising Incidence of Prostate Cancer," *Journal of the American Medical Association* 273 (1995): 548–52. This article concluded that "the recent dramatic epidemic of prostate cancer is likely the result of the increasing detection of tumors from increasing PSA screening . . . Changes in the intensity of medical surveillance is the most plausible explanation of this trend." Another study suggested that the "trend of increase is due primarily to the use of the prostate specific antigen." R. Y. Demers, "Prostate Cancer Trends in Southeast Michigan 1973–1992," *In Vivo* 8 (1994): 429–31.

23. B. L. Dalkin, F. R. Ahmann, and J. B. Kopp, "Prostate Specific Antigen Levels in Men Older than 50 Years without Clinical Evidence of Prostatic Carcinoma," *Journal of Urology* 150 (1993): 1837–39. "In their derivation of normal prostate specific antigen (PSA) levels (0 to 4.0 ng./ml.) Hybritech used almost exclusively men less than 60 years old."

24. See, for example, Ian Thompson, "Editorial: Prostate Cancer Diagnosis," *Journal of Urology* 152 (1994): 1180, and H. Ballentine Carter, "Editorial: Prostate Cancer Diagnosis," *Journal of Urology* 152 (1994): 1168–69.

25. A. R. Waldman and D. M. Osborne, "Screening for Prostate Cancer," *Oncology Nursing Forum* 21 (1994): 1513–17.

26. One 1993 article in the *Archives of Internal Medicine* noted that "[PSA] does not seem to be effective alone as a screening test for prostate cancer. Additionally, the efficacy of treatment for prostate cancer with radiation therapy or radical prostatectomy remains to be demonstrated . . . Education of the patient regarding the risks, benefits, and costs of PSA screening and subsequent treatment should be addressed before performing a PSA test." V. J. Dorr, S. K. Williamson, and R. L. Stephens, "An Evaluation of Prostate-specific Antigen as a Screening Test for Prostate Cancer," *Archives of Internal Medicine* 153 (1993): 2529–37.

27. Warren E. Leary, "Health Experts Urge Reduced Use of Some Medical Tests," *New York Times*, 13 December 1995, sec. A12, p. 3.

28. C. R. Tillyer et al., "Disagreement between the Roche Cobas and Hybritech TANDEM-E PSA Assays When Measuring Free, Complexed and Total Serum Prostate Specific Antigen," *Annals of Clinical Biochemistry* 31 (1994): 501–5. This article notes that "it is possible that the adoption of a universal standard for PSA will not completely resolve the disagreement between PSA assay on individual patient samples."

Index

Library of Congress Cataloging-in-Publication Data

Wailoo, Keith.
    Drawing blood : technology and disease identity in twentieth-century America /
Keith Wailoo.
        p.   cm. — (The Henry E. Sigerist series in the history of medicine)
    Includes bibliographical references and index.
    ISBN 0-8018-5474-1 (alk. paper)
    1. Anemia—United States—History.   2. Anemia—Social aspects—United States.
I. Title. II. Series.
    [DNLM: 1. Anemia—history—United States.   Technology, Medical—history—
United States.   3. Sociology, Medical—United States.   4. Technology Assessment,
Biomedical—United States.   WH 11 AA1 W13d 1997]
RC641.W34   1997
616.1'52'009—dc20
DNLM/DLC
for Library of Congress   96-27700
                                                   CIP